Nutrition and Bariatric Surgery

Nutrition and Bariatric Surgery

Edited by

Jaime Ruiz-Tovar

Bariatric Surgery Unit, Garcilaso Clinic, Madrid, Spain
Professor of Surgery, University Alfonso X, Madrid, Spain

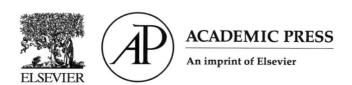

Academic Press is an imprint of Elsevier
125 London Wall, London EC2Y 5AS, United Kingdom
525 B Street, Suite 1650, San Diego, CA 92101, United States
50 Hampshire Street, 5th Floor, Cambridge, MA 02139, United States
The Boulevard, Langford Lane, Kidlington, Oxford OX5 1GB, United Kingdom

Copyright © 2021 Elsevier Inc. All rights reserved.

No part of this publication may be reproduced or transmitted in any form or by any means, electronic or mechanical, including photocopying, recording, or any information storage and retrieval system, without permission in writing from the publisher. Details on how to seek permission, further information about the Publisher's permissions policies and our arrangements with organizations such as the Copyright Clearance Center and the Copyright Licensing Agency, can be found at our website: www.elsevier.com/permissions.

This book and the individual contributions contained in it are protected under copyright by the Publisher (other than as may be noted herein).

Notices

Knowledge and best practice in this field are constantly changing. As new research and experience broaden our understanding, changes in research methods, professional practices, or medical treatment may become necessary.

Practitioners and researchers must always rely on their own experience and knowledge in evaluating and using any information, methods, compounds, or experiments described herein. In using such information or methods they should be mindful of their own safety and the safety of others, including parties for whom they have a professional responsibility.

To the fullest extent of the law, neither the Publisher nor the authors, contributors, or editors, assume any liability for any injury and/or damage to persons or property as a matter of products liability, negligence or otherwise, or from any use or operation of any methods, products, instructions, or ideas contained in the material herein.

Library of Congress Cataloging-in-Publication Data
A catalog record for this book is available from the Library of Congress

British Library Cataloguing-in-Publication Data
A catalogue record for this book is available from the British Library

ISBN: 978-0-12-822922-4

For information on all Academic Press publications visit our website at
https://www.elsevier.com/books-and-journals

Publisher: Charlotte Cockle
Acquisitions Editor: Megan R. Ball
Editorial Project Manager: Aleksandra Packowska
Production Project Manager: Bharatwaj Varatharajan
Cover Designer: Miles Hitchen

Typeset by TNQ Technologies

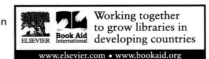

*In memoriam of Maria Celia Tovar, my mother.
Thanks for your teachings.
Everything I have and everything I am, I owe it to you.*

Contents

Contributors..xi
Preface...xv

CHAPTER 1 Preoperative nutritional deficiencies: epidemiology and prevalence of nutritional deficiencies among morbidly obese patients, specifying which ones should be supplemented..........................1
M. Lluch Escudero Pallardó, Carlos Sánchez Juan and Marcos Bruna Esteban
Introduction...2
Micronutrient deficiency...3
Macronutrient deficiency..6
Recommendations and methodology of patient performance...........6
References..12

CHAPTER 2 Nutritional evaluation and calculation of nutritional requirements in the preoperative course.................17
Jose Jorge Ortez Toro, Carlos Miguel Peteiro Miranda and Julia Ocón Bretón
Introduction..17
Nutritional assessment..18
Nutritional requirements calculation...................................24
References...32

CHAPTER 3 Preoperative diets: LCD, VLCD, and commercial supplements...35
Sonsoles Gutiérrez Medina, Carmen Aragón, Álvaro Sánchez and Clotilde Vázquez
Low-calorie and very low-calorie diets................................35
Commercial products..39
VLCD in bariatric surgery..40
References...43
Further reading..44

CHAPTER 4 Impact of preoperative nutritional intervention on comorbidities: type 2 diabetes, hypertension, dyslipidemia, and nonalcoholic fatty liver disease 45
Lorea Zubiaga and Jaime Ruiz-Tovar
Introduction 46
Types of dietary interventions in the preoperative time..................47
Impact of preoperative nutritional interventions in obesity's comorbidities 50
Wise associations' recommendations guidelines 53
Conclusions 58
References 59

CHAPTER 5 Fluid therapy during bariatric surgery 63
Esther García-Villabona and Carmen Vallejo-Lantero
Fluid management approaches 63
Guiding parameters for administering fluids 67
Conclusion 72
References 73

CHAPTER 6 Bariatric surgery options 75
Jaime Ruiz-Tovar and Lorea Zubiaga
Introduction 75
Restrictive procedures 76
Mixed procedures 78
Malabsorptive procedures 80
Conclusion 84
Acknowledgments 84
References 85

CHAPTER 7 Postoperative complications: indications and access routes for enteral and parenteral nutrition ... 87
E. Martín Garcia-Almenta, E. Martin Antona, O. Cano-Valderrama and A.J. Torres García
Early postoperative complications 89
Late postoperative complications 95
References 97

CHAPTER 8 Nutritional treatment in the critically-ill complicated patient 99
María Asunción Acosta Mérida, Pablo B. Pedrianes Martín and Gema M. Hernanz Rodríguez
Introduction 99
Calculation of nutritional requirements 100

Low-calorie high-protein diets 102
Micronutrient supplementation.. 104
Complications of artificial feeding.. 104
Considerations for support treatment in the critical obese patient.. 106
Key points.. 110
References... 110

CHAPTER 9 Nutritional recommendations after adjustable gastric banding.. 115
Amalia Paniagua Ruiz, Manuel Durán Poveda and Sonsoles Gutiérrez Medina

Introduction.. 116
Postoperative nutritional stages 117
Calorie goals... 121
Macronutrients 121
Micronutrients assessments and recommendations before and after bariatric surgery 122
Specific recommendations on LAGB and pregnancy................ 127
References... 127

CHAPTER 10 Nutritional recommendations after sleeve gastrectomy... 129
Raquel Sánchez Santos, Alicia Molina López and Marta López Otero

Sleeve gastrectomy: technique and patient selection................ 129
Recommendations in the immediate postoperative period 130
Nutritional recommendations in LSG at discharge.................. 131
Nutritional recommendations in LSG in the follow-up 131
Complications and nutritional issues in LSG 135
References... 138

CHAPTER 11 Nutritional recommendations after mixed procedures 141
Amador García Ruiz de Gordejuela, Alicia Molina López and Ramón Vilallonga Puy

Introduction.. 141
Recommendations in the immediate postoperative period 143
Long-term recommendations 146
Specific nutritional aspects in relation to gastric bypass.......... 148
Nutritional complications in the gastric bypass patient 149
Supplementation in the gastric bypass patient 153
References... 153

CHAPTER 12 Nutritional recommendations after hypoabsorptive procedures: OAGB, duodenal switch, SADI-S 155

Luciano Antozzi, Gisela Paola Latini, Joao Caetano Marchesini, Tamires Precybelovicz, Andres Sánchez Pernaute and Miguel Ángel Rubio-Herrera

Introduction 156
Preoperative nutritional evaluation and supplementation 157
Preoperative eating behavior screening and weight loss 158
Postoperative diet and supplementation 159
Gastrointestinal symptoms 167
Long-term follow up 168
Conclusions 169
References 169

CHAPTER 13 Postoperative vitamin and mineral supplementation 173

Ma Jose Castro Alija, Jose María Jiménez Perez and Ana García del Rio

Introduction 173
Nutritional deficiencies according to the different surgical techniques in bariatric surgery 174
Recommendations for vitamin and mineral supplementation after bariatric surgery 177
Implications and decision making. Supplementation, consensus, and evidence 181
References 184

CHAPTER 14 Special nutritional requirements in children and adolescents undergoing bariatric surgery 187

Pablo Priego

Introduction 187
Nutritional assessment 188
Nutrition education 189
Nutritional needs 190
Nutritional monitoring 194
Conclusion 196
References 197

CHAPTER 15 Special nutritional requirements in the elderly patient undergoing bariatric surgery............ 199
Andrei Sarmiento, Ramiro Carbajal and Rosa Lisson

Introduction.. 199
Preoperative clinical evaluation... 200
Nutritional profile.. 200
Aging-related changes in gastric function (could predispose to nutritional issues)... 201
Aging-related changes in small intestinal function (could predispose to nutritional issues)... 201
Vitamin D... 201
Calcium.. 202
Vitamin B12... 202
Iron... 202
Protein.. 202
Laparoscopic sleeve gastrectomy... 203
Roux-en-Y gastric bypass... 203
One anastomosis/mini gastric bypass... 204
Follow-up and supplementation in elderly patients..................... 204
Conclusion.. 204
References.. 205

CHAPTER 16 Special nutritional requirements in specific situations in women: pregnancy, lactancy, and postmenopausal status............................ 209
Irene Bretón Lesmes, Cynthia González Antigüedad and Clara Serrano Moreno

Introduction.. 209
Obesity and reproductive function in women.............................. 210
Bariatric surgery and pregnancy... 211
Bariatric surgery and menopause.. 217
Pregnancy, lactation, and menopause in women with previous bariatric surgery: summary of recommendations........................ 218
References.. 219

CHAPTER 17 Follow-up and screening of postoperative nutritional deficiencies 223
Natalia Pérez-Ferre, Clara Marcuello-Foncillas and Miguel Ángel Rubio-Herrera

Introduction.. 223
Pathophysiology of nutritional deficiencies after weight loss surgery.. 224
Micronutrient deficiencies after weight loss surgery................... 226

Iron 227
Vitamin D and calcium 228
Vitamin B12 (cobalamine) 230
Folic acid 230
Vitamin B1 (thiamin) 231
Fat-soluble vitamins: A, E, K 232
Trace elements 233
Selenium 236
Suggested protocol for the follow-up and screening of
nutritional deficiencies after weight loss surgery 236
Further reading 236

CHAPTER 18 Postoperative management of specific complications: anaemia, protein malnutrition and neurological disorders 239

Manuel Ferrer-Márquez, Mercedes Vázquez-Gutiérrez and Pablo Quiroga-Subirana

Anemia 240
Protein malnutrition 244
Neurological complications 245
References 253
Further reading 256

CHAPTER 19 The importance of a cookbook for patients who have bariatric surgery 257

Silvia Leite Faria and Mary O'Kane

Introduction 258
Practical challenges 258
Ongoing postoperative care 261
Other nutrients 265
Vitamin and mineral supplements 266
Vegetarian/vegan diet 266
Whole food plant-based diet 267
Side effect 268
IFSO cookbook 269
The contents of a bariatric cookbook 269
Cultural differences 269
Menu planning 270
Conclusion 270
Best recipes for normal phase by Sílvia Leite Faria 271
References 279
Resources 282

Index 283

Contributors

María Asunción Acosta Mérida
Esophagogastric, Endocrinometabolic and Obesity Surgery Division, Hospital Universitario de Gran Canaria "Dr. Negrin", Professor at the University of Las Palmas de Gran Canaria, Las Palmas de Gran Canaria, Canary Islands, Spain

Luciano Antozzi
Centro de Cirugías Especiales, Bahía Blanca, Buenos Aires, Argentina

Carmen Aragón
Department of Endocrinology, Fundacion Jimenez Diaz University Hospital, Madrid, Spain

Julia Ocón Bretón
University Clinical Hospital "Lozano Blesa", Endocrinology and Nutrition Department, Area of Nutrition, Zaragoza, Spain

Irene Bretón Lesmes
Department of Endocrinology and Nutrition, Hospital General Universitario Gregorio Marañón, Madrid, Spain

O. Cano-Valderrama
Department of Surgery, Hospital Clínico Universitario San Carlos, Madrid, Spain

Ramiro Carbajal
Hospital Nacional Edgardo Rebagliati Martins, Lima, Perú

Ma Jose Castro Alija
Faculty of Nursing, University of Valladolid, Valladolid, Spain; Endocrinology and Clinical Nutrition Research Center (ECNRC), Valladolid, Spain

Ana García del Rio
CIC bioGUNE, Bizkaia Technology Park, Derio, Spain

Marcos Bruna Esteban
General Surgery Department, La Fe University Hospital, Valencia, Spain

Silvia Leite Faria
Gastrocirurgia de Brasilia/University of Brasilia, Brasilia, Federal District, Brazil

Manuel Ferrer-Márquez
Bariatric Surgery Department, Hospital Universitario Torrecárdenas, Almería, Spain

Esther García-Villabona
Department of Anesthesiology, University Hospital La Princesa, Madrid, Spain

Cynthia González Antigüedad
Department of Endocrinology and Nutrition, Hospital General Universitario Gregorio Marañón, Madrid, Spain

Gema M. Hernanz Rodríguez
Department of Anesthesiology and Critical Care Medicine, Hospital Universitario de Gran Canaria "Dr. Negrin", Las Palmas de Gran Canaria, Canary Islands, Spain

Jose María Jiménez Perez
Faculty of Nursing, University of Valladolid, Valladolid, Spain; Endocrinology and Clinical Nutrition Research Center (ECNRC), Valladolid, Spain

Carlos Sánchez Juan
Endocrinology and Nutrition Department, General University Hospital, University of Valencia, Valencia, Spain

Gisela Paola Latini
Centro de Cirugías Especiales, Bahía Blanca, Buenos Aires, Argentina

Rosa Lisson
Hospital Nacional Edgardo Rebagliati Martins, Lima, Perú

Marta López Otero
Department of Surgery, Complejo Hospitalario Universitario de Vigo, Vigo (Pontevedra), Spain

Alicia Molina López
Department of Nutrition, Universitat Rovira i Virgili, Tarragona, Spain

Joao Caetano Marchesini
Clínica Doctor Caetano Marchesini, Curitiba, Brazil

Clara Marcuello-Foncillas
Endocrinology and Nutrition Department, Hospital Clinico San Carlos, Madrid, Spain

E. Martin Antona
Department of Surgery, Hospital Clínico Universitario San Carlos, Madrid, Spain

E. Martín Garcia-Almenta
Department of Surgery, Hospital Clínico Universitario San Carlos, Madrid, Spain

Sonsoles Gutiérrez Medina
Division of Endocrinology and Nutrition, Department of Medicine, Rey Juan Carlos University Hospital, Madrid, Spain

Alicia Molina López
Department of Nutrition and Dietetics, Hospital Universitari Sant Joan de Reus; Reus (Tarragona), Spain

Jose Jorge Ortez Toro
University Clinical Hospital "Lozano Blesa", Endocrinology and Nutrition Department, Area of Nutrition, Zaragoza, Spain

Mary O'Kane
Leeds Teaching Hospitals NHS Trust, Department of Nutrition and Dietetics, Leeds, United Kingdom

M. Lluch Escudero Pallardó
Faculty of Pharmacy, University of Valencia, Valencia, Spain

Pablo B. Pedrianes Martín
Department of Endocrinology and Nutrition, Hospital Universitario de Gran Canaria "Dr. Negrin", Las Palmas de Gran Canaria, Canary Islands, Spain

Natalia Pérez-Ferre
Endocrinology and Nutrition Department, Hospital Clinico San Carlos, Madrid, Spain

Andres Sánchez Pernaute
Hospital Clínico San Carlos, Madrid, Spain

Carlos Miguel Peteiro Miranda
University Clinical Hospital "Lozano Blesa", Endocrinology and Nutrition Department, Area of Nutrition, Zaragoza, Spain

Manuel Durán Poveda
Department of Surgery, Faculty of Health Sciences, Rey Juan Carlos University, Madrid, Spain; Department of General Surgery, Rey Juan Carlos University Hospital, Madrid, Spain

Tamires Precybelovicz
Clínica Doctor Caetano Marchesini, Curitiba, Brazil

Pablo Priego
Division of Esophagogastric and Bariatric Surgery, Ramón y Cajal University Hospital, Madrid, Spain; Surgery, University Alcalá de Henares, Madrid, Spain

Ramón Vilallonga Puy
Bariatric Surgery Unit, Vall de Hebron University Hospital, Barcelona, Spain

Pablo Quiroga-Subirana
Neurology Department, Hospital Universitario Torrecárdenas, Almería, Spain

Miguel Ángel Rubio-Herrera
Endocrinology and Nutrition Department, Hospital Clinico San Carlos, Madrid, Spain

Jaime Ruiz-Tovar
Bariatric Surgery Unit, Garcilaso Clinic, Madrid, Spain; Department of Surgery, University Alfonso X, Madrid, Spain

Amalia Paniagua Ruiz
Division of Endocrinology and Nutrition, Department of Medicine, Rey Juan Carlos University Hospital, Madrid, Spain; Department of Medicine, Section of Endocrinology and Nutrition, Faculty of Health Sciences, Rey Juan Carlos University, Madrid, Spain

Amador García Ruiz de Gordejuela
Bariatric Surgery Unit, Vall de Hebron University Hospital, Barcelona, Spain

Álvaro Sánchez
Department of Endocrinology, Fundacion Jimenez Diaz University Hospital, Madrid, Spain

Raquel Sánchez Santos
Department of Surgery, Complejo Hospitalario Universitario de Vigo, Vigo (Pontevedra), Spain

Andrei Sarmiento
Surgery at Universidad Privada San Juan Bautista, Lima, Perú

Clara Serrano Moreno
Department of Endocrinology and Nutrition, Hospital General Universitario Gregorio Marañón, Madrid, Spain

A.J. Torres García
Department of Surgery, Hospital Clínico Universitario San Carlos, Madrid, Spain

Carmen Vallejo-Lantero
Department of Anesthesiology, University Hospital La Princesa, Madrid, Spain

Clotilde Vázquez
Department of Endocrinology, Fundacion Jimenez Diaz University Hospital, Madrid, Spain

Mercedes Vázquez-Gutiérrez
Endocrinology and Clinical Nutrition Department, Hospital Universitario Torrecárdenas, Almería, Spain

Lorea Zubiaga
Lille University, Institut National de la Santé et de la Recherche Médicale (INSERM)-U1190, EGID, CHU Lille, Lille, France

Preface

Obesity is actually considered a "pandemia" in developed and developing countries, representing a relevant health burden. Obesity is not only an image problem, but it is also a health problem, reducing expectancy and quality of life. These are mostly associated with metabolic disorders, such as type 2 diabetes mellitus, dyslipidemia, hypertension, sleep apnea-hypopnea syndrome, liver steatosis… The term "morbid" means that obesity itself represents a disease.

Bariatric surgery is the best therapeutic option to achieve a significant and maintained weight loss for morbidly obese patients. Actually, thousands of bariatric procedures are performed all around the world. Diverse techniques have been developed since the first bariatric approaches were performed 60 years ago. Nowadays, all these techniques can be classified into restrictive, malabsorptive, or mixed procedures, depending on their mechanism of action to induce the weight loss. Restrictive approaches tend to reduce the gastric volume and consequently decrease the amount of food intake, whereas malabsorptive ones aim to bypass segments of the small bowel, reducing the absorption of nutrients.

Though bariatric techniques are mostly focused on reducing the calories intake, the absorption of essential nutrients is often hindered, including vitamins, minerals and proteins. Thus, inadequate postoperative diets and the lack of close follow-up schemes of bariatric patients can lead to the development of nutritional deficiencies, which can become health problems.

The different bariatric techniques may imply different nutritional carencies, based on the mechanism of action and the anatomical modification induced. In addition, the requirements can significantly change depending of the type of population (elderly, adolescents, child-bearing women…). Moreover, nutritional counseling must not begin after surgery, but even in the preoperative course, as a correct nutritional status reduces intra- and postoperative adverse events.

In summary, the nutritional support is an essential point for the success of bariatric surgery, not only for achieving a correct weight loss and remission of comorbidities, but also for reducing the risk of nutritional sequelae. Therefore, the formation of multidisciplinary teams is mandatory with a correct collaboration between bariatric surgeons, endocrinologists, and dietitians, for the election of the most appropriate technique, but also for a correct nutritional counseling, vitamin and mineral supplementation, and early diagnosis and treatment of nutritional deficiencies.

This book aims to assess the most relevant aspects of the nutrition of the bariatric patients in the pre- and postoperative course. The different bariatric approaches are separately considered. I hope that this book, based on the current evidence in nutrition and bariatric surgery, can be helpful in the clinical practice. However, we must always keep in mind that bariatric surgery is continuously changing, and actual evidence can be outdated next year, requiring future updates.

Finally, I want to thank to all the contributing authors, all of them, friends and experts in the field of bariatric surgery and nutrition, their availability, their time, and efforts to write all the chapters.

Jaime Ruiz-Tovar, MD, PhD
Editor

CHAPTER 1

Preoperative nutritional deficiencies: epidemiology and prevalence of nutritional deficiencies among morbidly obese patients, specifying which ones should be supplemented

M. Lluch Escudero Pallardó[1], Carlos Sánchez Juan[2], Marcos Bruna Esteban[3]

[1]*Faculty of Pharmacy, University of Valencia, Valencia, Spain;* [2]*Endocrinology and Nutrition Department, General University Hospital, University of Valencia, Valencia, Spain;* [3]*General Surgery Department, La Fe University Hospital, Valencia, Spain*

Chapter outline

Introduction 2
Micronutrient deficiency 3
    Vitamins 3
        Preoperative vitamin B1 deficiency 3
        Preoperative vitamin B12 deficiency 3
        Preoperative vitamin D deficiency 4
        Preoperative vitamin B9 deficiency 4
        Another preoperative vitamin deficiency 5
    Minerals 5
        Preoperative iron deficiency 5
        Preoperative selenium deficiency 5
        Preoperative zinc deficiency 6
Macronutrient deficiency 6
    Proteins 6
Recommendations and methodology of patient performance 6
    Evaluation 6
    Preparation of the surgical patient 9
        Treatment of protein deficiency 10

Treatment of vitamin B1 deficiency 10
Treatment of vitamin B12 deficiency 10
Treatment of vitamin D and calcium deficiency 10
Treatment of acid folic deficiency 11
Treatment of iron deficiency 11
Treatment of selenium deficiency 11
Treatment of zinc deficiency 11
References 12

Introduction

Obesity is a global pandemic, in 1997, World Health Organization draws up a report that warns of a new epidemic that can expose the world's population to the development of noncommunicable diseases, thus referring to obesity. This organization estimates that the prevalence of obesity has tripled in the last 3 decades; currently, there are 1900 million overweight adults and more than 650 million with obesity. In 2016, 13% of the world's population is considered obese (11% of men and 15% of women) and approximately 2.8 million people die annually due to problems arising from overweight and obesity [1].

The increasing prevalence of obesity forces to establish intervention criteria in two clearly differentiable but complementary fields, prevention and therapeutics [2].

Once obesity has been established, pharmacological treatments produce very discrete results with a very low long-term maintenance rate, considered insufficient tools. Therefore, the only treatment with proven long-term efficacy on weight loss and treatment of associated comorbidities in patients with severe obesity is bariatric surgery [3,4]. Despite their advantages, some of the bariatric procedures can be accompanied by micronutrient deficiencies and other related metabolic complications. It is common to think that vitamin and mineral deficiencies in the western world are rare due to the wide variety of foods, their accessibility, and low prices, but this is wrong in western society. Instead at any time, the trend is for many people to eat foods that are "unhealthy" and have inappropriate eating behavior, favoring foods with high energy density and low micronutrient content [5]. In addition to a poorly balanced diet, obesity patients have other factors, such as alcohol consumption, chronic subclinical inflammation, several diseases (diabetes, hypertension, hypothyroidism, renal, and liver disease), and medications that can impact blood levels of micronutrients [6].

Micronutrient deficiency is common in obese patients admitted for bariatric surgery, especially, a considerable prevalence of low levels of vitamin D, folic acid, vitamin B1, vitamin B12, vitamin A, vitamin E, zinc, iron, and selenium has been seen [7–9].

This higher prevalence of micronutrient deficiencies in obese people could also promote postoperative diet-related complications [10] and postoperative nutritional deficiencies [11]. In addition, patients who are going to undergo bariatric surgery are at risk of suffering postoperative nutrient deficiencies due to several mechanisms: reduced food intake, anatomical changes that cause nutrient malabsorption, a reduction of hydrochloric acid secretion and intrinsic factors due to surgery, postoperative nausea and vomiting, poor food choices, or poor tolerance of certain foods [11−13]. That is why it is important to know what is the prevalence of nutritional deficiency among patients before bariatric surgery, and which patients have a higher risk of such deficiencies. In this way, better preoperative preparation of the patient could be done.

Each of the deficits that usually appear in those patients who are candidates for bariatric surgery is detailed below.

Micronutrient deficiency
Vitamins
Preoperative vitamin B1 deficiency
Vitamin B1 (Thiamine) serves as a coenzyme in a wide variety of intricate biochemical pathways, making it vital for proper tissue and organ function [14]. Deficiency of this essential vitamin may lead to serious metabolic derangements causing cardiovascular and neurological manifestations, like cerebral dysfunctions, peripheral polyneuropathy, or Wernicke encephalopathy (WE) [15].

Vitamin B1 is not stored in large amounts in any tissue and may become depleted within a few weeks. It is rapidly destroyed in the process of food preparation and when ingested with ethanol.

An increase in the vitamin requirements caused by strenuous physical activity, major surgery, major trauma, fever, pregnancy, lactation, and adolescent growth may accelerate the clinical manifestations of deficiency, that is why WE can occur after all types of bariatric surgical procedures. Predisposing risk factors for WE associated with bariatric surgery are vomits and regurgitations after surgery, excessive alcohol consumption, rapid postbariatric weight loss, or long-term parenteral nutrition. Various medical conditions and medications such as diuretics may increase vitamin B1 requirements induce vitamin B1 loss in the urine [15].

One study that evaluated the preoperative nutritional status of various nutrients in morbidly obese patients indicated that 29% of the patients suffered from preoperative vitamin B1 deficiency [5]. This study notes that males had a greater tendency for deficiency, but in the study conducted by Carrodeguas et al. (2005), the authors observe that male patients presented with greater mean preoperative vitamin B1 levels (3.2 μg/dL) than female patients (2.4 μg/dL). In this study, the incidence of this deficiency in the race is also analyzed: a greater deficit was demonstrated in Hispanic patients, followed by African Americans and Caucasian patients [7].

Preoperative vitamin B12 deficiency
Vitamin B12 (cobalamin) is involved in the synthesis of methionine and thymidine, fundamental for DNA duplication and acetyl-CoA synthesis for system myelination central nervous [16]. Vitamin B12 deficiency could be a cause of macrocytic (megaloblastic) anemia and, in advanced cases, pancytopenia, paresthesia, peripheral

neuropathy, demyelination of the corticospinal tract and dorsal columns, psychiatric disorders, including impaired memory, irritability, depression, dementia and, rarely, psychosis, and also combined vitamin B12 and folate deficiency causes hyperhomocysteinemia, which is an independent risk factor for atherosclerotic disease [17].

Vitamin B12 is absorbed in the terminal ileum, for which it requires that the stomach, pancreas, and terminal ileum be anatomically and functionally intact. Gastric level, acidity, and digestive enzymes separate the vitamin from its strong binding to food proteins and parietal cells secrete the factor intrinsic, fundamental for absorption in the ileum. Pancreatic trypsin and bicarbonate facilitate digestion and absorption. In the case of patients with obesity, a prevalence of low levels of vitamin B12 has been seen in 13% of patients [18].

The most important causes of vitamin deficiency B12 in the general population are as follows [19]:

- Deficit in contribution: long vegetarian diet evolution.
- Digestion deficit: inability to release vitamin B12 from food, particularly in hypochlorhydria and atrophic gastritis.
- Malabsorption: due to resection/disease of the terminal ileum.
- Drug interactions: neomycin, metformin, colchicine, anticonvulsants, etc.

Preoperative vitamin D deficiency

Vitamin D can be made in the skin from exposure to sunlight, which is the major source of vitamin D for most humans. Vitamin D_2 or ergocalciferol is formed by the action of ultraviolet radiation on the ergosterol steroid in plants and vitamin D_3 is generated in the skin of higher animals by the effect of exposure to ultraviolet rays from sunlight, from 7-dehydrocholesterol. Regardless of the origin of circulating vitamin D (food, skin, or drug) during its passage through the liver it is hydroxylated in position 25. 25 OH-vitamin D is processed through sunlight in humans, and therefore, it has a significant relationship with physical activity [20]. In addition, vitamin D is sequestered in the large body fat reserve and, therefore, its bioavailability is reduced in this type of patient [21].

Hypovitaminosis D is common among the general population and frequent in people with morbid obesity before bariatric surgery (25% of patients). For this reason, it is essential to look for nutritional deficiencies in each patient, before the operation [22,23]. These patients are at risk of subsequent deficiencies due to restrictive surgical techniques and especially malabsorption and some authors recommend oral vitamin D supplementation even before any bariatric operation. Calcium is absorbed by active vitamin D-mediated transport in the duodenum and proximal jejunum. It can also be absorbed passively throughout the small intestine. Therefore, it is important to assess a possible calcium deficiency together with vitamin D deficiency [24].

Preoperative vitamin B9 deficiency

Vitamin B9 (folic acid/folate) (the anion form) is a water-soluble vitamin, and it is a member of the vitamin B group. Folate deficiency has severe metabolic and clinical consequences, like anemia or defects of the neural tube. Folate and vitamin B12 have interdependent roles in nucleic acid synthesis, and their deficiencies can cause megaloblastic anemia [25]. Although the incidence is not high, it can appear in morbidly obese people due to different factors, and one of the most important is the quality of the diet. In this case, there is a 6% prevalence of deficit in patients with obesity [26].

Another preoperative vitamin deficiency
Vitamin A (retinol) is one of the fat-soluble vitamins, and its deficiency can lead to night blindness, reduced infection control, and problems in reproduction. Vitamin A can be found in fruits and vegetables, milk, liver, and eggs [27]. Vitamin A deficiency is more frequent in underdeveloped countries and in people with defects in liver storage, a prevalence of deficit has been observed in 11% of obese patients [26].

Some studies show that there may be a deficiency of vitamins E and C in obese patients, and, therefore, they should be studied and monitored from the preoperative time [26].

Minerals
Preoperative iron deficiency
Iron has a fundamental role in the homeostasis, participating in many vital cellular processes, such as oxygen transportation, energy production, cell growth, and synthesis of neurotransmitters, among others.

Dietary iron is classified as heme iron (animal origin), in its ionic form Fe^{2+} (ferrous), easily absorbed in the duodenum and proximal jejunum, and as nonheme iron, being the form more present in the Western diet. In the latter, the oxidized iron (Fe^{3+}), which is less absorbable, is the form that predominates, Heme iron (Fe^{2+}) is 2—6 times more bioavailable from the diet than nonheme iron [5].

Transferrin is the protein that transports iron in plasma. Under normal conditions, 20%—50% of the binding sites of iron in transferrin are occupied. Low levels may be present in iron deficiency anemia, malnutrition, and some chronic diseases [28]. Because no single iron status marker is a definitive determinant for the diagnosis of iron deficiency, the preferred screening approach is based on a combination of markers that should include low serum iron concentration, low levels of serum ferritin (implying depleted iron stores), and low transferrin saturation.

Iron deficiency is considered the most common mineral deficiency among humans and in candidates for bariatric surgery. Anemia caused by iron deficiency has been described in 5.5%—21.9% of severely obese patients before bariatric surgery [29]. On the other hand, the chronic inflammatory process induced by obesity increases the production of hepcidin by the liver and in adipose tissue via IL-6, which decreases the availability of systemic iron [30]. Many deficiencies will remain subclinical but could become clinically evident in stressful situations such as surgery; furthermore, preoperative iron deficiency has been associated with an increased risk of developing an iron deficiency in the postoperative period [31].

Preoperative selenium deficiency
Selenium is an essential element with important biological roles, including regulation of antioxidants activities, improvement of immune functions, normal growth,

and body maintenance [32]. A low selenium level is an independent risk factor for cardiovascular disease, high homocysteine levels, and some types of cancers. Selenium intake is on average 24% and 31% lower by obese subjects as compared to nonobese men and women, respectively [33].

Preoperative zinc deficiency

Zinc is the second most common trace element found in the human body. It plays an essential role in more than 300 enzymatic reactions and cellular function and metabolism [34,35], protecting cells from radical damage free [36]. This mineral is part of the metabolism of hormones involved in the pathophysiology of obesity, and it seems to be related to the mechanisms of insulin resistance commonly present in obesity. A prevalence of deficit has been found in 28% of obese patients [26].

Macronutrient deficiency
Proteins

Sarcopenia is a pathological disorder characterized by the generalized loss of lean mass and skeletal muscle function. For this reason, it was considered a risk factor, affecting the quality of life of the bariatric patient [37]. This pathology is also associated with diabetes, metabolic syndrome, cardiovascular disease, and fibrosis or steatosis in patients with nonalcoholic fatty liver disease. Sarcopenia has been primarily studied in older adults and individuals with chronic conditions but emerging evidence suggests that "healthy," younger individuals are also at risk for presenting with this condition. Therefore, it is a factor to take into account those patients who are candidates for bariatric surgery. In fact, the term "sarcopenic" obesity has already been established [38]. Depending on the age, gender, or habits of the patient, the prevalence of sarcopenia among the obese population ranges from 0% to 45% [39].

The problem with this condition is the diagnosis. For this reason, to avoid the risk of sarcopenic obesity, the diagnosis of obesity requires the utilization of various methods, including body composition evaluation, metabolic, functional, and a genetic approach [40]. Albumin and transferrin levels, also, are used in many studies as potential indicators of protein status [23]. These levels do not always reflect the actual state of protein intake, as they are affected by other conditions such as inflammation, liver disease, and nephrotic syndrome [41]. Some studies reflect an albumin deficit, so it is advisable to guide the patient and give him nutritional education from the preoperative period [10].

Recommendations and methodology of patient performance
Evaluation

Before the intervention, the evaluation of the patient with morbid obesity should be considered from a multidisciplinary perspective that includes various health professionals such as endocrinologists, surgeons, nutritionists, anesthetists, psychologists and psychiatrists, pulmonologists, digestologists, radiologists, educators, and other specialists who deemed necessary. The Interdisciplinary European Guidelines on Metabolic and Bariatric Surgery [42] recommend that the team that provides this assessment should be specialized in obesity management and bariatric surgery.

In obesity, as in any disease, it is important to conduct an anamnesis where the interrogation that corresponds to obesity is deepened. The patient will be asked about aspects such as family history, dietary and toxic habits, comorbidities (diabetes, dyslipidemia, high blood pressure, etc.) medications, weight loss evolution, and sedentary habit. This section will also study the context in which obesity develops, knowing the professional and family limitations, the degree of support from relatives or closest people, the degree of motivation of the patient, or those difficulties that may present themselves to the time to make a lifestyle change.

Obese people often displace nutritious foods with high-calorie foods that are rich in refined carbohydrates and fats; these diets also have deficiencies [10]; for this reason, it is vitally important to know the patient's eating habits through an assessment method, such as the frequency of consumption questionnaire [43].

In addition, the evolution of obesity should be studied in depth, recording the age of onset, evolution of weight (maximum and minimum weight) together with a record of previous failures and possible triggering causes (changes in the home, in work or marital status, anxious pictures, physical exercise, etc.) [44].

ASMBS made a recommendation for preoperative micronutrient screening. All candidates for bariatric surgery undergo preoperative nutritional evaluation, including micronutrient measurements, firstly, to optimize clinical conditions at the time of surgery, and secondly, because bariatric procedures can increase micronutrient deficiencies (Table 1.1) [45,46].

These nutritional deficiencies also can make obese patients prone to short-term complications after surgery, as it can decrease the patient's ability to fight infections or to develop the necessary healing cascade mechanisms that require energy, amino acids, minerals, and vitamins. Am and Nm (2003) [47] conclude that preoperative micronutrient deficiencies should be diagnosed and treated properly before performing surgery on the patient.

Table 1.1 Preoperative blood tests to be undertaken on patients undergoing all bariatric procedures.

Hemogram and nutritional (proteins, albumin, calcium, etc.)
Full blood count ferritin
Folate
Vitamin B12
25 hydroxy-vitamin D calcium
Parathyroid hormone
Liver function test (bilirubin, GOT, GPT, GGT
Urea and electrolytes (sodium, potassium, etc.)
Fasting glucose
HbA1c
Lipid profile

The process of nutritional detection and the subsequent identification of micronutrient deficiencies can also affect the selection of the bariatric procedure, thus choosing the best technique for each patient.

Keeping in mind the recommendations of several authors, reference ranges established for each of the nutrients or micronutrients and the treatment if any deficit is shown in Table 1.2.

Table 1.2 Level diagnosis of vitamin and mineral deficiencies and recommendations to treat them procedures [48].

	Diagnosis	Deficiency	Patients who are diagnosed with low levels before surgery
Thiamine	2.8–8.5 µg/dL	<2.5 µg/dL	Oral route: 100 mg, 2–3 times a day until symptoms resolve. Intravenous route: 200 mg, 3 times a day up to 500 mg, 1 or 2 times a day for 3–5 days. Followed by 250 mg/d for 3–5 days or until symptoms resolve.
Vitamin B12	400–800 pg/mL	<400 pg/mL	1000 mcg/day cobalamin orally. Intramuscular: 1000 mcg monthly until normal levels are reached.
Vitamin D (serum 25 OH)	30–80 ng/mL	<30 ng/mL	Vit D3 at least 2000 IU/up to 6000 IU/day or 50,000 IU of vit D2, 1–3 times/week. Vit D3 is a better treatment alternative.
Folic acid	3–17.0 ng/mL	<3 ng/mL	Folic acid tablets 5 mg daily given for about 3–4 months corrects the deficiency.
Iron	60–160 ug/dL	<50 ug/dL	150–200 mg/day of elemental iron with a maximum of 300 mg/day divided into 2–3 times a day. If oral therapy is not sufficient, intravenous iron infusion may be required.
Selenium	90–120 µg Se L^{-1}	<90 Se L^{-1}	100 µg/day
Zinc	74–110 ug/dL	<70 ug/dL in women <74 ug/dL in men	The administration of a polyvitamin is sufficient in this case.
Calcium	9–10.5 mg/d	<9 mg/dL, patients without kidney disease.	1200 mg/day

Preparation of the surgical patient

After a global evaluation, patients with a potential risk or demonstrable nutrient and micronutrient insufficiencies or deficiencies should be treated with the respective nutrient-micronutrient.

The guidelines on perioperative and postoperative biochemical monitoring and micronutrient replacement for patients undergoing bariatric surgery made by British Obesity and Metabolic Surgery Society in September 2014 [49] state that a multivitamin and mineral supplement may be necessary as the diets carried out by patients before surgery are not always nutritionally complete.

Clinical guidelines recommend that nutritional intervention should start before the surgical procedure as preoperative [45]. Benaiges et al. (2019) observed that most of the changes in dietary habit 1 year after surgery had been taught before surgery. In this study, through group meetings, patients were taught to include new nutrient-dense foods and to eliminate processed foods from their diet, reducing portion sizes. In addition, nutrition education on strict meal planning was encouraged [50].

A nutritional intervention adapted to each candidate patient must be planned, bearing in mind that this diet must be complete and cover all requirements (Table 1.3) and correcting any kind of deficit.

Table 1.3 Dietary reference intakes (IDR) of different countries of the European Union, the United States, and the World Health Organization [51].

Nutrients	Recommended daily intakes for adults
Vitamin B12,	1—1.5 g
Vitamin D	5—15 g
Biotin	60 g
Iodine, selenium	100 g
Folate, molybdenum	200—400 g
Vitamin A, B1, B2, B6, fluorine, copper	1.2—2 mg
Pantothenate, manganese	5—10 mg
Vitamin E, zinc, iron	15 mg
Vitamin C	50—100 mg
Magnesium	300—420 mg
Calcium, phosphorus	1—1.3 g
Sodium, essential fatty acids	1—5 g
Potassium	450—470 mg
Dietary fiber	20—40 g
Protein	15%—20%
Available carbohydrates	45%—55%
Water	>1 L

Treatment of protein deficiency
An intake of 15%–20%/day should be recommended with foods based on a diet rich in egg and dairy (added to purees, creams, salads, smoothies, etc.).

Some protein powder may be prescribed to enrich the diet in case the recommendations cannot be reached with natural foods or hypoproteinemia. If the clinical situation does not improve, it will be necessary to use parenteral nutrition [48].

To prevent sarcopenia, the patient should also be reminded of the importance of physical exercise and outdoor activities [20,21]. Early instauration of adequate nutritional support in combination with physical activity is a major anabolic stimulus for muscle protein synthesis and prevention of sarcopenia occurrence [52].

Treatment of vitamin B1 deficiency
Dietary sources include only limited quantities in a variety of animal and vegetable products, and it is abundant only in a small number of foods such as yeast, whole grain, beef, lean pork, and legumes (beans and peas). It is absent from fats, oils, and refined carbohydrates. Certain foods such as tea and coffee contain thiaminase, which is able to destroy the vitamin during food storage, preparation, or during passage in the gastrointestinal tract [53].

Current guidelines for bariatric surgery suggest preventive suppletion (12 mg) in multivitamin treatment for all patients undergoing surgery, but higher doses for patients with suspicion for deficiency [54]. In patients who are diagnosed with low levels before surgery, 100 mg of vitamin B1 orally twice daily must be recommended until their levels are satisfactory (Table 1.2) [45,55]. In recalcitrant or recurrent cases of vitamin B1 deficiency, the addition of antibiotics for small intestine bacterial overgrowth should be considered [15].

Treatment of vitamin B12 deficiency
In the event of vitamin B12 deficiency, a diet rich in this micronutrient is established, teaching the patient to follow a dietary guideline that includes foods rich in this vitamin. In addition, an oral contribution is established, which, if insufficient, will be replaced by an intramuscular contribution (1000 mcg monthly until normal levels are reached). High concentrations of vitamin B12 can be found in animal products, especially viscera such as liver, kidneys, and brain (50–100 mcg/100 g), followed by egg yolk, clams, oysters, crab, sardines, salmon (5–50 mcg/100 g) and finally lean meats, dairy, and fish such as cod, hake, sole, or tuna (0.2–5 mcg/100 g) [56].

Treatment of vitamin D and calcium deficiency
Good sources of vitamin D3 are fish (not only fatty fish), egg yolk, and offal such as liver. Meat contains a small amount of vitamin D3. In addition, some wild mushrooms may contain significant amounts of vitamin D2 [57]. Some foods are fortified with vitamin D in some countries [58].

It is recommended to supplement the diet with 1200 mg of calcium and vitamin D3, 800 U/day, or 16,000 U two times a month [24].

Treatment of acid folic deficiency
Folic acid is prevalent in leafy vegetables, wholemeal products, and legumes and is characterized by low storage capacity. Dietary folate is found in the highest concentrations in liver and leafy green vegetables. Lower plasma levels are most likely due to decreased consumption of the respective nutrients. Fortified foods provide a good additional dietary source in countries with folic acid food fortification practice [59].

In general, to obtain normal levels, the administration of a polyvitamin is sufficient or with the administration of Folic acid tablets 5 mg daily given for about 3—4 months [48].

Treatment of iron deficiency
In this case, nutritional education is important, where the intake of foods rich in heme and nonheme iron will be recommended, stressing the importance of the latter being accompanied by foods rich in vitamin C. The richest sources of iron are cereals, vegetables, nuts, eggs, fish, and meat [60]. Iron is also added to food as a fortificant in many countries [61,62]. Prophylaxis of iron deficiency with oral supplements is very effective, using a polyvitamin or an iron preparation, especially in ferrous form, in doses of 45—60 mg of elemental iron, together with vitamin C.

If prophylaxis is not effective, patients with preoperative anemia due to iron deficiency or chronic disease may receive preoperative treatment with oral or intravenous iron, depending on the time before surgery, oral iron tolerance, and the state of iron metabolism. The treatment should be oral iron, 100 mg of elemental iron, three times a day. In the case of nonresponse, intravenous iron is established as a protocol [48].

Treatment of selenium deficiency
The selenium content of each food depends on the selenium content of the soil where plants are grown or animals are raised. Animals that eat grains or plants that were grown in selenium-rich soil have higher levels of selenium in their muscles. Selenium also can be found in seafood. In the United States, meats and bread are common sources of dietary selenium. Some nuts also contain selenium, especially Brazilian nuts [32].

In the event of not reaching an adequate level through diet, oral supplements may be recommended (100 μg/day) [48].

Treatment of zinc deficiency
Large amounts of zinc can be found in lamb, leafy and root vegetables, crustaceans, beef kidney, liver, heart, and mollusks. Other foods with moderate amounts of this micronutrient are whole grains, pork, poultry, milk, low-fat cheese, yogurt, eggs, and nuts [63]. The administration of a polyvitamin is sufficient in case of deficiency.

In addition, it has recommended a good strategy to ensure the acquisition of good habits during preoperative time and their maintenance in the postsurgery follow-up. The organization of working groups with candidates for bariatric surgery is highly recommended, including a dietary habit and nutritional status evaluation.

For all this, the preoperative stage is essential for the good management of the morbidly obese patient, as nutritional deficiencies can be found in the population that are candidates for bariatric surgery. All these deficiencies are capable of being corrected with an adequate supplement and management of the preoperative diet.

References

[1] WHO. Descriptive note No. 311. WHO | obesity and overweight. 2016.
[2] Kushner RF. Weight loss strategies for treatment of obesity. Prog Cardiovasc Dis 2014; 56(4):465–72.
[3] Li Z, Maglione M, Tu W, Mojica W, Arterburn D, Shugarman LR, et al. Metaanalysis: pharmacologic treatment of obesity. Ann Intern Med 2005;142(7):532–46.
[4] Buchwald H, Avidor Y, Braunwald E, Jensen MD, Pories W, Fahrbach K, et al. Bariatric surgery: a systematic review and meta-analysis. J Am Med Assoc 2004;292(14): 1724–37.
[5] Kaidar-Person O, Rosenthal RJ. Commentary regarding flancbaum L, belsley S, Drake V, colarusso T, Tayler E. Preoperative nutritional status of patients undergoing roux-en-Y gastric bypass for morbid obesity. J Gastrointest 2007;10(7):1033–7.
[6] Aasheim ET, Hofsø D, Hjelmesaeth J, Birkeland KI, Bøhmer T. Vitamin status in morbidly obese patient: a cross-sectional study. Am J Clin Nutr 2008;87:362–9.
[7] Carrodeguas L, Kaidar-Person O, Szomstein S, Antozzi P, Rosenthal R. Preoperative thiamine deficiency in obese population undergoing laparoscopic bariatric surgery. Surg Obes Relat Dis 2005;1(6):517–22.
[8] Frame-Peterson LA, Megill RD, Carobrese S, Schweitzer M. Nutrient deficiencies are common prior to bariatric surgery. Nutr Clin Pract 2017;32(4):463–9.
[9] Schweiger C, Weiss R, Berry E, Keidar A. Nutritional deficiencies in bariatric surgery candidates. Obes Surg 2009;20(2):193–7.
[10] Moizé V, Deulofeu R, Torres F, de Osaba, Vidal J. Nutritional intake and prevalence of nutritional deficiencies prior to surgery in a Spanish morbidly obese population. Obes Surg 2011;21(9):1382–8.
[11] Ben-Porat T, Elazary R, Yuval JB, Wieder A, Khalaileh A, Weiss R. Nutritional deficiencies after sleeve gastrectomy: can they be predicted preoperatively? Surg Obes Relat Dis 2015;11(5):1029–36.
[12] Snyder-Marlow G, Taylor D, Lenhard MJ. Nutrition care for patients undergoing laparoscopic sleeve gastrectomy for weight loss. J Am Diet Assoc 2010;110(4):600–7.
[13] Stein J, Stier C, Raab H, Weiner R. Review article: the nutritional and pharmacological consequences of obesity surgery. Aliment Pharmacol Ther 2014;40(6):582–609.
[14] Goodwin DW. The Wernicke-Korsakoff syndrome: a clinical and pathological study of 245 patients, 82 with post-mortem examinations. J Am Med Assoc 1972;219(3):389.
[15] Singh S, Kumar A. Wernicke encephalopathy after obesity surgery: a systematic review. Neurology 2007;68(11):807–11.
[16] Hvas AM, Nexo E. Diagnosis and treatment of vitamin B12 deficiency: an update. Haematologica 2006;91(11):1506–12.
[17] Nygård O, Nordrehaug JE, Refsum H, Ueland PM, Farstad M, Vollset SE. Plasma homocysteine levels and mortality in patients with coronary artery disease. N Engl J Med 1997;337(4):230–7.

References

[18] Hamoui N, Anthone G, Crookes PF. Calcium metabolism in the morbidly obese. Obes Surg 2004;14(1):9–12.

[19] Oh R, Brown DL. Vitamin B12 deficiency. Am Acad Fam Physicians 2003;67(5): 979–86.

[20] Holick MF. Vitamin D deficiency. N Engl J Med 2007;357:266–81.

[21] Wortsman J, Matsuoka LY, Chen TC, Lu Z, Holick MF. Decreased bioavailability of vitamin D in obesity. Am J Clin Nutr 2000;72(3):690–3.

[22] Krzizek E-C, Brix JM, Herz CT, Kopp HP, Schernthaner G-H, Schernthaner G, Ludvik B. Prevalence of micronutrient deficiency in patients with morbid obesity before bariatric surgery. Obes Surg 2017;28(3):643–8.

[23] Al-Mutawa A, Anderson A, Alsabah S, Al-Mutawa M. Nutritional status of bariatric surgery candidates. Nutrients 2018;10(1):67.

[24] Ducloux R, Nobécourt E, Chevallier J-M, Ducloux H, Elian N, Altman J-J. Vitamin D deficiency before bariatric surgery: should supplement intake be routinely prescribed? Obes Surg 2011;21(5):556–60.

[25] Arenas BC. Interrelacion entre vitamina B12 y acido folico. Avances 2011;8:10–5.

[26] Madan AK, Orth WS, Tichansky DS, Ternovits CA. Vitamin and trace mineral levels after laparoscopic gastric bypass. Obes Surg 2006;16(5):603–6.

[27] Cañete A, Cano E, Muñoz-Chápuli R, Carmona R. Role of vitamin A/retinoic acid in regulation of embryonic and adult hematopoiesis. Nutrients 2017;9(2):159.

[28] Salazar-Lugo R. Metabolismo del hierro, inflamación y obesidad. Saber 2015;27(1): 5–16.

[29] Salgado W, Modotti C, Nonino CB, Ceneviva R. Anemia and iron deficiency before and after bariatric surgery. Surg Obes Relat Dis 2014;10(1):49–54.

[30] Miret S, Simpson RJ, McKie AT. Physiology and molecular biology of dietary iron absorption. Annu Rev Nutr 2003;23(1):283–301.

[31] Van der Beek ESJ, Monpellier VM, Eland I, Tromp E, van Ramshorst B. Nutritional deficiencies in gastric bypass patients; incidence, time of occurrence and implications for post-operative surveillance. Obes Surg 2014;25(5):818–23.

[32] Surai PF. Natural antioxidants in poultry nutrition: new developments. In: Proc 16th European symposium on poultry nutrition, Strasbourg, France, 26–30 August 2007; 2007. p. 669–76.

[33] Wang Y, Gao X, Pedram P, Shahidi M, Du J, Yi Y, Sun G. Significant beneficial association of high dietary selenium intake with reduced body fat in the CODING study. Nutrients 2016;8(1):24.

[34] Chimienti F, Aouffen M, Favier A. Zinc homeostasis- regulating proteins: new drug targets for triggering cell fate. Curr Drug Targets 2003;4:323–38.

[35] King JC. Determinants of maternal zinc status during pregnancy. Am J Clin Nutr 2000; 71:1334–43.

[36] Powell SR. The antioxidant properties of zinc. J Nutr 2000;130:1447–54.

[37] Batsis JA, Mackenzie TA, Barre LK, Lopez-Jimenez F, Bartels SJ. Sarcopenia, sarcopenic obesity and mortality in older adults: results from the National Health and Nutrition Examination Survey III. Eur J Clin Nutr 2014;68(9):1001–7.

[38] Baumgartner RN. Body composition in healthy aging. Ann N Y Acad Sci 2000;904: 437–48.

[39] Cauley JA. An overview of sarcopenic obesity. J Clin Densitom 2015;18(4):499–505.

[40] Romero-Corral A, Somers VK, Sierra-Johnson J, Thomas RJ, Collazo-Clavell ML, Korinek J, Lopez-Jimenez F. Accuracy of body mass index in diagnosing obesity in the adult general population. Int J Obes 2008;32(6):959—66.
[41] Mahan L, Escott-Stump S. Krause's food nutrition therapy. 12th ed. St. Louis, MO, USA: Saunders/Elsevier; 2008. p. 84—5.
[42] Fried M, Yumuk V, Oppert J-M, Scopinaro N, Torres AJ, Weiner R, Frühbeck G. Interdisciplinary European guidelines on metabolic and bariatric surgery. Obes Facts 2013; 6(5):449—68.
[43] Flegal KM, Larkin FA, Metzner HL, Thompson FE, Guire KE. Counting calories: partitioning energy intake estimates from a food frequency questionnaire. Am J Epidemiol 1988;128(4):749—60.
[44] Rubio MA, Moreno C. Implicaciones nutricionales de la cirugía bariátrica sobre el tracto gastrointestinal. Nutr Hosp 2007;22(2):124—34.
[45] Mechanick JI, Youdim A, Jones DB, Garvey WT, Hurley DL, McMahon MM, Brethauer S. Clinical practice guidelines for the perioperative nutritional, metabolic, and nonsurgical support of the bariatric surgery patient-2013 update: cosponsored by American Association of Clinical Endocrinologists, The Obesity Society, and American Society of Obesity. Obesity 2013;21(S1):S1—27.
[46] Thibault R, Huber O, Azagury DE, Pichard C. Twelve key nutritional issues in bariatric surgery. Clin Nutr 2016;35(1):12—7.
[47] Am Q, Nm K. Nutrition in wound care management: a comprehensive overview. 2015.
[48] Palma Moya M, Quesada Charneco M, Fernández Soto ML. Trastornos nutricionales tras cirugía bariátrica y su tratamiento. Endocrinol Nutr 2007;54:42—7.
[49] British Obesity and Metabolic Surgery Society. BOMSS guidelines on peri-operative and postoperative biochemical monitoring and micronutrient replacement for patients undergoing bariatric surgery. Available from: https://www.bomss.org.uk/wp-content/uploads/2014/09/BOMSS-guidelines-Final-version1Oct14.pdf. [Accessed 11 March 2020].
[50] Benaiges D, Parri A, Subirana I, Pedro-Botet J, Villatoro M, Ramon JM, Goday A. Most of qualitative dietary changes observed one year post-bariatric surgery can be achieved with a preoperative dietary intervention. Endocrinol Diabetes Nutr 2019;67(1):20—7.
[51] Cuervo M, Corbalan M, Baladia E, Cabrerizo L, Formiguera X, Iglesias C, et al. Comparativa de las Ingestas Dieteticas de Refe- rencia (IDR) de los diferentes paises de la Union Europea, de Estados Unidos (EEUU) y de la Organizacion Mundial de la Salud (OMS). Nutr Hosp 2009;24(4):384—414.
[52] Robinson SM, Reginster JY, Rizzoli R, Shaw SC, Kanis JA, Bautmans I, Rueda R. Does nutrition play a role in the prevention and management of sarcopenia? Clin Nutr 2018; 37(4):1121—32.
[53] Davis RE, Icke GC. Clinical chemistry of thiamin. Adv Clin Chem 1983;(23):93—140.
[54] Zafar A. Wernicke's encephalopathy following roux on Y gastric bypass surgery. Saudi Med J 2015;36(12):1493—5.
[55] Kaidar-Person O, Person B, Szomstein S, Rosenthal RJ. Nutritional deficiencies in morbidly obese patients: a new form of malnutrition? Obes Surg 2008;18(7):870—6.
[56] Green R, Allen LH, Bjørke-Monsen A-L, Brito A, Guéant J-L, Miller JW, Yajnik C. Vitamin B12 deficiency. Nat Rev Dis Primers 2017;3:17040.
[57] Mattila P. Analysis of cholecalciferol, ergocalciferol and their 25-hydroxylated metabolites in foods by HPLC. Dissertation, EKT Series 995. University of Helsinki; 1995.

[58] Jan Y, Malik M, Yaseen M, Ahmad S, Imran M, Rasool S, Haq A. Vitamin D fortification of foods in India: present and past scenario. J Steroid Biochem Mol Biol 2019;193: 105417.
[59] Bailey LB, Stover PJ, McNulty H, Fenech MF, Gregory JF, Mills JL, Raiten DJ. Biomarkers of nutrition for development—folate review. J Nutr 2015;145(7):1636S—80S.
[60] Samaniego-Vaesken M, Partearroyo T, Olza J, Aranceta-Bartrina J, Gil Á, González-Gross M, Varela-Moreiras G. Iron intake and dietary sources in the Spanish population: findings from the ANIBES study. Nutrients 2017;9(3):203.
[61] Hurrell RF. Preventing iron deficiency through food fortification. Nutr Rev 1997;55(6): 210—22.
[62] FFI. Wheat Flour Fortification Status. Map of global progress. Countries with mandatory wheat flour fortification regulations. Flour Fortification Innitiative (FFI); December 2016. Available from, http://www.ffinetwork.org/global_progress/index.php. [Accessed 16 March 2020].
[63] Pennington JAT. Bowes & Church's food values of portions commonly used. 17th ed. Philadelphia: Lippincott; 1998.

CHAPTER 2

Nutritional evaluation and calculation of nutritional requirements in the preoperative course

Jose Jorge Ortez Toro, Carlos Miguel Peteiro Miranda, Julia Ocón Bretón
University Clinical Hospital "Lozano Blesa", Endocrinology and Nutrition Department, Area of Nutrition, Zaragoza, Spain

Chapter outline

Introduction	17
Nutritional assessment	18
Sarcopenic obesity	23
Nutritional requirements calculation	24
Energy intake	25
Recall of food eaten	25
Food records	25
Food frequency questionnaires	26
New technologies	26
Total energy expenditure	26
Resting metabolic rate	28
Physical activity energy expenditure	31
Thermic effect of food	31
Protein requirements	32
References	32

Introduction

Obesity is a major public health burden of pandemic proportions and represents a major health challenge because it increases the risk of diseases such as type 2 diabetes mellitus, fatty liver disease, hypertension, myocardial infarction, stroke, dementia, osteoarthritis, obstructive sleep apnea, and several cancers. Surgery is the most effective treatment for morbid obesity in terms of sustainable weight loss along with a reduction in mortality and obesity-related comorbidities [1].

Bariatric surgery elicits a series of reactions including the release of stress hormones and inflammatory mediators. This systemic inflammatory response syndrome causes protein catabolism and loss of muscle tissue that implies a worse clinical evolution and greater morbidity and mortality [2].

In the perioperative period, usually occurs an alteration in nutritional status as a consequence of anorexia, nausea/vomiting, fasting, and prolonged prostration (additionally to the increase of protein catabolism). Inflammation in obesity favors the decrease in muscle mass and strength. Therefore, to decrease perioperative morbidity and mortality, the optimization of nutritional status and body composition becomes an important action before surgery [2].

It is necessary to obtain a medical history, clinical evaluation of comorbidities and secondary causes of obesity. Anamnesis must include a comprehensive history with data on ethnicity, family history, dietary habits, weight-loss history, physical activity, frequency eating pattern, and the possible presence of eating disorders. The presence of depression and other mood disorders, previous treatments for obesity, patient expectations, and motivation for change must be evaluated. Moreover, a physical examination, anthropometric measurements, and a routine laboratory test (including fasting blood glucose and lipid panel, kidney function, liver profile, urine analysis, and prothrombin time/INR) must be performed to assess surgical risk. In addition, psychosocial assessment is conducted to assess mood, social and family support, substance use, cognitive function, and psychosocial status [3].

Last but not least, the diagnosis and treatment of obesity cannot be separated from a nutritional history, measurement of energy expenditure, and, above all, body composition assessment, with a particular interest in body fat mass percentage [4].

Nutritional assessment

All bariatric patients must undergo nutritional evaluation and micronutrient measurements before any bariatric procedure. Evidence supports the need to identify and correct preoperative nutritional deficiencies as part of the comprehensive preoperative evaluation. Nutrient screening with iron studies, B12 vitamin and folic acid (RBC folate, homocysteine, methylmalonic acid optional), and 25-vitamin D (vitamins A and E optional) should be done. More extensive testing should be considered in patients undergoing malabsorptive procedures [3].

Obesity can be associated with altered nutritional status. The causes of malnutrition in obesity are multifactorial and include the following: a high intake of calorically dense foods with low nutritional quality, limited bioavailability of some nutrients (vitamin D), chronic inflammation status, and small intestinal bacterial overgrowth resulting in lack of uptake of micronutrients. That leads to altered body composition and body cell mass leading to diminished physical and mental function and impaired clinical outcomes [5].

The available evidence suggests that disease-related malnutrition is associated with increased morbidity, mortality and costs. Consequently, in obesity, it is necessary to make an adequate screening and assessment of malnutrition before bariatric surgery, to improve perioperative morbidity. Currently, there are several risk screening tools in use such as Nutrition Risk Screening-2002 (NRS-2002), Malnutrition Universal Screening Tool (MUST), Nutritional Assessment (MNA) either in its full or short form (MNA-SF), Malnutrition Screening Tool (MST), and the Short Nutritional Assessment Questionnaire (SNAQ). These tools are all compiled of various combinations of registered or measured body mass index (BMI), weight loss, food intake, disease severity, and age. Therefore, they are not considered good tools for nutritional risk evaluation in obese patients [6]. Consequently, to establish the diagnosis of malnutrition in this group of patients, the use of Global Leadership Initiative on Malnutrition diagnostic criteria is recommended, which requires at least a phenotypic criteria (involuntary weight loss or BMI or reduced muscle mass) and etiologic criteria (reduced food intake or assimilation and inflammation) [7].

The visceral adipose tissue is an endocrine organ that synthesizes hormones and cytokines (adiponectin, TNF-α, leptin, IL-6). Chronic inflammation contributes to malnutrition through associated altered metabolism with an elevation of resting energy expenditure, increased protein catabolism, and muscle depletion [6].

The world health organization (WHO) defines obesity as a condition in which percentage body fat (PBF) is increased. Therefore, due to the endocrine and inflammatory role of the adipose tissue, it is necessary to classify obesity condition on the basis of body fat composition and distribution, rather than the increase of body weight. Currently, PBF turns out to be the better tool for a correct diagnosis of obesity, universally valid [8].

Anthropometric-based stratification allows us to economically and easily evaluate not only total body fat but also its regional distribution, however, prone to measurement errors. Body mass index, waist circumference, waist/hip ratio, waist height ratio, and skinfold thickness are the common measures of the degree of body fat used in routine clinical practice:

- Body mass index: According to the classification based on BMI, the ratio between weight in kilograms and height in meters squared (kg/m^2), a patient is considered overweight for BMI values greater than 25 kg/m^2 and obesity is classified when BMI is greater than 30 kg/m^2. BMI is currently the most widely used criteria to identify and classify obesity. Its popularity stems in part from its convenience, safety, and minimal cost, but leads to a large error and misclassification.

BMI does not measure the PBF directly and poorly distinguishes between total body fat and total body lean, or bone mass. It is not useful for obesity diagnosis in certain conditions such as fluid retention, muscularity, sarcopenia, spinal deformities, physical disabilities, and transcultural differences. Currently, there are different methods to diagnosis obesity (Table 2.1) [8].

A person's body fat percentage can be indirectly estimated by using the CUN-BAE (Clínica Universidad de Navarra-Body Adiposity Estimator), as follows [9]:

$$BF\% = -44.988 + (0.503 \times age) + (10.689 \times sex) + (3.172 \times BMI) \\ - (0.026 \times BMI^2) + (0.181 \times BMI \times sex) - (0.02 \times BMI \times age) \\ - (0.005 \times BMI^2 \times sex) + (0.00021 \times BMI^2 \times age)$$

where male = 0 and female = 1 for sex.

Table 2.1 Obesity evaluation.

	Obesity evaluation		
BMI	• 30.00–34.99 kg/m^2: Class I obesity. • 35–39.9 kg/m^2: Class II obesity. • 40–49.9 kg/m^2: Class III or morbid obesity. • $\geq$ 50 kg/m^2: Class IV or extreme obesity.		
Fat mass (gold standard)	PBF > 25% (♂) PBF % > 33% (♀)		
Visceral Adiposity	WC	WC > 102 cm (♂) WC > 88 cm (♀)	
	TC (L3)	VAT > 130 cm^2/m^2	

- Waist circumference (WC): It is recommended to measure WC in adults with BMI below 35 kg/m^2, to further assess disease risk. WC, separately or in combination with BMI, is positively associated with morbidity and mortality independent of age, sex, and ethnicity. Progressively higher values of WC is associated with a progressive elevation in metabolic markers of cardiovascular disease risk [10]. Currently, no consensus exists on the optimal protocol for the measurement of WC. In the most often used protocol National Institutes of Health, WC is measured in the horizontal plane midway in the distance of the superior iliac crest and the lower margin of the last rib [10].
- Waist hip ratio (WHR): WHR, separately or in combination with BMI, was associated with increased risk of death and cardiovascular disease. However, recent evidence indicated that, compared with the WHR, waist circumference alone was more strongly associated with the absolute amount of visceral fat [10].
- Waist height ratio (WHtR): The WHtR, calculated by dividing the WC by height, has recently gained attention as an anthropometric index for central adiposity. A meta-analysis of studies evaluating different indices of adiposity indicates that WHtR is a better predictor of diabetes, hypertension, dyslipidemia, metabolic syndrome, and other cardiovascular outcome measures than BMI or waist circumference in both men and women [11].
- Midupper arm circumference (MUAC): MUAC is used to identify chronic energy deficiency and can also be used to predict BMI for when height or weight is unavailable [11]:

$$\text{Male}: \text{BMI} \,(\text{kg/m}^2) = 1.01 \times \text{MUAC (cm)} - 4.7$$
$$\text{Female}: \text{BMI} \,(\text{kg/m}^2) = 1.01 \times \text{MUAC (cm)} - 6.7$$

- Midarm muscle circumference (MAMC): MAMC can be used to evaluate fat-free mass or lean components of the body in nutritional assessment and is also viewed as an outcome measure to evaluate nutritional interventions It is calculated from Ref. [9]:

$$\text{MAMC (cm)} = \text{MUAC (cm)} - [\text{TSF (mm)} \times 0.3142]$$

Alternatively, midarm muscle area (MAMA) can be used to evaluate fat-free mass and, similar to MUAC to address the original but incorrect assumptions that the midarm and midarm muscle are circular, TSF is twice the rim diameter of fat and to take account of the area occupied by bone [11]:

$$\text{MAMA} = \frac{(\text{MUAC (cm)} - [\text{TSF (mm)} \times 0.3142])^2}{12.57} - K$$

where k equals 10 in men and 6.5 in women.
- Skinfold anthropometry: Tricipital (TSF), bicipital, subscapular, and suprailiac are the most used skinfolds. Total body fat can be estimated from the skinfolds using the Durnin—Womersley equation:

$$D = C - M \times \log{(PT + PB + PS + PA)}$$

$C = 1.1143$ (men) and 1.1278 (women). $M = 0.0618$ (men) y 0.0775 (women). Diagnosis, therapy, and follow-up of all subtypes of obesity must not be based only on body weight parameters, but body composition parameters are required. Currently, we have different methods for analyzing body composition, the use of which will depend on cost, availability, and facility of use (Tables 2.2 and 2.3) [12]:

- *Bioimpedance (BIA):* BIA measures the opposition of electrical current through body tissues, which can then be used to estimate total body water and body composition. Fat mass can be calculated by subtracting fat-free mass (FFM) from the total body weight.
BIA is a noninvasive, low cost, and useful bedside method for body composition assessment in clinical and nonclinical settings. Its accuracy is limited by a lack of validation for individuals aged >80 or obese patients (BMI >35 kg/m^2).

Table 2.2 Body composition analysis.

		Body composition analysis
BIA	Advantages	Inexpensive, no radiation exposure, accessible, and can be performed at the bedside.
	Limitations	Equations and algorithms that require further refinement for the clinical population. Affected by fluid retention and obesity (BMI>35 kg/m^2).
TC	Advantages	Accurate. Ability to identify muscle radiodensity to determine ectopic fat accumulation in muscle.
	Limitations	Cost. High ionizing radiation exposure.
US	Advantages	Safe, easy, and inexpensive. No radiation exposure. Differentiate abnormal muscle from normal muscle.
	Limitations	Reproducibility is unknown.
DXA	Advantages	Safe, inexpensive, and readily available, reproducible, and low radiation exposure.
	Limitations	Failure to differentiate water from muscle.

Table 2.3 Nutritional assessment of prebariatric surgery.

Nutritional assessment pre-bariatric surgery	
Anthropometric assessment	Body weight, BMI, WC, skinfold thickness, MUAC, MAMC, and MAMA.
Biochemical assessment	Fasting blood glucose and lipid panel, kidney function, liver profile, urine analysis, and prothrombin time/INR. Iron studies, B12 vitamin and folic acid (homocysteine, methylmalonic acid optional), and 25-vitamin D (vitamins A and E optional). For evaluating inflammation C-reactive protein (CRP), albumin, or prealbumin.
Body composition and functional assessment	DXA, BIA (BMI < 35 kg/m^2), TC (muscle mass, VAT, SAT, and myosteatosis), and US. Grip strength and physical performance for functional assessment.
Comorbidities evaluation	Type 2 diabetes, metabolic syndrome, dyslipidemia, hyperuricemia, fatty liver disease, hypertension, cardiovascular disease, obstructive sleep apnea syndrome, asthma, dementia, depressive disorder, osteoarthritis, polycystic ovary syndrome, gastrointestinal reflux disease, and cancer (postmenopausal breast, endometrial, prostate, and colorectal cancer).

Phase angle, which is a derived measure obtained from direct measurement of resistance and reactance, can be interpreted as an indicator of membrane integrity and water distribution between intracellular and extracellular spaces. Phase angle has been noted to be a prognostic indicator, with studies revealing a positive association with survival in multiple pathologies [13].

- *Computed tomography (CT)*: CT and magnetic resonance imaging are gold-standard techniques to quantify body composition. A single abdominal cross-sectional computed tomography image at the third lumbar vertebra provides an accurate estimate of whole-body skeletal muscle. CT imaging can further define these compartments with abdominal adipose tissue being delineated into visceral (VAT), intramuscular (muscle quality), and subcutaneous adipose tissue (SAT). The use of CT and magnetic resonance imaging, although considered gold standard methods for accurate body composition analysis, is primarily limited to research settings due to high costs, limited availability, and radiation exposure in the case of CT.

- *Dual-energy x-ray absorptiometry (DXA)*: DXA studies body composition in a model of three compartments (fat mass, lean, and bone). DXA allows quantifying total fat and lean soft tissue. The newly released software is able to extrapolate the visceral fat mass thus applying a body composition method to the evaluation of cardiovascular risk.

  DXA can be used in obese subjects undergoing bariatric surgery to monitor lean and fat mass changes. Furthermore, DXA analysis can also be used to evaluate sarcopenia, which is considered a risk factor for metabolic disease.

The technical limits of DXA are the maximum weight limit (200 kg) and the restrictions for height compromise the accuracy of the measurement with DXA for subjects outside normality range and wide of the individual examined (197 × 66 cm).

- *Ultrasound (US)*: US is a promising low-cost, low-risk, noninvasive, and portable technique. It has been used to assess body composition, with most studies focusing on visceral and subcutaneous adiposity, although it has been increasingly used for the assessment of skeletal muscle mass.
An advantage of US for skeletal muscle assessment includes the quantification of muscle quantity and quality through different parameters. Currently, the major setback for its universal use is the lack of standardized measurement protocols, including which parameters to analyze.

Sarcopenic obesity

Sarcopenia has been defined as a progressive and generalized skeletal muscle disorder that involves the accelerated loss of muscle strength and muscle mass or quality. Sarcopenia is associated with increased adverse outcomes including falls, functional decline, frailty, and mortality (Table 2.4) [14].

Sarcopenic obesity is usually identified when both low muscle mass and increased adiposity are present in an individual leading to adverse outcomes. Sarcopenia and obesity share some underlying pathophysiological pathways such as

Table 2.4 Sarcopenia diagnosis criteria.

Sarcopenia diagnosis criteria		
Muscle strength	Grip strength	<27 kg (♂) <16 kg (♀)
	Chair stand	>15 s for five rises
Muscle mass and quality	DXA	ASMI < 7 kg/m^2 (♂) y < 5.7 kg/m^2 (♀)
	BIA	ASMI < 7 kg/m^2 (♂) y < 5.4 kg/m^2 (♀)
	TC (L3)	SMI < 55 cm^2/m^2 (♂) y < 39 cm^2/m^2 (♀) Attenuation (Quality): BMI > 25 kg/m^2: <41 HU BMI >25 kg/m^2: <33 HU
	MAMA	♂ < 32 cm^2 ♀ < 18 cm^2
Physical performance (severity)	Gait speed	≤0.8 (m/s)
	TUG	≥20 s
	SPPB	≤8 point score
	400 m walk	Noncompletion or ≥6 min for completion

ASMI, *Appendicular skeletal muscle mass;* HU, *Hounsfield unit;* MAMA, *Midarm muscle area;* SMI, *Skeletal muscle index;* SPPB, *Short physical performance battery;* TUG, *Timed Up and Go test.*

increased proinflammatory cytokines, oxidative stress, insulin resistance, hormonal changes, and decreased physical activity [15].

Epidemiologic studies have shown that sarcopenic obesity is associated with an increased risk of disability, frailty, cardiometabolic disease, hospitalization, loss of independence, impaired quality of life, and mortality. Furthermore, muscle loss can also increase the risks of death and disability during weight loss in individuals with obesity. For this reason, to avoid the risk of sarcopenic obesity, the diagnosis of obesity requires the utilization of various methods, including body composition evaluation, metabolic and functional approach obesity [16].

The updated "Sarcopenia, revised European consensus on definition and diagnosis" (EWGSOP2) proposed a gradual approach to the diagnosis of sarcopenia. Diagnosis starts with a measure of muscle strength, usually grip strength. If grip strength is below the reference values, then sarcopenia should be suspected. The second step is the measurement of muscle mass with body composition techniques (TC, BIA, DXA, and US) or MAMA by anthropometry. Finally, physical performance should be considered as a measure of the severity of sarcopenia [17].

In brief, optimizing body composition, physical function, and nutritional status before bariatric surgery can minimize catabolism and support anabolism throughout surgical treatment allowing patients to recover substantially better and faster. Therefore, programs for fast track surgery later developed into preoperative enhanced recovery after bariatric surgery have been created and consist of a combined series of clinical pathways to minimize stress and facilitate recovery, improving postoperative outcomes [18].

Nutritional requirements calculation

Estimation of energy requirements is always one of the most difficult duties on clinical nutrition and in this particular area of obesity, it becomes a highly complex task. Usually, the most used method to do these are the prediction equations but we also have other options that we need to know.

Obesity is fundamentally a mismatch between energy intake and energy expenditure that results in changes in body weight and composition, as we can see in Fig. 2.1. Due to the worldwide obesity pandemic, efforts have been made to determine which factors increase energy intake relative to expenditure. Special interest exists in identifying interindividual factors that explain differential susceptibility to weight gain but is a very difficult task. Several methods for the assessment of these components are available. Each method carries issues that, if not considered, may lead to equivocal results and interpretations, we are going to make a brief review of each method [19,20].

Noteworthy, there are many terms to define the resting metabolic rate (RMR), like basal metabolic rate (BMR) or resting energy expenditure (REE), what is truly "basal" is really hard to measure, throughout this chapter we will use RMR as a synonym of BMR or REE, indicating basal or resting values.

Nutritional requirements calculation

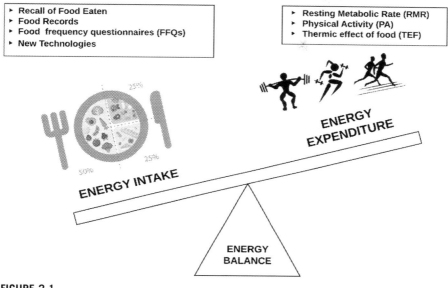

FIGURE 2.1

Body weight regulation.

Energy intake

Defined as the total energy consumed by an individual, provided by the major sources of dietary energy (carbohydrate, protein and fat). Finding a precise, homogeneous and objective method to measure this, has always been a true challenge. Now we will present the most used methods in routine clinical practice and also the newest and innovative food and energy intake assessment tools.

Recall of food eaten

This approach quantitatively assesses recent food intake. The method comprises the collection of foods consumed during the last day. Although easy to administer, the main issue is that a single 24-h recall may not reflect habitual intake. Thus, some authors recommend that three 24-h recalls should be applied to estimate energy intake [21].

Food records

This method consists in weighing the food and drinks consumed over a time frame, usually 3—7 days, food records are considered the most accurate method of dietary assessment. However, the trouble of weighing and recording intake over several days makes subjects to alter their dietary pattern as well as under-report their intake [21].

Food frequency questionnaires

It estimates the usual frequency of consumption of certain foods, with a specific size during a given period of time (1 year, 1 month). They are easier and more reliable for the memory because the usual ingestion is usually remembered. However, it does not capture short-term within-person variation to allow for investigation of diurnal variation or timing [22].

New technologies

Many upgrades in technology have been developed in recent years to improve the limitations of energy intake measurement [21]. In obesity, measuring changes in energy intake is critical for assessing the efficacy of dietary interventions and current methods as counting calories, estimating portion size and using food labels or diet history to estimate human energy intake have considerable constraints, thus research on new technologies has been encouraged to mitigate the present weakness [23].

For a better understanding, we classified the novel methods in three groups, first devices that monitor intake through sensors, second smartphone-based photographic methods linked to food databases and third, a predictive equation based on frequent measurements of body weight over extended periods [21,23]. In Table 2.5 we sum up some of the novel methods.

However, the major challenge of these methods is that they rely on self-reported data. Human memory is not 100% accurate in recalling past behavior; consequently, these measurements do not directly or objectively measure dietary intake or EI. The main issue of these methods is the underestimation of EI when compared to total energy expenditure (TEE) measured with double water label technique (gold standard). In conclusion, 24h food recalls were associated with a lower degree of misreporting and less variation in the degree of under-reporting compared to other assessments [20–22,24].

Total energy expenditure

The factors that determine daily energy expenditure are RMR, physical activity, and the thermic effect of food (TEF). These factors account for about 60%, 30%, and 10% of daily energy expenditure, respectively [21]. Noteworthy that the gold standard for measure TEE is doubly labeled water (DLW), which is a very complicated technique that determines CO_2 production by using uncommon and nonradioactive isotopes of oxygen and hydrogen in water. Subjects ingest water labeled with 2H and 18O (i.e., doubly labeled water) to enrich their body water compartment then the difference between both represents VCO_2 (the total volume of carbon dioxide that you breathe out). Consequently, this technique allows determining VCO_2 rate over the course of 1–2 weeks [24,25]. We sum up and schematize all these in the diagram in Fig. 2.2.

There are many equations commonly used for calculating TEE, they are very inaccurate, and there is no consensus on its use, despite that, they are very used in daily clinical practice; in Table 2.6, we summarize two of them [26].

Table 2.5 Novel methods for measure EI.

Monitoring devices and tools	Automated Wrist Motion Tracking	Also called a "bite counter" is worn like a watch and automatically tracks wrist motion for monitoring eating in humans
	Automatic Ingestion Monitor (AIM)	Uses integrated hand gestures, jaw motions and accelerometer sensors to detect food intake in free-living individuals
	Intelligent Food-Intake Monitor	It integrates multisensor monitors to track chewing speed, and images of the type and amount of food consumed.
Camera-scan-sensor based technologies	Remote Food Photography Method	Participants send images taken on their smartphone wirelessly to a Food Photography Application©, which is linked to the Food and Nutrient Database for Dietary Studies 3.0
	Real-Time Food Recognition System	The user uses the mobile camera at the food plate for the recognition process. After the selection of the food from a database and indication of its approximate volume, the calorie and nutrition values are displayed.
	"Snap-n-Eat"	A photo of the food plate is captured. The analytical system is based on predefined EI and nutritional density for each food category
	GoCARB	The user photographs their food the images are segmented and recognized and their carbohydrate content is estimated.
Mathematical Algorithm	A different, novel approach to assess EI	It is a formula validated thru DLW/DXA measurements collected over 2 years in 140 free-living from the CALERIE study [24].

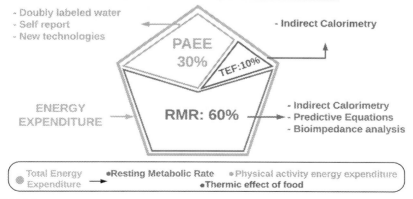

FIGURE 2.2

Components of daily energy expenditure.

Table 2.6 Predictive equations for TEE.

Harris−Benedict (kcal/day)

TEE = RMR × IF × AF × TF
RMR woman: 655.1 + 9.5 × weight (kg) + 1.8 × height (cm)−4.7 × age (years)
RMR man: 66.5 + 13.8 × weight (kg) + 5 × height (cm)−6.8 × age (years)
Activity factor (AF): bedridden: 1.2/bedridden + mobile: 1.25/walking: 1.3
Thermal factor (TF): 38°C: 1.1/39°C: 1.2/40°C: 1.3/41°C: 1.4
Injury factor (IF): uncomplicated patient (1), postoperative oncology: (1.1), long bone fracture (1.2), moderate sepsis (1.3), peritonitis (1.4), polytrauma in rehabilitation: (1.5), polytrauma + sepsis (1.6), 30%−50% burn (1.7), 50%−70% burn (1.8), 70%−90% burn (2)

Pocket formula (kcal/day)

TEE for weight loss: 20−25 kcal/kg of weight
TEE for weight maintenance: 25−30 kcal/kg of weight
TEE for weight gain: 30−35 kcal/kg of weight

Resting metabolic rate

RMR represents the energy needed to maintain bodily functions like breathing, circulating blood, organ/cellular functions, and basic neurological functions at rest and accounts for most daily energy expenditure [26]. We are going to discuss the most used methods to approach RMR.

- **Indirect calorimetry**

    Indirect calorimetry involves the measurement of gas exchange (O_2 consumption [VO_2] and CO_2 production [VCO_2]) to estimate substrate oxidation, and thus calculate energy expended [19]. It is a respiratory test that measures the patient's production of CO_2 and consumption of oxygen for approximately 30 min until steady a state is achieved. Results are worked into the modified Weir equation of heat output [27].

$$RMR = [(3.796 \times VO_2) + (1.214 \times VCO_2)] \times 1440 \text{ min/day}$$

where RMR = resting metabolic rate (kcal/day); VO_2 = oxygen consumption (L/min); CO_2 = CO_2 exhaled (L/min).

The result indicates the number of kilocalories the patient consumes in 24 h and also provides information on macronutrient utilization through the respiratory quotient (RQ).

$RQ = VCO_2/VO_2$ and provides information on the type of substrate being used. The RQ for the metabolism of fat, protein, and carbohydrate are 0.7, 0.83, and 1.0, respectively. Overfeeding will result in an RQ > 1.0 as a result of increased CO_2 production associated with lipogenesis [20,27].

The most used devices are metabolic carts because they are "user-friendly" and allow us to assess energy expenditure over shorter periods of time (from minutes to hours) and are relatively inexpensive devices. With metabolic carts, we can measure the RMR and in some cases diet-induced thermogenesis, which when combined with an estimated physical activity level provides a broad estimation of TEE [19].

We also have whole room metabolic chambers (room calorimeters) that allow the participant to be self-sufficient for at least 24 h (up to 7—14 days) with food delivered through air-tight doors, and this is also used to assess TEE [19,25].

Nowadays "metabolic cart" is the most used method in research, becoming almost in a gold standard because of its versatility, availability, and inexpensive price compared with other methods like doubly labeled water (real gold standard assessing TEE).

- **Predictive equations**

Estimating TEE and RMR in overweight and obese individuals raises questions about accuracy. First, most commonly used RMR equations have been developed in study populations that included few obese individuals. Second, and of particular relevance to RMR, the main variable used in most equations (e.g., body weight) does not adequately reflect the changes in body composition that accompany weight gain as a result of excess fat. Despite all of these, prediction equations are widely used in clinical practice and that is why we summarized the most important ones in Table 2.7.

Table 2.7 Predictive equations for RMR.

Mifflin formula [28]
Woman: REE = (10 × kg) + (6.25 × height (cm))−(5 × age) + 161 Man: REE = (10 × kg) + (6.25 × height (cm))−(5 × age) + 5
Schofield formula [29] *MegaJoules (MJ)

Age 18—30 years: Men RMR (MJ) = 0.063 weight−0.042 height (m) + 2.953
       Women RMR (MJ) = 0.057 weight + 1.84 height (m) + 0.411
Age 30—60 years: Men RMR EE (MJ) = 0.048 weight−0.011 height (m) + 3.670
       Women RMR (MJ) = 0.034 weight + 0.006 height (m) + 3.530
Age ≥60 years: Men RMR (MJ) = 0.038 weight + 4.068 height (m)−3.491
       Women RMR (MJ) = 0.033 weight + 1.917 height (m) + 0.074

WHO formula [29] *KiloJoules (kJ)

Age 18—30 years: Men RMR (kJ) = 64.4 weight−113.0 height (m) + 3000
       Women RMR (kJ) = 55.6 weight + 1397.4 height (m) + 146
Age 30—60 years: Men RMR (kJ) = 47.2 weight + 66.9 height (m) + 3769
       Women RMR (kJ) = 36.4 weight−104.6 height (m) + 3619
Age ≥60 years: Men RMR (kJ) = 36.8 weight + 4719.5 height (m)−4481
       Women RMR (kJ) = 38.5 weight + 2665 height (m)−1264

Henry formula [29]

Age 18—30 years: Men RMR (MJ) = 0.0600 weight + 1.31 height (m) + 0.473
       Women RMR (MJ) = 0.0433 weight + 2.57 height (m)−1.18
Age 30—60 years: Men RMR (MJ) = 0.0476 weight + 2.26 height (m)−0.574
       Women RMR (MJ) = 0.0342 weight + 2.10 height (m) −0.0486
Age ≥60 years: Men RMR (MJ) = 0.0478 weight + 2.26 height (m)−1.07
       Women RMR (MJ) = 0.0356 weight + 1.76 height (m) + 0.0448

Some studies recommend WHO equations for groups with mixed BMI ≥ 25 kg/m^2 because they offer the most accurate prediction, whereas Mifflin equations are most accurate for groups with a BMI 30—39.9 and Henry's equations for those groups with BMI ≥ 40 kg/m^2 [29].

Nevertheless, according to a recent review Mifflin equation provides the more precise estimation of RMR in most individuals with a BMI 30—39.9 and ≥ 40 kg/m^2 compared to other equations [30]. For healthy and obese adolescents, the Schofield equation provides a more accurate and precise RMR estimation [25]

- **Bioimpedance analysis**

We already explained this technique previously and its importance, nevertheless its ability to calculate RMR, is still controversial. There are many studies trying to identify the best equation using raw-BIA variables as bioimpedance index (direct an accurate proxy of FFM) and phase angle (related to body mass) but there is still no conclusive information [31].

General considerations of RMR

Body composition is the major determinant of RMR and accounts for 65%—90% of interindividual variation. Body composition comprises fat mass (i.e., all body lipids, which is predominantly located in adipose tissue) and FFM (i.e., including nonlipid components of skeletal muscle and vital organs). Adipose tissue is less metabolically active than FFM, although it is not metabolically inert. FFM is metabolically heterogeneous and some tissues within this compartment are more active than others. For example, brain and visceral organs comprise 5% of body weight but account for 70%—80% of RMR, whereas skeletal muscle comprises 35% of body weight but accounts for only 20% of RMR. In obesity, weight gained is mainly adipose tissue and, although this is metabolically less active than other tissues, it still contributes to an overall increase in energy expenditure. FFM also increases with weight gain in obesity and thus contributes to increased energy requirements [21].

This results in a curvilinear increase in RMR as body weight rises as a result of increased fatness. Thus, absolute RMR is higher in obese compared to lean individuals and rises with increasing BMI. However, RMR is lower when expressed per kg body weight thus impacting the accuracy of RMR prediction equations based on body weight [21,26].

Obesity also influences TEE through two opposing mechanisms that make accurate predictions difficult. First, the additional energy costs associated with moving excess adipose tissue may contribute to an increase in TEE, although this is relatively small compared to the associated increase in RMR. Second, TEE may be reduced as a result of lower levels of physical activity resulting from the practical difficulties of moving a heavy bodyweight when BMI exceeds ≥ 35 kg/m^2 [21,26].

Despite these factors that confound the estimation of energy expenditure in obesity, energy prediction equations are widely used in clinical and public health practice and there is little consensus on which equation is most appropriate for use with people who are obese.

Physical activity energy expenditure
Which can be broadly divided into energy expenditure due to intentional and non-intentional activity. Physical activity energy expenditure (PAEE) includes exercise; sports; occupational, leisure-time, and household activities; personal care; and transportation. Such multiple activities make it difficult to recall and then categorize PAEE. It is the most variable component of daily energy expenditure. PAEE is often overreported and the percent of overreporting varies with race, degree of overweight, and weight loss. The most common methods to measure PAEE are DLW, self-report, and accelerometers [19]

- **Doubly labeled water**

    DLW technique is considered the gold standard for the measurement of TEE under free-living conditions, although it is expensive and impractical in clinical practice [19,24].

    DLW is also a very precise method to measure PAEE but it does it by subtracting the RMR and the TEF from the TEE, which means that this method is highly influenced by accurate estimation of TEF and RMR [21]

- **Self-report**

    PAEE can be calculated using self-reports of the physical activity performed on a typical day. The main issue is that people tend to overreport PAEE. Here, the energy cost (intensity) of activities is expressed as metabolic equivalents (MET). The MET is the ratio between the rate of energy expended during an activity to the rate of energy expended at rest. For instance, an activity of 1.5 MET requires a rate of energy expenditure 50% higher than the rate of energy expenditure at rest. The product of the activity MET times the minutes spent in the activity is an index of energy expended [21,32].

    It is a very inaccurate method and not recommended for research purposes but there are more conservative groups that are trying to improve its precision through different methods.

- **New technologies**

    Technological advancements in portable sensing devices such as pedometers and accelerometers have made it possible to determine physical activity objectively in real time. However, for a given activity and duration, the expended energy may differ by body weight and efficiency of motion. Thus, approaches such as the combination of accelerometry with heart rate monitoring or additional movement measures have remarkably improved the accuracy of determining PAEE when compared against the DLW technique [21].

Thermic effect of food
TEF represents the energy required for ingestion and digestion of food, along with absorption, transport, and storage of nutrients. It is the smallest component of total energy expenditure, accounting for $\approx 10\%$ over the entire day [21].

Indirect calorimetry is used to measure TEF. The main issues with IC are the caloric content and composition of the test meal and duration of the measurement period. The caloric content of the meal directly influences TEF. Proteins and lipids show the highest and lowest thermogenic effect, respectively [19,21].

Protein requirements

Patients with obesity have a higher protein turnover and greater catabolism due to obesity-associated insulin resistance altering the anabolic effect of insulin on protein synthesis. Both insufficient protein intake and protein overconsumption can have adverse health consequences.[33]

Weight loss causes a decrease in total body mass due to a decrease in both fat mass and lean mass. Consuming a high-protein diet during weight loss diminishes the weight loss-induced reduction of lean mass and muscle mass. The results of several systematic reviews and meta-analyses demonstrate that high (defined as >1.0 g/kg per day) compared with normal (0.8 g/kg per day) protein intake prevents a loss of lean mass during moderate weight loss.[33] The available evidence seems to indicate that an initial protein intake of 2 g/kg body weight (IBW)/day be given to those with a BMI 30–39.9 kg/m^2 and 2.5 g/kg IBW/day for patients with a BMI ≥40 kg/m^2 [22].

Protein or mixed meal ingestion inhibits muscle protein breakdown and increases the muscle protein synthesis rate because it stimulates insulin secretion and activates anabolic signaling pathways that stimulate amino acid incorporation into muscle proteins. In another way, the relationship between protein intake and the postprandial muscle protein synthesis rate is saturable, reaching a maximum of 30 g of protein. Amino acids from protein consumed in excess of this amount are degraded and oxidized. Postprandial net muscle protein accretion can therefore not be increased by eating more protein [33].

References

[1] Colquitt J, Pickett K, Loveman E, Frampton G. Surgery for weight loss in adults (review) summary of findings for the main comparison. Cochrane Database Syst Rev 2014. https://doi.org/10.1103/PhysRevB.86.184510.

[2] Weimann A, Braga M, Carli F, et al. ESPEN guideline: clinical nutrition in surgery. Clin Nutr 2017. https://doi.org/10.1016/j.clnu.2017.02.013.

[3] Mechanick JI, Apovian C, Brethauer S, et al. Clinical practice guidelines for the perioperative nutrition, metabolic, and nonsurgical support of patients undergoing bariatric procedures — 2019 update: cosponsored by American Association of Clinical Endocrinologists/American College of Endocrinology. Endocr Pract 2019;25(12):1346–59. https://doi.org/10.4158/GL-2019-0406.

[4] Lorenzo D, Transl J, Lorenzo A De, et al. Why primary obesity is a disease? J Transl Med 2019:1–13. https://doi.org/10.1186/s12967-019-1919-y.

References

[5] Sherf Dagan S, Goldenshluger A, Globus I, et al. Nutritional recommendations for adult bariatric surgery patients: clinical practice. Adv Nutr An Int Rev J 2017. https://doi.org/10.3945/an.116.014258.

[6] Cederholm T, Barazzoni R, Austin P, et al. ESPEN guidelines on definitions and terminology of clinical nutrition. Clin Nutr 2017. https://doi.org/10.1016/j.clnu.2016.09.004.

[7] Cederholm T, Jensen GL, Correia MITD, et al. GLIM criteria for the diagnosis of malnutrition — a consensus report from the global clinical nutrition community. J Cachexia Sarcopenia Muscle 2019;10(1):207—17. https://doi.org/10.1002/jcsm.12383.

[8] De Lorenzo A, Soldati L, Sarlo F, Calvani M, Di Lorenzo N, Di Renzo L. New obesity classification criteria as a tool for bariatric surgery indication. World J Gastroenterol 2016. https://doi.org/10.3748/wjg.v22.i2.681.

[9] Gómez-Ambrosi J, Silva C, Catalán V, et al. Clinical usefulness of a new equation for estimating body fat. Diabetes Care 2012. https://doi.org/10.2337/dc11-1334.

[10] Ross R, Neeland IJ, Yamashita S, et al. Waist circumference as a vital sign in clinical practice: a consensus statement from the IAS and ICCR working group on visceral obesity. Nat Rev Endocrinol 2020. https://doi.org/10.1038/s41574-019-0310-7.

[11] Madden AM, Smith S. Body composition and morphological assessment of nutritional status in adults: a review of anthropometric variables. J Hum Nutr Diet 2016. https://doi.org/10.1111/jhn.12278.

[12] Sheean P, Gonzalez MC, Prado CM, McKeever L, Hall AM, Braunschweig CA. American Society for Parenteral and Enteral Nutrition Clinical Guidelines: the validity of body composition assessment in clinical populations. J Parenter Enteral Nutr 2020;44(1):12—43. https://doi.org/10.1002/jpen.1669.

[13] Molina Vega M, García Almeida JM, Vegas Aguilar I, et al. Revisión sobre los fundamentos teórico-prácticos del ángulo de fase y su valor pronóstico en la práctica clínica. Nutr Clin Med 2017. https://doi.org/10.7400/NCM.2017.11.3.5055.

[14] Cruz-Jentoft AJ, Sayer AA. Sarcopenia. Lancet 2019;393(10191):2636—46. https://doi.org/10.1016/S0140-6736(19)31138-9.

[15] Batsis JA, Villareal DT. Sarcopenic obesity in older adults: aetiology, epidemiology and treatment strategies. Nat Rev Endocrinol 2018. https://doi.org/10.1038/s41574-018-0062-9.

[16] Koliaki C, Liatis S, Dalamaga M, Kokkinos A. Sarcopenic obesity: epidemiologic evidence, pathophysiology, and therapeutic perspectives. Curr Obes Rep 2019;8(4):458—71. https://doi.org/10.1007/s13679-019-00359-9.

[17] Cruz-Jentoft AJ, Bahat G, Bauer J, et al. Sarcopenia: revised European consensus on definition and diagnosis. Age Ageing 2019. https://doi.org/10.1093/ageing/afy169.

[18] Mannaerts GHH, van Mil SR, Stepaniak PS, et al. Results of implementing an enhanced recovery after bariatric surgery (ERABS) protocol. Obes Surg 2016. https://doi.org/10.1007/s11695-015-1742-3.

[19] Lam YY, Ravussin E. Indirect calorimetry: an indispensable tool to understand and predict obesity. Eur J Clin Nutr 2017;71(3):318—22. https://doi.org/10.1038/ejcn.2016.220.

[20] Blasco Redondo R. Resting energy expenditure; assessment methods and applications. Nutr Hosp 2015;31:245—54. https://doi.org/10.3305/nh.2015.31.sup3.8772.

[21] Fernández-Verdejo R, Aguirre C, Galgani JE. Issues in measuring and interpreting energy balance and its contribution to obesity. Curr Obes Rep 2019;8(2):88—97. https://doi.org/10.1007/s13679-019-00339-z.

[22] Dickerson RN, Patel JJ, McClain CJ. Protein and calorie requirements associated with the presence of obesity. Nutr Clin Pract 2017;32(1_suppl):86S–93S. https://doi.org/10.1177/0884533617691745.

[23] Herrera MCA, Chan CB. Narrative review of new methods for assessing food and energy intake. Nutrients 2018;10(8):1–19. https://doi.org/10.3390/nu10081064.

[24] Sanghvi A, Redman LM, Martin CK, Ravussin E, Hall KD. Validation of an inexpensive and accurate mathematical method to measure long-term changes in free-living energy intake. Am J Clin Nutr 2015;102(2):353–8. https://doi.org/10.3945/ajcn.115.111070.

[25] Chima L, Mulrooney HM, Warren J, Madden AM. A systematic review and quantitative analysis of resting energy expenditure prediction equations in healthy overweight and obese children and adolescents. J Hum Nutr Diet 2020;(2):1–13. https://doi.org/10.1111/jhn.12735.

[26] Mazzo R, Ribeiro FB, Vasques ACJ. Accuracy of predictive equations versus indirect calorimetry for the evaluation of energy expenditure in cancer patients with solid tumors — an integrative systematic review study. Clin Nutr ESPEN 2020;35(xxxx):12–9. https://doi.org/10.1016/j.clnesp.2019.11.001.

[27] Rosenthal MD, Vanzant EL, Brakenridge SC. Nutritional assessment, parenteral, and enteral nutrition. 7th ed. Elsevier; 2018. https://doi.org/10.1016/B978-0-323-47873-1.00009-7.

[28] Mifflin MD, St Jeor ST, Hill LA, Scott BJ, Daugherty SA, Koh YO. A new predictive equation for resting energy expenditure in healthy individuals. Am J Clin Nutr 1990;51(2):241–7. https://doi.org/10.1093/ajcn/51.2.241.

[29] Madden AM, Mulrooney HM, Shah S. Estimation of energy expenditure using prediction equations in overweight and obese adults: a systematic review. J Hum Nutr Diet 2016;29(4):458–76. https://doi.org/10.1111/jhn.12355.

[30] Itani L, Tannir H, Kreidieh D, El Masri D, El Ghoch M. Validation of predictive equations for resting energy expenditure in treatment-seeking adults with overweight and obesity: measured versus estimated. J Popul Ther Clin Pharmacol 2020;27(1):e32–47. https://doi.org/10.15586/jptcp.v27i1.653.

[31] Marra M, Cioffi I, Sammarco R, et al. Are raw BIA variables useful for predicting resting energy expenditure in adults with obesity? Nutrients 2019;11(2). https://doi.org/10.3390/nu11020216.

[32] Dhurandhar NV, Schoeller D, Brown AW, Heymsfield SB, Thomas D, et al. Energy balance measurement: when something is not better than nothing. Int J Obes 2015;39(7):1109–13. https://doi.org/10.1038/ijo.2014.199.

[33] Bettina M, Klein S, Fontana L. A word of caution against excessive protein intake. Nature Rev Endocrinol 2020;16:59–66. https://doi.org/10.1038/s41574-019-0274-7.

CHAPTER 3

Preoperative diets: LCD, VLCD, and commercial supplements

Sonsoles Gutiérrez Medina[1], Carmen Aragón[2], Álvaro Sánchez[2], Clotilde Vázquez[2]

[1]*Division of Endocrinology and Nutrition, Department of Medicine, Rey Juan Carlos University Hospital, Madrid, Spain;* [2]*Department of Endocrinology, Fundacion Jimenez Diaz University Hospital, Madrid, Spain*

Chapter outline

Low-calorie and very low-calorie diets 35
   Definition 35
   Indications 36
   Contraindications 36
   Instructions for use of VLCD diets 36
      VLCD alone 36
      Meal replacement 37
   Regulations 37
   Clinical efficacy 37
   Side effects 38
Commercial products 39
VLCD in bariatric surgery 40
References 43
Further reading 44

Low-calorie and very low-calorie diets
Definition

Diet is considered the cornerstone of obesity treatment. There is a wide variety of diets that differ according to the energy intake and distribution of macronutrients.

    Depending on caloric contribution, they are classified as follows: isocaloric diets, used in phases of weight maintenance, moderately hypocaloric diets (LCD) that provide >1200 kcal per day (12–20 kcal/kg of ideal weight/day), which represent a daily deficit of 500–1000 kcal with respect to total energy expenditure, and very low-calorie diets (VLCD) that provide 800–1200 kcal per day (<12 kcal/kg of ideal weight/day; 0.8–1.5 g/kg ideal weight of high biological value proteins) to achieve weight reduction and preserve lean mass [1].

An alternative definition of VLCD has also been proposed as one that provides less than 50% of the subject's daily energy requirements [2].

The concept of VLCD was developed to overcome the poor results obtained with LCDs. However, an intake of less than 800 kcal/day does not provide benefits in weight loss, variation in body composition, appetite, and physical and psychological symptoms [3].

Indications

VLCD can be recommended in patients between 18 and 65 years old with a body mass index (BMI) above 30 kg/m^2, who have previously failed under an LCD diet, and remain motivated to ensure postoperative compliance with the diet.

Other situations where rapid weight loss before surgery is required, such as severe respiratory failure or major comorbidities (poor controlled type 2 diabetes, sleep apnea Hypopnea syndrome, dyslipidemia, disabling arthrosis, etc.) may also benefit from a VLCD.

As VLCDs can cause more adverse effects and require closer monitoring than LCDs, they should be reserved for cases where the health risks of excess weight are high and require rapid weight loss. However, these types of diets can be considered safe and effective if used properly, on well-selected individuals and under close medical supervision.

Contraindications

Before the initiation of a VLCD, an appropriate assessment should be made to evaluate the risks and rule out contraindications. These include the following [1]:

- Pregnancy and lactation.
- Systemic diseases, cancer, infection.
- Heart diseases: recent myocardial infarction, cardiac conduction disorder, history of cardiogenic syncope.
- Recent cerebrovascular disease.
- History of renal or hepatic disease: renal failure, hepatic cirrhosis, or severe hepatopathies.
- Psychiatric diseases: eating disorders, substance abuse, major depression, autolytic attempts.
- Type 2 diabetes mellitus.
- Cholelithiasis.

Adolescents and elderly people should be considered as relative contraindications to VLCD use because of the risk of altering energy requirements for growth or health maintenance. The use of these diets is not recommended for periods longer than 16 weeks [1,2].

Instructions for use of VLCD diets

VLCD alone

It is based on replacing all meals with commercial formulas, providing a caloric intake of less than 800 kcal per day. Very prolonged use is not recommended as it can lead to malnutrition. In addition, the withdrawal rate is high, reaching up to 50%.

Meal replacement

It is the most common form of use of VLCDs. It consists of replacing one or more of the main meals of the day with commercial formulas (they provide around 200 kcal per intake).

In any case, VLCDs should always be accompanied by recommendations for permanent lifestyle changes, to promote weight loss and avoid regaining lost weight.

Regulations

The European Commission, with Directive 96/8/EC, regulated foodstuffs intended for use in energy-restricted diets with the objective of weight loss. In Spain, it was incorporated into the legal system by means of a specific technical health regulation that governs these products (Royal Decree 1430/1997, of 15 September, BOE of 24 September) [4].

The provisions established in Regulation (EU) No. 609/2013 are mandatory as of July 20, 2016, with Royal Decree 1430/1997 of September 15, 1997 continuing to be in force, as well as the list of substances contained in the annex to Regulation (EC) No. 953/2009, regarding substitutes for the complete diet for weight control until the date of application of Commission Regulation (EU) No. 2017/1798 of June 2, 2017, which complements Regulation (EU) No. 609/2013 of the European Parliament and of the Council as regards specific compositional and information requirements for replacements for the complete diet for weight control.

Clinical efficacy

In a review of VLCDs and long-term weight maintenance, it was reported that 90% of patients who followed VLCDs lost at least 10 kg, compared to 60% of those who maintained LCDs. The rate of weight loss with VLCD was higher than with LCD (1.5—2 kg/week in women and 2—2.5 kg/week in men versus 0.4—0.5 kg/week) being higher in the first 4—6 weeks and slowing down to 0.8 kg/week in the following 6 months [5]. A more recently published meta-analysis of the efficacy of meal replacements in weight loss revealed that the group assigned to partial replacement diets lost more weight than those assigned to the conventional diet group: −1.44 kg (−2.48 to −0.39 kg; I 2 = 38%). These differences were greater if accompanied by a structured support program [6].

However, the results beyond 1 year of follow-up in most studies are similar to those of moderately low-calorie diets. For this reason, and considering the side effects, there are authors who discourage VLCDs in the long term. In addition, the dropout rate is usually higher with VLCDs than with traditional low-calorie diets. Therefore, the higher rate of initial weight loss with VLCD is not a predictor of subsequent maintenance. As is widely known, maintenance of weight loss improves when dietary treatment is accompanied by exercise programs, behavioral therapy, and drugs.

In terms of changes in body composition, VLCDs contribute to the loss of fat mass (75%), especially of the abdominal compartment. Lean mass decreases up to 25% [7]. In the first week a negative nitrogen balance occurs, as glycogen and fluids are mainly mobilized, reaching a neutral balance after 3—4 weeks. Adequate protein intake and regular physical exercise can contribute to the preservation of lean mass.

VLCDs have beneficial effects on the lipid profile. Studies have shown significant reductions in total cholesterol, LDL cholesterol, triglycerides, and apo-B100, with controversial results in HDL cholesterol [8].

Regarding carbohydrate metabolism, several studies have reported a decrease in fasting plasma glucose levels and an improvement in insulin resistance, independent of weight reduction [9]. The increase in insulin sensitivity at the peripheral level has been studied by euglycemic-hyperinsulinemic clamp and HOMA-IR. In addition, the decrease in serum insulin and C-peptide levels experienced by patients following VLCD has also been related to the partial recovery of pancreatic β-cell function, with the improvement of the first and second phases of insulin secretion [10].

In hypertensive patients, a drop in systolic and diastolic blood pressure has been observed, which has been associated with improved endothelial function, changes in vagal nerve activity, and improved insulin resistance, as no changes in diuresis, natriuresis, aldosterone, or plasma renin activity have been observed [11].

It has been described that the use of VLCDs contributes to the reduction of liver volume, by decreasing its fat content, which makes them very attractive in the preoperative phase of bariatric surgery [12]. In addition, they lead to a 40% reduction in endogenous glucose production and in hepatic resistance to insulin, improvement in the proinflammatory profile, and a reduction in C-reactive protein levels.

In patients with sleep apnea hypopnea syndrome (SAHS), the use of these diets has been associated with fewer episodes of desaturation and improvement in residual capacity and expiratory reserve volume [13]. This benefit is greater in cases of severe SAHS and is maintained for up to 2 years.

From the psychological point of view, multiple studies have published improvements in depression and anxiety scales, as well as in several quality-of-life parameters such as vitality, physical function, health perception, and emotional state [14,15].

Side effects

Among the most important side effects are

- General symptoms: asthenia, cold, anxiety, dizziness, hunger, ketosis breath, skin dryness, hair loss.
- Digestive complications: nausea, vomiting, and alteration of the intestinal transit. Constipation is the most common. To prevent this, foods rich in fiber such as vegetables are recommended. In the more severe cases, fiber supplements should be added.

- Orthostatic hypotension, probably secondary to dehydration.
- Cholelithiasis: it is caused both by the release of cholesterol from the adipose tissue due to rapid weight loss, which makes the bile more lithogenic, and by the low contribution of fat in the diet, which leads to incomplete emptying of the gallbladder. It affects 11%—28% of cases.
- Hyperuricemia: in patients with a history of gout it can trigger a gouty crisis.
- Reduction of bone mass: energy restriction and ketosis can lead to a negative calcium balance.

Given the risk of hypoglycemia in diabetic patients receiving treatment with insulin or oral hypoglycaemic drugs such as sulfonylureas or methylglinides, a reduction in their dose and close monitoring is recommended to make appropriate dose adjustments. In addition, titration of diuretics and other antihypertensive drugs may be necessary for hypertensive patients to avoid possible dehydration and hypotension.

Commercial products

The VLCDs are usually prescribed as commercial products, whose regulation in Spain dates from 1997 (Royal Decree Num 1430/1997). In addition, the Scientific Commission for Food-related Matters (SCOOP Expert Group of the European Union) set up in 2001 recommendations on the requirements to be met by VLCDs-commercial products, based on scientific experience.

The composition of macronutrients recommended in VLCD diets according to RD 1430/1997 is summarized in Table 3.1.

In terms of micronutrients, these products must provide 100% of the RDA of vitamins and minerals (Table 3.2). The RDA in Spain is regulated in the RD N 1275/2003.

There is no recommended amount of fiber in food substitutes; however, they usually provide between 3% and 5%. Several studies have shown that these products favor the sensation of satiety and gastric fullness in the 3 h following intake. The sensation of

Table 3.1 Recommended composition of very low calorie diets RD 1430/1997.

Nutrient	Recommendatión
Energy	800—1200 kcal/day
Proteíns	25%—50% of total energy intake (maximum 125 g/day)
Fat	Maximum 30% of the total caloric content Ácido linoleico: mínimo 4.5 g/día
Fiber	10—30 g/day
Minerals	100% of daily recommendations
Vitamins	100% of daily recommendations
Oligoelements	100% of daily recommendations

Table 3.2 CRD vitamins and minerals (RD 1430/1997).

Vitamins		Minerals	
Vitamin A (µg)	700	Sodium (mg)	575
Vitamin D (µg)	5	Chlorine (g)	2
Vitamin E (µg)	10	Potassium (g)	4.7
Vitamin K (µg)	60–80	Phosphorus (mg)	550
Vitamin C (µg)	45	Calcium (mg)	700
Vitamin B1 (mg)	1.4	Magnesium (mg)	150
Vitamin B2 (mg)	1.6	Iron (mg)	9.5
Vitamin B3 (mg)	1.8	Zinc (mg)	15
Vitamin B6 (mg)	1.5	Magnesium (mg)	1–2.3
Vitamin B9 (mg)	200	Copper (g)	900
Vitamin B12 (mg)	1.4	Iodine (µg)	150
Biotin (mg)	0.15	Selenium (µg)	50–70
Pantoténico acid (mg)	6	Molybdenum (µg)	45
		Chromium (µg)	20–35
		Fluor (mg)	3–4

hunger reaches its minimum expression half an hour after consuming the preparation and does not return to the initial values within 3 h of taking the product [16].

The composition of the food substitutes and enteral nutrition formulas used as VLCD, currently marketed in Spain, are summarized in Table 3.3.

VLCD in bariatric surgery

VLCDs and LCDs have been widely used to achieve preoperative weight loss. Many health centers state that any candidate for bariatric surgery must meet a weight loss goal, as a way to demonstrate the ability to adhere to nutritional prescription after bariatric surgery. It can also help reduce the risk of perioperative complications and achieve greater postsurgical weight loss, although there is no consensus so far on the benefits of the latter two aspects [17].

The scientific literature on VLCDs and LCDs before bariatric surgery describes the results of comparing treatment approaches with or without meal replacement nutritional preparations. Schouten and coworkers [18] in a 2016 study compared VLCD with regular foods versus diet alone with meal replacements. They found no statistically significant differences in weight loss and surgery outcomes; however, diet tolerance and acceptance were better in the group that received usual foods.

Most patients who are candidates for bariatric surgery have nonalcoholic fatty liver disease that causes an increase in liver size, which in turn makes access to the gastroesophageal region difficult and increases the risk of bleeding. Holderbaum et al. [12] in a recent systematic review describe the effects of VLCDs on liver volume. The patients included in this review received diets between 400 and 800 Kcal, mostly

Table 3.3 Composition of food substitutes and low-calorie special medical purpose foods available in Spain.

	Presentation	TCV	Protein (g) %	Fat (g) %	Carbohydrates (g) %	Fiber (g) %
Food substitutes						
OPTIFAST NestléHealthScience	Packet 55 g	216	20 37%	6.1 25%	19 35%	3.6 3%
BIMANAN	Packet 50 g	206	14	6.5	22	2.7
Enteral nutrition formulas used as VLCD						
OPTISOURCE NestléHealthScience	Packet 50 g	210	15 29%	4.5 19%	27.4 52%	0
OPTISOURCE PLUS NestléHealthScience	Brick 250 mL	218	17.6 32%	4.5 19%	25 46%	3.75 3%
VEGESTART Complet Vegenat	Brick 200 mL	204	17 33%	3.6 16%	21 43%	8.4 8%
Bi1 Bíficare Adventia	Brick 200 mL	200	18 36%	422 19%	20 40%	6 5%

based on commercial preparations with or without conventional foods. The period of administration of the diets varied between 10 days and 12 weeks. All patients achieved weight loss and reduction of liver volume ranging from 5% to 20% from the initial volume. The studies with longer follow-ups observed a greater reduction in liver volume from the second to the fourth week. The systematic review found no greater reduction in liver volume in relation to increased dietary maintenance or increased caloric restriction. No difference was found in perioperative complications. Dr. Salas Salvadó's group published a paper [19] comparing the outcomes of VLCD's with LCDs in terms of achieving liver size reduction and reducing perioperative complications. They found that both types of diet reduced liver volume equally and that the factor associated with the greatest reduction was a basal liver volume greater than 3L. In addition, they found no difference in perioperative complications. Compliance with both diets was good and the only difference found in terms of tolerance was that patients with VLCD referred more frequent feelings of weakness.

Regarding the influence of preparatory weight loss on the results of long-term bariatric surgery, the work of Tang and collaborators [20] studied postsurgical weight loss as a function of the effect achieved by the VLCD performed the previous 14 days. Interestingly, those patients with presurgical weight loss of less than 5% had greater weight loss after surgery, although when measuring total weight loss and the percentage of excess body mass index lost, the results were better in those who lost 5% or more of their weight with the VLCD.

Sun and collaborators in a 2020 paper [21] investigated the relationship between baseline weight and preparatory weight loss with mortality at 30 days of bariatric surgery. They obtained data from more than 400,000 patients who had undergone surgery at centers of excellence in the United States and Canada. They found that those patients with a higher presurgical BMI had a higher risk of 30-day mortality (for BMI greater than or equal to 55 the OR for mortality was 5.29) and that presurgical weight loss behaved as a protective factor (OR for weight loss greater than 10% 0.56).

The influence of VLCDs on the postsurgical healing process has been rarely studied. It is possible to assume that a diet that is deficient in energy, and therefore catabolic, could negatively affect the collagen repair processes and therefore predispose to the appearance of fistulas. To evaluate this hypothesis, Chakravartty and his group [22] studied the expression of collagen genes in 18 patients, 9 of them undergoing 4 weeks of preoperative VLCD versus 9 patients who continued their usual diet. They found that at the time of surgery the expression of collagen I, collagen III, and elastin genes was lower in the VLCD group. After 1 week of the surgery, the expression of collagen type I was still decreased, but no differences were found in the histological processes of healing. There were no differences in surgical times or average hospital stay.

The North American guidelines [23] for the management of the bariatric surgery candidate recommends preoperative weight loss for the reduction of liver volume, although it makes no mention of the type of diet or duration [24]. However, the latest version of the European multidisciplinary guide does not mention this weight loss. The latest update of the European Association of Endoscopic Surgery's guide to bariatric surgery, endorsed by the IFSO [25], recommends preoperative nutritional intervention because of its effect on the results of surgery. The Spanish Society of

Obesity Surgery in its recommendations for clinical practice in bariatric and metabolic surgery [26] includes the need for preoperative weight loss because of its benefits in reducing liver volume and improving associated comorbidities, such as diabetes or sleep-disordered breathing. Moreover, the clinical recommended procedures [27] of the same society, highlights the benefits of preoperative weight loss with VLCD (between 2 and 6 weeks) and LCD (between 6 and 12 weeks).

References

[1] Vilchez López FJ, Campos Martín C, Amaya García MJ, Sánchez Vera P, Pereira Cunill JL. Very low calorie diets in clinical management of morbid obesity. Nutr Hosp 2013;28(2):275—85.

[2] Tsai GA, Waden TA. Systematic review: an evaluation of major commercial weight loss programs in the United States. Ann Intern Med 2005;142:56—66.

[3] Foster GD, Wadden TA, Peterson FJ, Letizia K, Bartlett SJ, Conill AM. A controlled comparison of three very-low calorie diets: effects on weight, body composition, and symptoms. Am J Clin Nutr 1992;55:811—7.

[4] Rubio MA, Moreno C. Dietas de muy bajo contenido calórico: adaptación a nuevas recomendaciones. Rev Esp Obes 2004;2:91—8.

[5] Saris WHM. Very low calorie diets and sustained weight loss. Obes Res 2001;9(Suppl. 4):295S—301S.

[6] Astbury NM, Piernas C, Hartmann-Boyce J, Lapworth S, Aveyard P, Jebb S. A systematic review and meta-analysis of the effectiveness of meal replacements for weight loss. Obes Rev 2019;20(4):569—87.

[7] National Task Force on the Prevention and Treatment of Obesity. Very low-calorie diets. J Am Med Assoc 1993;270:967—74.

[8] Hong K, Li Z, Wang HJ, Elashoff R, Heber D. Analysis of weight loss outcomes using VLCD in black and white overweight and obese women with and without metabolic syndrome. Int J Obes 2005;29:436—42.

[9] Malandrucco I, Pasqualetti P, Giordani I, Manfellotto D, De Marco F, Alegiani F, et al. Very-low-calorie diet: a quick therapeutic tool to improve cell function in morbidly obese patients with type 2 diabetes. Am J Clin Nutrition 2012;95:609—13.

[10] Foo J, Krebs J, Hayes MT, Bell D, Macartney-Coxson D, Croft T. Studies in insulin resistance following very low calorie diet and/or gastric bypass surgery. Obes Surg 2011;21:1914—20.

[11] Xydakis AM, Case CC, Jones PH, Hoogeveen RC, Liu MY, Smith EO, et al. Adiponectin, inflammation, and the expression of the metabolic syndrome in obese individuals: the impact of rapid weight loss through caloric restriction. J Clin Endocrinol Metab 2004;89:2697—703.

[12] Holderbaum M, Casagrande D, Sussenbach BC. Effects of very low calorie diets on liver size and weight loss in the preoperative period of bariatric surgery: a systematic review. Surg Obes Relat Dis 2018;14(2):237—44.

[13] Johansson K, Neovius M, Trolle Lagerros Y, Harlid R, Rössner S, Granath F, et al. Effect of a very low energy diet on moderate and severe obstructive sleep apnoea in obese men: a randomised controlled trial. BMJ 2009;3:339—47.

[14] Kaukua J, Pekkarinen T, Sane T, Mustajoki P. Health-related quality of life in WHO class II-III obese men losing weight with very low-energy diet and behaviour modification: a randomised clinical trial. Int J Obes Relat Metab Disord 2002;26:487—95.

[15] De Luis DA, Izaola O, García Alonso M, Aller R, Cabezas G, De la Fuente B. Effect of a hypocaloric diet with a commercial formula in weight loss and quality of life in obese patients with chronic osteoarthritis. Nutr Hosp 2012;27(5):1648−54.

[16] Moizé V, et al. Obesity, 2006;14:166−529.

[17] Rubio Herrera MA, Sánchez-Vilar Burdiel O, Aragón Valera, C. Nutrición y tratamiento quirúrgico de la obesidad. Gil A. Tratado de Nutrición ISBN 9788491101956.

[18] Schouten R, van Der Kaaden I, vant Hof G, Feskens P. Comparison of preoperative diets before bariatric surgery: a randomized, single-blinded, non-inferiority trial. Obes Surg 2016;26:1743−9.

[19] Gils Contreras A, Bonada Sanjaume A, Montero Jaime M, et al. Effects of two preoperatory weight loss diets on hepatic volume, metabolic parameters, and surgical complications in morbid obese bariatric surgery candidates: a randomized clinical trial. Obes Surg 2018;28(12):3756−68.

[20] Tan SYT, Loi PL, Lim CH, et al. Preoperative weight loss via very low caloric diet (VLCD) and its effect on outcomes after bariatric surgery. Obes Surg 2020;30(6):2099−107.

[21] Sun Y, Liu B, Smith JK, et al. Association of preoperative body weight and weight loss with risk of death after bariatric surgery. JAMA Netw Open 2020;3(5):e204803. Published 2020 May 1.

[22] Chakravartty S, Vivian G, Mullholland N, et al. Preoperative liver shrinking diet for bariatric surgery may impact wound healing: a randomized controlled trial. Surg Obes Relat Dis 2019;15(1):117−25.

[23] Mechanick JI, Apovian C, Brethauer S, et al. Clinical practice guidelines for the perioperative nutrition, metabolic, and nonsurgical support of patients undergoing bariatric procedures - 2019 update: cosponsored by American association of clinical endocrinologists/American college of endocrinology, the obesity society, American society for metabolic & bariatric surgery, obesity medicine association, and American society of anesthesiologists - executive summary. Endocr Pract 2019;25(12):1346−59.

[24] Fried M, Yumuk V, Oppert JM, et al. Interdisciplinary European guidelines on metabolic and bariatric surgery. Obes Surg 2014;24(1):42−55.

[25] Di Lorenzo N, Antoniou SA, Batterham RL, et al. Clinical practice guidelines of the European Association for Endoscopic Surgery (EAES) on bariatric surgery: update 2020 endorsed by IFSO-EC, EASO and ESPCOP. Surg Endosc 2020;34(6):2332−58.

[26] Díez I, Martínez C, Sánchez-Santos R, Ruiz JC, Frutos MD, De la Cruz F, Torres AJ. Recomendaciones de la SECO para la práctica de cirugía bariátrica y metabólica. (Declaración de Victoria-Gasteizt 2015). BMI-2015, 5.3.3, 842−845.

[27] Martín García-Almenta E, Ruiz-Tovar Polo J, Sánchez Santos R. Vía Clínica de Cirugía bariátrica. 2017. ISBN: 978-84-697-7104-4.

Further reading

[1] Vidal Casariego A, Calleja Fernández A, Ballesteros Pomar MD. Dietas de muy bajo contenido calórico. En Rubio Herrera MA. Manual de obesidad mórbida. 2nd ed. Madrid: Editorial Médica panamericana; 2015. p. 107−12.

[2] Dwyer JT, Melanson KJ. Dietary Treatment of Obesity. C. 18 de Obesity ed. JF Caro. http://www.Endotext.com.

CHAPTER 4

Impact of preoperative nutritional intervention on comorbidities: type 2 diabetes, hypertension, dyslipidemia, and nonalcoholic fatty liver disease

Lorea Zubiaga[1], Jaime Ruiz-Tovar[2,3]

[1]*Lille University, Institut National de la Santé et de la Recherche Médicale (INSERM)-U1190, EGID, CHU Lille, Lille, France;* [2]*Bariatric Surgery Unit, Garcilaso Clinic, Madrid, Spain;* [3]*Department of Surgery, University Alfonso X, Madrid, Spain*

Chapter outline

Introduction	46
Types of dietary interventions in the preoperative time	47
Low calories diet	49
Very low calories diet	49
Low carbohydrate diets	49
Impact of preoperative nutritional interventions in obesity's comorbidities	50
Preoperative nutritional intervention and type 2 diabetes	50
Preoperative nutritional intervention and hypertension	51
Preoperative nutritional intervention and dyslipidemia	52
Preoperative nutritional intervention and NAFLD	52
Wise associations' recommendations guidelines	53
The American societies for metabolic and bariatric surgery guidelines	54
General preoperative conditions	54
T2D preoperative conditions	55
HTN preoperative conditions	55
DLP preoperative conditions	55
NAFLD preoperative conditions	55
The European societies for metabolic and bariatric surgery guidelines	56
General preoperative conditions	56
T2D preoperative conditions	57

> *HTN preoperative conditions* 57
> *DLP preoperative conditions* 57
> *NAFLD preoperative conditions* 58
> **Conclusions** 58
> **References** 59

Introduction

Obesity is a major global health issue leading to the main cause of morbidity and mortality in the 21st century [1]. As the most effective and enduring treatment for morbid obesity, metabolic surgery provides a relief solution for this epidemic due to the capacity of these different surgical procedures for shifting physiological and metabolic processes in the body [2]. Thanks to these shifts it is possible to induce larger amounts of sustainable weight loss, reducing the adiposity and achieving the improvement of other entities such as type 2 diabetes (T2D), hypertension (HTN), dyslipidemia (DLP), and nonalcoholic fatty liver disease (NAFLD), among others. However, metabolic surgery is not entirely risk-free and carries potential complications, even death. Thankfully, these risks have decreased considerably in the last decades, due to the technological improvements and to an increased knowledge of the disease [2].

To reduce the surgical risks, one of the measures recommended in most guidelines is to support a preoperative weight loss [3]. The goal for these measures is basically to reduce the risk of perioperative complications such as bleeding, thrombosis, liver damage, respiratory problems, and rhabdomyolysis. In particular, the visceral fat, thicker abdominal wall, and the liver volume are particularly challenging for surgeons during the performance of the procedures in the operating room [4]. For surgeries on the upper abdomen, the hepatomegaly (with or within steatohepatitis) is a complex condition. The elevation and manipulation of the hepatic left lobe of a large and fatty liver during laparoscopic procedures is a tricky scenario. In fact, the fatty liver is the main condition increasing the conversion ratio from laparoscopic to laparotomy procedures [5]; consequently, the probability of increasing the risk of wound infections, abdominal hernias, and length of hospital stay, rises. Moreover, within the cohort of patients with BMI ≥ 50 kg/m^2 exists an increased rate of complications compared to patients with a lower BMI. Likewise in this cohort, the conventional metabolic surgery procedures have been demonstrated to be significantly less effective without other interventions [3]. For this reason, several bridging options between the basal situation of the patients, and the access to technically challenging surgical metabolic procedures are developed. There are widely different programs and recommendations depending on the support of wise societies, countries, centers, or surgeons. The options offered to patients vary from the specific preoperative nutritional interventions (more frequently used); passing through some medical therapies (e.g., orlistat, liraglutide, thiazolidinedione, naltrexone, etc.) or endoscopic techniques (e.g., intragastric balloon or endo-sleeve), and finally by suggesting some restrictive techniques such as laparoscopic adjustable banding or the laparoscopic sleeve gastrectomy (LSG) to reduce the weight and the surgical risk. The selection of one of these options can differ a lot from an specialist to other because there is no strong consensus regarding the best option [4].

To make this situation worse, some insurance companies in the United States and other countries require an important preoperative weight loss before surgery allowing coverage for surgery [6]. Although coverage of metabolic surgery has expanded in the last years (particularly in regard to LSG), many insurance companies limit access to these surgical procedures by requiring an additional attempt at nonsurgical weight loss before the operation. Similarly, some bariatric and metabolic centers prescribe mandatory successful adherence to diet programs to accept patients for operation, and these required programs can last between 3 and 12 months [7]. However, multiple studies [8–12] have shown there to be no definitive perioperative or postoperative advantage for patients who participate in all of these weight-loss requirements. It is necessary to recognize that mandated weight loss programs for a long specified time frame (more than 12 weeks and especially those aimed at achieving a 1-year diet due to waiting lists) might worsen the patient's initial condition. Some physicians are convinced that these programs are only obstacles to delay unnecessarily the surgery, increase some risks of morbi-mortality, and undermine the patient's will [7]. In this sense, the intention of these programs changed from a set time period to a more goal-oriented approach. The goal of the preoperative nutritional interventions must strive for a specific amount of weight loss (usually who could lose $\geq$ 5% of the basal weight). A goal per weight objective is shown to be associated with better outcomes, both in the weight loss results and in the patient's mentality [4]. Likewise, it must be accepted that some patients are not going to lose weight by any means other than metabolic surgery.

Although questions remain about whether preoperative nutritional interventions can modify operative risk complications or impact in the surgery outcomes, a widespread idea is that these dietary options involve the patient in the treatment of the disease and make them aware of their condition [13]. Thus, conversely to insurance-mandated weight loss management programs, surgeon managed preoperative weight loss solutions (normally by diet interventions) have been proposed to be more specifically adapted to anatomical, physiological, and psychological features of each patient and thus to achieve better outcomes after surgery. In fact, rather than reducing surgical risks or outcomes, it was being suggested that these preoperative diets can help to modify some emotional impact and lifestyle changes specifically associated with metabolic surgery [14]. In this chapter, we will discuss some of the nutritional option results before metabolic surgery.

Types of dietary interventions in the preoperative time

A preoperative nutritional intervention to weight loss is defined as the variation of diet depending on their caloric intake and/or their composition to reduce weight and volume. Depending on the caloric contribution, the diets are usually classified on isocaloric diets (for weight maintenance), low-calorie diets (LCD) (800−1200 kcal/day), and very low caloric value diets (VLCD) (<800 kcal/day) [15,16]. By contrast, regarding the nutrients composition, the diets are classified as low fat, low carbohydrates, or low protein diets. Here, the three most widely used diets in metabolic surgery weight loss programs will be described, and a comparative scheme of these three options is shown in Table 4.1.

Table 4.1 Differences between LCD, VLCD, and LCKD [17].

Type of diets	LCD	VLCD	LCKD
Kcal[a]	800−1200	<800	<600
Lipids[b]	33	30	24
Carbohydrates	145	55	15
Proteins	60	80	80
Food and portion adjustment	Yes	Yes, closely supervision	Not necessary but requires strict monitoring
Meal substitutes	Allowed	Recommended	Mandatory
Examples	Breakfast 200 g of semiskimmed milk, 50 g of bread, or low-fat/unsweetened yogurt Lunch Free consumption of vegetables (minimum 250 g) or 100 g of fruit or <80 g of wholemeal carbs (pasta, rice, bread) Dinner Free consumption of vegetables (min 250 g), 100 g of fruit 150 g of lean meat (turkey/chicken) or 200 g of fish or 100 g of low-fat cheese,	Breakfast 200 g of semiskimmed milk, 20 g of bread, or low-fat/unsweetened yogurt Lunch Free consumption of vegetables (minimum 250 g), 100 g of fruit 150 g of lean meat (turkey/chicken) or 200 g of fish, Dinner 100 g of low-fat cheese, free consumption of vegetables (min 250 g), 100 g of fruit	Breakfast 2 scoops and 2 tablets of multiminerals Lunch 2 scoops and 2 tablets of multivitamins + free consumption of vegetables (500 g/day) Dinner 2 scoops and 2 tablets of omega 3 → snacks (mid-morning, mid afternoon, after dinner): one scoop
Time (suggested)	2−12 weeks	2−4 weeks	<2 weeks

Limit physical activity and excessive stress and take at least 2 L of liquids per day (water or infussions not sweetened or sparkilin drinks. Take 8−9* scoops of special formulas (regular size: 200 mL one scoop = 10 g. Composition: 0.3 g of carbohydrates; 8.2 g of protein; 0.4 g of fats) and oral supplements.
[a] In all forbidden sweets and industrial bakery.
[b] Allowed until 20 g of extra virgin olive oil per day.

Low calories diet

The LCD is a controlled low calorie, carbohydrate, and fat diet, between 800 and 1200 kcal. Normally, it is based on control of the food available in each medium, attending fundamentally to energy criteria. This option is usually used for a short period of time with a maximum extension of 12 weeks to achieve good compliance [12]. In fact, this diet helps establish healthy eating and portion control helping prepare for eating postsurgery. It can be indicated to encourage routine and portion control to avoid eating disorders, vomiting, or anxiety to patients in the postoperative time because at the beginning they do not understand the body's new signals of restriction or malabsorption.

Very low calories diet

The VLCD, which provides between <800 kcal per day, is a type of diet with very or extremely low daily food energy consumption. This kind of diet is based on controlling the portions of the food eaten, but it can use regulated formulations. On these types of diets strict vigilance is mandatory for monitoring the content of the recommended daily requirements for vitamins, minerals, trace elements, essential fatty acids, protein, and electrolyte balance to obtain a significant weight reduction and adequate nutrition with the conservation of the lean mass [8]. VLCD usually can replace one or two regular meals by liquid or powder formula diets. This option can also be used as "crash" therapy before surgery. Sometimes, in patients with BMI ≥ 50 kg/m^2, the VLCD is used for longer times with the intention of starting to accustom the body to the impact it will receive with the surgery (ketogenic changes due to malabsorptive techniques that are usually applied in these patients).

Low carbohydrate diets

Another variant of diets that can be used in preoperative programs is LCDs at the expense of carbohydrates. These diets that have lowered the percentage of dietary carbohydrate and/or the glycemic index of the carbohydrate have consistently shown improvements in glycemic control and cardiovascular risk. However, low-carbohydrate diets (especially ketogenic diets) should be closely monitored because they have a high risk of inducing adverse responses (electrolytic disorders, ketogenic conditions, asthenia, weariness, hypotension, constipation, kidney's problems, etc.) or risky hypoglycemic events [16,17].

One of the examples of these diets is the low carbohydrate ketogenic diet (LCKD), which has become very fashionable in recent years. The LCKDs are defined as those diets where the daily consumption of carbohydrates is fewer than 50 g, regardless of fat, protein, or caloric intake. However, in the low carbohydrates formulations, if the glucides are drastically reduced or entirely absent, they should be substituted for a portion of the protein (0.8—1.5 g of high biological value protein per kilogram). In this sense, these diets are also called "fattening" diets. Modified fasting or protein-saving diets, as they attempt to achieve weight loss comparable to that obtained with fasting diets, but minimizing the side effects of the body's protein losses [16–18]. These kinds of diets must be followed during short periods and closely supervised because they can seriously affect the patient's mood due to monotony. Likewise, the VLCD and the LCKD also have a high risk of "rebound" phenomena, that is, when patients start adding more calories, they can regain weight very quickly.

Impact of preoperative nutritional interventions in obesity's comorbidities

Increased BMI has been related to a greater number of surgical complications (wound infection, sepsis, pneumonia, pulmonary embolism, etc.) preceding metabolic surgery. It has been raised in different studies that decreasing patient BMI before these procedures it is possible to reduce surgical complications, especially in super-obese patients (BMI ≥ 50 kg/m^2), in whom laparoscopic procedures are technically challenging [12]. In fact, depending on the surgeon or the volume of the center, patients with very high BMI are sometimes considered to be nonsurgical candidates [4]. Therefore, weight loss measures before metabolic surgery, using nutritional interventions, would help mitigate some barriers and make this kind of surgery more accessible to patients. In addition, it is demonstrated that the majority of these nutritional interventions achieve the control and even the remission of obesity's comorbidities. The main benefits obtained in the most frequent comorbidities are described below.

Preoperative nutritional intervention and type 2 diabetes

Patients with obesity and T2D usually have their diets checked long before any measure preoperative intervention is decided. The goal of reducing the carbohydrate intake in these patients is more of an obligation than a recommendation since dietary carbohydrate control is the major determinant of postprandial glucose levels [7]. In fact, the postprandial levels are now considered one of the primary factors to be evaluated in the genesis and progression of T2D [19]. Also, several clinical studies have shown that low-carbohydrate diets improve glycemic control per-se as long as the patients have good compliance [16,17]. Obesity plus T2D is an insulin-resistance condition, and it seems that LCKD diets may achieve better results than in patients who are still insulin sensitive, in whom LCD and VLCD diets are more appropriate. But an adjustment to each case is necessary because there are many variables to consider beyond reducing HbA1c.

The improvement of T2D due to nutritional intervention remains around 63% of the cases [4]. These patients also reduced insulin requirements or medication doses. However, it is not strong to demonstrate that patients who exhibit significant glycemic amelioration to these programs are more likely to achieve earlier remission of their diabetes or get long outcomes in the postoperative period [20]. But in terms of coping with the surgery, there is no doubt that good glycemic control helps not only to avoid episodes of hypoglycemia due to treatment mismatches but also to reduce complications due to micro- and macrovascular disorders associated with T2D [21].

There is an obvious need for closed monitoring of glucose control and adjustments of concomitant hypoglycemic therapy in patients with T2D both before and after metabolic surgery. In fact, in patients prescribed a preoperative nutritional intervention (especially in those with LCKD diets) any glucose-lowering drugs will most likely need to be adjusted [17]. Patients should be instructed about the hypoglycemic symptoms of alarm and how to adjust their drug doses (especially insulin) if repeated plasma glucose <90 mg/dL occurs. Generally, first-line drugs in the treatment of T2D are retained until surgery (metformin, GLP-1 analogs, inhibitors of dipeptidyl peptidase 4, acarbose, etc.).

Typically, all patients that underwent 2 weeks of nutritional programs before surgery were also treated with metformin (or other hypoglycemic drugs) to control the fasting blood glucose values. For this reason, it is difficult to separate the effect of the diet from that of the medicaments. Health centers not using glycemic control or LCD's protocols have not reported a dramatic worsening of postoperative outcomes, but more randomized control trials are needed [8].

T2D is a chronic disease, and for the most part it is not frequent to achieve a remission with the preoperative diets. Moreover, over the years, it has been observed that when weight stability is achieved—usually 12 months after surgery—some patients might relapse with increased glucose levels [22]. Recent publications support that the nutritional and lifestyle interventions in conjunction with medical treatment can prevent relapse of T2D or mitigate the effects of it. Finally, it is important to note that a positive preoperative glycemic response to a preoperative nutritional intervention can be used to tailor diabetic treatment after surgery in a manner that prevents risky hypoglycemic episodes or delay relapses [23].

Preoperative nutritional intervention and hypertension

Patients with obesity are much more likely to require more than three antihypertensive drugs. The HYDRA study (hypertension and diabetes risk screening and awareness) found that a >5-fold greater probability of requiring three antihypertensive medicaments to achieve adequate blood pressure control <140/90 mmHg in those individuals who have a BMI >40 kg/m^2 [24]. The patients with HTN have a significantly increased risk of cardiovascular events and they must be rapidly submitted to preventive strategies that include reinforcement of lifestyle measures with a special focus on diet adequacy, opting for low sodium and low trans fat diets. Preoperative nutritional interventions in candidates to metabolic surgery can improve their blood pressure around 75% of the cases [4]; but in any case, reducing these values is considered conditioning factors to delay the surgical procedure. Intensive medical intervention to reduce tension peaks is mandatory regardless of the indication for surgery in all phases of the perioperative phase [25].

Lack of response or even relapses can also be seen in HTN patients undergoing metabolic surgery. Therefore, the control of blood pressure, dietary measures, and pharmacological resources must continue to be implemented during follow-up [23].

Preoperative nutritional intervention and dyslipidemia

Obesity is often associated with altered levels of lipids profile characterized by high total cholesterol, low HDL-cholesterol, elevated LDL-cholesterol, and hypertriglyceridemia (TG). Moreover, disturbances in transfer proteins and lipase functions (such as lipoprotein lipase and hepatic lipase) are also associated and all these conditions are also called "*atherogenic dyslipidemia*," which is considered a strong predictive factor for cardiovascular events [26]. To actually lower the cardiovascular risk in patients with obesity, the improvement of the lipid profile must be constant and maintained over time, something that is only succeeded after metabolic surgery. However, preoperative nutritional interventions have been shown to reduce TG and LDL levels and increase HDL, which are desirable conditions in any patient and more so in those who will be under surgical stress [27].

DLP improvement through dietary interventions undoubtedly decreases the risk of cardiovascular events (intra- and postoperative) [12]. However, studies evaluating how these dietary regimes can decrease atherogenic criteria (such as reduction of carotid intima thickness) have not been formally conducted so the benefit in reducing cardiovascular events is more assumed than confirmed. Conversely, a conflictive situation in the preoperative programs is the discussion as to which diet is more effective in reducing lipid values. And contrary to popular belief, low-carbohydrate diets seem to be more effective than low-fat diets, since carbohydrates are the main driver of atherogenic dyslipidemia [26,28].

One of the most beneficial consequences of reducing lipid values is the reduction of the preinflammatory state of obesity and metabolic syndrome. Very high cholesterol and triglyceride values (as well as blood glucose) predispose to a chronic state of inflammation, which is not recommended before any surgery. But in severe cases of DLP (with a high genetic component of the disease), it is likely that dietary intervention will not be sufficient to improve the values and therefore it is recommended to initiate as soon as possible the medical treatment using drugs such as fibrates or statins. These drugs are introduced according to the cardiovascular risk (see Table 4.2) and it is recommended that before any surgical intervention (not only metabolic surgery) the goals of reducing hyperlipidemia should be prioritized [29].

Preoperative nutritional intervention and NAFLD

Previous studies regarding the use of a VLCD before metabolic surgery have focused on the impact of this protocol in the intraoperative and postoperative complications, particularly with regard to reducing hepatomegaly. An enlarged and fatty liver is the most common cause requiring conversion of a laparoscopic gastric bypass or band surgery to an open procedure [8,12,30].

Table 4.2 Score of cardiovascular risk and dyslipidemia's therapy [26].

Cardio vascular risk (Score) %	LDL-C levels				
	< 70 mg/dL < 1,8 mmol/L	70 to < 100 mg/dL 1,8 to < 2,5 mmol/L	100 to < 155 mg/dL 2,5 to < 4 mmol/L	155 to < 190 mg/dL 4 to < 4,9 mmol/L	> 190 mg/dL > 4,9 mmol/L
< 1					
≥ 1 to < 5					
> 5 to < 10, or hight risk					
≥ 10 or very hight risk					

- None intervention
- Diet and lifestyle intervention
- Diet and lifestyle intervention and consider drugs if uncontrolled values
- Diet and lifestyle intervention and consider drugs (mandatory in patients with miocardial infarction)
- Diet and lifestyle intervention immediate drug intervention

There is evidence showing that a 2-week LCD before metabolic surgery is associated with significant improvement in steatosis, inflammation, and hepatocellular ballooning in NAFLD [30]. In these patients, the good results in the preoperative time were associated with improved excess weight loss and liver function after surgery. It is an important highlight that high-salt and high-fructose diets have been implicated in the development of NAFLD and associated with the increased prevalence of NAFLD in clinical studies. Thus, NAFLD patients should pursue any of the dietary approaches and adhere to a low-sodium and low-fructose diet [31].

LCKD also has been proposed as a treatment for NAFLD. It became popular several years ago in morbidly obese patients who were to undertake metabolic surgery because of its rapid effect of weight loss. The LCKD induces a higher consumption of body fat deposits in the liver as the main energy source. In other words, it shifts metabolism from a glycolytic state to a lipolytic one as a consequence of carbohydrate shortage, and it uptakes fat as the main source of energy. However, even though this diet has been shown to contribute to body weight loss and liver volume diminution, it has been questioned for inconveniences such as the poor adherence of patients to this regime due to multiple food restrictions and the high requirements of vitamin and mineral supplementation need to be followed [16,32].

Wise associations' recommendations guidelines

As the current literature is very diverse in terms of defining the advantages or disadvantages of nutritional interventions before metabolic surgery, a mandatory policy has not yet been approved for the preoperative phase [33]. However, the beneficial results appear to outweigh the negative ones, which have led to various scientific associations around the world to establish some guidelines. These guidelines require physician supervision and typically 6–12 months of recent documentation of dietary attempts and recent complementary studies (blood analysis, renal and respiratory function, or psychological evaluation depending on the case) to choose the diet most suited to the needs of each patient [34]. However, patients often must assume the cost of the preoperative nutritional diets (as an average in a range from $108 USD to $2120 USD [4,35]) and these programs lasting for more than 1 month can discourage them. Otherwise, multiple reviews have shown that the weight lost during a long diet program is often regained, and in some cases, the weight gain after ending such a program is greater than the initial loss. Furthermore, obese patients often go through this cycle of weight loss and gain multiple times, leading to the rebound phenomenon, a condition associated with increased risk of cardiovascular diseases [36,37].

The American societies for metabolic and bariatric surgery guidelines

These societies support the team approach to perioperative care and confirm that this activity is mandatory with special attention to nutritional and metabolic issues. However, the guidelines of this association are more focused on postsurgical nutritional interventions. In fact, these societies are fighting against the unreasonable demands of insurers emphasized that the nutritional measures required for a time were inappropriate, capricious, and counterproductive, given the complete absence of a reasonable level of medical evidence to support the exigencies as a condition sine qua non to approve a metabolic surgery [34,38]. In this sense, this society frequently updates medical-evidence-based recommendations. These recommendations are set out below, according to the subject matter of nutrition and comorbidities in the preoperative phase.

General preoperative conditions

Patients must undergo a preoperative exhaustive analysis of the causes of obesity, with special attention directed to those elements that could influence a suggestion for metabolic surgical procedures (Grade A). The initial evaluation must include an exhaustive medical and psychosocial history, physical examination, and appropriate laboratory testing to assess possible surgical risks (Grade A). A lifestyle medicine checklist should be completed for all candidates to metabolic surgery (Grade D). Preoperative nutritional interventions for weight loss by different diets, medical or other therapies may be recommended to patients in selected cases but there is not a consensus. However, it is recommended that all patients should undergo an evaluation of their ability to incorporate nutritional and behavioral changes before and after any metabolic surgical procedure (Grade C). In fact, all patients must undergo an appropriate nutritional evaluation, including micronutrient measurements in all techniques but with extensive nutritional evaluations in case of malabsorptive techniques (Grade A) [34,39].

T2D preoperative conditions

The glycemic control must be optimized by extensive diabetes control programs, including nutritional measures, physical activity, and, as needed, hypoglycemic drugs (Grade A). Reasonable targets for preoperative blood glucose levels control (associated with shorter hospital stays and improved technical outcomes) include an HbA1C value of $\leq 6.5\%-7.0\%$, a fasting blood glucose level of ≤ 110 mg/dL, and a 2-h postprandial blood glucose concentration of ≤ 140 mg/dL (Grade A). Pre-operative Hb1Ac values of 7%—8% are accepted in patients with long-standing diabetes, advanced diabetes-related micro- or macrovascular complications, and extensive comorbid conditions, evolved disease or those who are unable to safely achieve lower targets in which the general goal has been difficult to attain despite intensive efforts (Grade A) [34]. These recommendations do not specify the best nutritional approach on sugar-free or low sugar-free diets before surgery, or suggest advice for LCKD-type diets.

HTN preoperative conditions

In general, the nutritional recommendations of any person with obesity and HTN include a reduced intake of sodium, saturated and trans fats, and red meat. However, the goal to apply special nutritional interventions on these patients is to reduce weight because it was estimated that there is almost 1 mmHg rise of blood pressure per kilogram of weight loss. In addition to obesity, age is a high-risk factor and the goals must change in subjects older than 60 years of age since the baseline values are already elevated in these patients (Grade C) [40].

DLP preoperative conditions

The fat consumption control has a cardiovascular risk prevention approach, rather than the regulation of the cholesterol level by itself. A fasting lipid panel should be obtained in all patients with obesity (Grade A). Treatment should be initiated according to available data and the current programs of cardiovascular wise societies (Grade D) [29,34]. No comparisons are specified between low-fat diets or LCD, VLCD, LCKD regimes.

NAFLD preoperative conditions

Preoperative nutritional interventions to weight loss can reduce liver volume and function probably helping to improve the technical aspects of surgery [30]. In general, dietary regimes are recommended to patients with hepatomegaly or fatty liver disease detected in the image test before the surgery (Grade B). No specific diets are suggested. It should also be noted that routine imaging studies are not recommended to screen liver's disease (Grade B) [34]. Abdominal ultrasound is indicated to evaluate symptomatic biliary disease and elevated liver function tests (Grade C) but could be useful (as well as the elastography) to identify NAFLD. The liver biopsies remain the gold standard. Liver biopsies in the preoperative time is a difficult test [30], but these biopsies can be performed at the time of the operation to document steatohepatitis and/or cirrhosis that may otherwise be unknown due to normal appearance on imaging and/or liver function tests (Grade C). A comprehensive evaluation is recommended in those patients with clinically significant and persistent abnormal liver function tests (Grade A) [34].

The European societies for metabolic and bariatric surgery guidelines

Although the European associations are consistent with the recommendations of the American guidelines, their interventions are not so subordinated to the restrictions made by the health insurance companies. In many countries, metabolic surgery is covered by public health systems (in some cases 100% of pre- and postoperative treatment) [41,42]. This scenario implies certain autonomy in bridging programs that advocate more for the patient to be involved in the treatment of their disease from the preoperative phase with the idea of being consistent in the postsurgical follow-up. Therefore, the recommendations are more lax in terms of scientific evidence and are more supported by experience, since so far the quality studies supporting preoperative nutritional programs have not demonstrated a greater benefit from them. These societies are more inclined to face the fact that the metabolic procedures induce significant and long-lasting changes in nutritional habits and eating behavior. The anatomical and functional modifications of the gastro-intestinal tract produced by the principal techniques always require the adaptation of patients' eating behavior to the new gastro-intestinal physiology, and procedure-specific nutritional problems and symptoms may occur [14].

General preoperative conditions

The European societies consider that decades of bariatric and metabolic surgery have proven that the outcomes and success with metabolic surgery are largely dependent on technically perfect surgery. However, these associations believe success depends more significantly on patient long-term compliance with previous and follow-up regimens [14]. The studies until now show that the overall quality of evidence was very low for the recommendation of a nutritional intervention for weight loss to reduce the postoperative complications. This low quality is mainly due to the heterogeneity of preoperative interventions and duration in the follow-up. However, apparently a pronounced postoperative weight loss was observed in general in those patients who underwent these interventions. No difference in the postoperative complications was found. In fact, consultation with a specialist panel favored a strong recommendation for the nutritional approach of the candidates to metabolic surgery [43]. The panel considered this practice feasible, requiring moderate human and financial resources, and being acceptable to stakeholders. An important component of successful and long-lasting weight loss is the adherence to nutrient-dense foods, containing sufficient amounts of lean proteins and fibers (fruits and vegetables). This is especially true in longer term after metabolic surgery when the stomach volume slowly, however inexorably, expands and appetite begins to increase. High-volume foods like vegetables and fruits can contribute substantially to weight regain prevention. However, these recommendations are not supported by robust clinical trials. Preoperative evaluation enables the identification of interventions that can enhance long-term compliance and weight maintenance [14].

T2D preoperative conditions
Independent of the weight loss goal suggested prior surgery, the preoperative glucose control is required in any candidate for metabolic surgery. It has been suggested that diabetic patients are at greater risk for infections and healing problems that can increase the risk of perioperative complications; although there are not enough scientific studies to support this evidence [43]. Ideally, metabolic control should be optimized to achieve HbA1c levels of 6.5%–7%, fasting glucose levels <110 mg/dL, and 2-h postload glucose < 140 mg/dL. In individuals with long-lasting diabetes, complications derived from micro and macropathologic lesions and poor glucose control, HbA1c levels <8% are acceptable. However, levels >8% must be closely supervised by a multidisciplinary team [14,44]. For patients treated with an LCD or VLCD before surgery, cessation of sulfonylureas, and GLP-1 agonist, reduction of basal insulin should be considered, with strict follow-up of daily glycemia. Individual considerations and follow-up are needed for each patient [13,14].

HTN preoperative conditions
Different European Cardiology associations considered, due to the results of several recent meta-analyses, that establishing a goal below 120–129/<80 mmHg, and 130–139/<80 mmHg in patients less than 65 years old and those aged ≥65 years, respectively, for the majority of the hypertensive population, was enough to maintain the disease controlled. Usually, to achieve these goals, dietary restrictions are not sufficient and pharmacological interventions are usually needed. However, the LCD and VLDC have demonstrated to help to decrease the blood pressure levels, and the principal recommendations in the patients with these interventions are the precautions in the moment of take diuretics for the high risk of dehydration. Daily pressure monitoring and initiation of drug therapy as quickly as necessary is recommended according to guidelines adapted to cardiovascular risk [13,43].

DLP preoperative conditions
Most patients undergoing bariatric surgery have a lipid profile characterized by increased levels of atherogenic small-dense LDL particles. In the preoperative phase, while lowering LDL-cholesterol is associated with reduced risk of cardiovascular disease, it remains unclear whether treatment of high triglyceride level and low HDL cholesterol improves cardiovascular outcomes. In humans, the fattening diets have been associated with significant reductions in total cholesterol, triglycerides levels, and LDL-cholesterol levels, and conversely increase the HDL-cholesterol

values. However, to achieve these results, the low-carbohydrate diets must avoid saturated trans fats if the goal is to reduce the cardiovascular risk by decreasing atherogenicity [45].

NAFLD preoperative conditions

Regarding the targets to be controlled in patients with NALFD before surgery through nutritional interventions, there are no special references in these guidelines, probably, because studies of these interventions associated with histological studies (before and after the diet) are infrequent. In fact, the impact of nutritional interventions is considered the same ones that have been done as in cases of hepatomegaly and fatty liver, where the goal was to reduce the liver volume and improve liver function. Patients with a higher BMI had a greater reduction in a liver volume regardless of the type of nutritional intervention performed. In fact, it was reported a reduction of 14.4% of the hepatic volume in patients with VLCD regimen while the LCD group was 11.3%, values that do not differ significantly from each other and as long as the initial liver volume less than 3 L [12].

Conclusions

Based on the current evidence, there are several gaps in the knowledge of the effectiveness of preoperative nutritional interventions for weight loss before metabolic surgery. Indeed, it is difficult to make any definitive evidence-based conclusions because the formal studies so far evaluate very different variables. Apparently, diets consisting of moderate/low carbohydrate, low fats, and high-protein contents may induce an acceptable weigh loss over 3 weeks. LCKD may achieve the initial target within a shorter duration, but its safety for the metabolic surgery candidates remains uncertain. In fact, the main advantage of applying these measures is the significant reduction of abdominal adiposity, which is mainly lodged in the liver. Patients with a higher BMI (≥ 50 kg/m^2) had a greater reduction in the liver volume regardless of the type of dietary intervention. This condition is especially desirable for surgeons to improve their performance skills in the operating room. The benefits of preoperative nutritional interventions are more associated with reducing conversion rates from laparoscopic surgery to open procedures and reduce surgical time than benefits associated with reducing surgical complications such as bleeding or leaks. In some studies, the nutritional intervention also implies a better decrease in BMI and weight maintenance after surgery, but the results are variable and the long-term cohort studies are still insufficient to achieve strong evidence. For this reason, the wise associations only make recommendations insofar as these interventions can be performed without increasing costs or preventing patients from accessing surgery. Likewise, preoperative interventions alone are helpful in the improvement of obesity-related comorbidities such as T2D, HTN, DLP, and NALFD. However, it is worth noting that nutritional interventions are only a bridge between the baseline situation and surgery and in no way replace the indication of this last one.

References

[1] American Society for Metabolic, Surgery B. Estimate of bariatric surgery numbers, 2011−2017. Gainesville: American Society for Metabolic and Bariatric Surgery; 2018.

[2] Schauer PR, Bhatt DL, Kirwan JP, et al. Bariatric surgery versus intensive medical therapy for diabetes - 5-year outcomes. N Engl J Med 2017;376(7):641−51.

[3] Stefura T, Dros J, Kacprzyk A, et al. Influence of preoperative weight loss on outcomes of bariatric surgery for patients under the enhanced recovery after surgery protocol. Obes Surg 2019;29(4):1134−41.

[4] Lee Y, Dang JT, Switzer N, Malhan R, Birch DW, Karmali S. Bridging interventions before bariatric surgery in patients with BMI $\geq$ 50 kg/m^2: a systematic review and meta-analysis. Surg Endosc 2019;33(11):3578−88.

[5] van Wissen J, Bakker N, Doodeman HJ, Jansma EP, Bonjer HJ, Houdijk AP. Preoperative methods to reduce liver volume in bariatric surgery: a systematic review. Obes Surg 2016;26(2):251−6.

[6] Kim JJ, Rogers AM, Ballem N, et al. ASMBS updated position statement on insurance mandated preoperative weight loss require- ments. Surg Obes Relat Dis 2016;12(5): 955−9.

[7] Naseer F, Shabbir A, Livingstone B, Price R, Syn NL, Flannery O. The efficacy of energy-restricted diets in achieving preoperative weight loss for bariatric patients: a systematic review. Obes Surg 2018;28(11):3678−90.

[8] Chakravartty S, Vivian G, Mullholland N, et al. Preoperative liver shrinking diet for bariatric surgery may impact wound healing: a randomized controlled trial. Surg Obes Relat Dis 2019;15(1):117−25.

[9] Baldry E, Aithal G, Kaye P, et al. Effects of short-term energy restriction on liver lipid content and inflammatory status in severely obese adults: results of a randomised controlled trial (RCT) using two dietary approaches. Diabetes Obes Metabol 2017; 19(8):1179−83.

[10] Schouten R, van der Kaaden I, van't Hof G, et al. Comparison of preoperative diets before bariatric surgery: a randomized, single-blinded, non-inferiority trial. Obes Surg 2016;26(8):1743−9.

[11] Heinberg LJ, Schauer PR. Pilot testing of a portion-controlled, commercially available diet on presurgical weight loss and metabolic outcomes in patients undergoing bariatric surgery. Obes Surg 2014;24(10):1817−20.

[12] Gils Contreras A, Bonada Sanjaume A, Montero Jaime M, et al. Effects of two preoperatory weight loss diets on hepatic volume, metabolic parameters, and surgical complications in morbid obese bariatric surgery candidates: a randomized clinical trial. Obes Surg 2018;28(12):3756−68.

[13] Fried M, Yumuk V, Oppert JM, et al. Interdisciplinary European Guidelines on metabolic and bariatric surgery. Obes Facts 2013;6(5):449−68.

[14] Busetto L, Dicker D, Azran C, et al. Practical recommendations of the obesity management task force of the European association for the study of obesity for the post-bariatric surgery medical management. Obes Facts 2017;10(6):597−632.

[15] Gerber P, Anderin C, Thorell A. Weight loss prior to bariatric surgery: an updated review of the literature. Scand J Surg 2015;104(1):33−9.

[16] Leonetti F, Campanile FC, Coccia F, et al. Very low-carbohydrate ketogenic diet before bariatric surgery: prospective evaluation of a sequential diet. Obes Surg 2015;25(1): 64−71.

[17] Matarese LE, Pories WJ. Adult weight loss diets: metabolic effects and outcomes. Nutr Clin Pract 2014;29(6):759—67.
[18] Davenport L, Johari Y, Klejn A, et al. Improving compliance with very low energy diets (VLEDs) prior to bariatric surgery-a randomised controlled trial of two formulations. Obes Surg 2019;29(9):2750—7.
[19] Zeevi D, Korem T, Zmora N, et al. Personalized nutrition by prediction of glycemic responses. Cell 2015;163(5):1079—94.
[20] Tan SYT, Loi PL, Lim CH, et al. Preoperative weight loss via very low caloric diet (VLCD) and its effect on outcomes after bariatric surgery obes surg. 2020 [published online ahead of print, 2020 Feb 19].
[21] Rometo D, Korytkowski M. Perioperative glycemic management of patients undergoing bariatric surgery. Curr Diabetes Rep 2016;16(4):23.
[22] Aminian A, Brethauer SA, Andalib A, et al. Individualized metabolic surgery score: procedure selection based on diabetes severity. Ann Surg 2017;266(4):650—7.
[23] Aminian A, Vidal J, Salminen P, et al. Late relapse of diabetes after bariatric surgery: not rare, but not a failure. Diabetes Care 2020;43(3):534—40.
[24] Pareek M, Bhatt DL, Schiavon CA, Schauer PR. Metabolic surgery for hypertension in patients with obesity. Circ Res 2019;124(7):1009—24.
[25] de la Sierra A. New American and European hypertension guidelines, reconciling the differences. Cardiol Ther 2019;8(2):157—66.
[26] Bajer B, Radikova, Havranov A, et al. Effect of 8-weeks intensive lifestyle intervention on LDL and HDL subfractions. Obes Res Clin Pract 2019;13(6):586—93.
[27] Pilone V, Tramontano S, Renzulli M, et al. Metabolic effects, safety, and acceptability of very low-calorie ketogenic dietetic scheme on candidates for bariatric surgery. Surg Obes Relat Dis 2018;14(7):1013—9.
[28] Hu T, Mills KT, Yao L, et al. Effects of low-carbohydrate diets versus low-fat diets on metabolic risk factors: a meta-analysis of randomized controlled clinical trials. Am J Epidemiol 2012;176(Suppl. 7):S44—54.
[29] Nordestgaard BG, Chapman MJ, Humphries SE, Ginsberg HN, Masana L, Descamps OS, et al. Familial hypercholesterolemia is underdiagnosed and undertreated in the general population: guidance for clinicians to prevent coronary heart disease: consensus statement of the European Atherosclerosis Society. Eur Heart J 2013;34: 3478—3490a.
[30] Wolf RM, Oshima K, Canner JK, Steele KE. Impact of a preoperative low-calorie diet on liver histology in patients with fatty liver disease undergoing bariatric surgery. Surg Obes Relat Dis 2019;15(10):1766—72.
[31] Hsu CC, Ness E, Kowdley KV. Nutritional approaches to achieve weight loss in nonalcoholic fatty liver disease. Adv Nutr 2017;8(2):253—65. Published 2017 Mar 15.
[32] Yancy Jr WS, Westman EC, McDuffie JR, et al. A randomized trial of a low-carbohydrate diet vs orlistat plus a low-fat diet for weight loss. Arch Intern Med 2010;170(2):136—45.
[33] Roman M, Monaghan A, Serraino GF, et al. Meta-analysis of the influence of lifestyle changes for preoperative weight loss on surgical outcomes. Br J Surg 2019;106(3): 181—9.
[34] Mechanick JI, Apovian C, Brethauer S, et al. Clinical practice guidelines for the perioperative nutrition, metabolic, and nonsurgical support of patients undergoing bariatric procedures - 2019 update: cosponsored by American association of clinical endocrinologists/American college of endocrinology, the obesity society, American

society for metabolic & bariatric surgery, obesity medicine association, and American society of anesthesiologists. Surg Obes Relat Dis 2020;16(2):175−247.

[35] Spielman AB, Kanders B, Kienholz M, Blackburn GL. The cost of losing: an analysis of commercial weight-loss programs in a metropolitan area. J Am Coll Nutr 1992;11: 36−41.

[36] Deb S, Voller L, Palisch C, et al. Influence of weight loss attempts on bariatric surgery outcomes. Am Surg 2016;82(10):916−20.

[37] Strohacker K, Carpenter KC, McFarlin BK. Consequences of weight cycling: an increase in disease risk? Int J Exerc Sci 2009;2:191−201.

[38] Tewksbury C, Williams NN, Dumon KR, Sarwer DB. Preoperative medical weight management in bariatric surgery: a review and reconsideration. Obes Surg 2017; 27(1):208−14.

[39] Frame-Peterson LA, Megill RD, Carobrese S, Schweitzer M. Nutrient deficiencies are common prior to bariatric surgery. Nutr Clin Pract 2017;32(4):463−9.

[40] Shariq OA, McKenzie TJ. Obesity-related hypertension: a review of pathophysiology, management, and the role of metabolic surgery. Gland Surg 2020;9(1):80−93.

[41] Sánchez-Santos R, Sabench Pereferrer F, Estévez Fernandez S, et al. Is the morbid obesity surgery profitable in times of crisis? A cost-benefit analysis of bariatric surgery. Cir Esp 2013;91(8):476−84.

[42] von Lengerke T, Krauth C. Economic costs of adult obesity: a review of recent European studies with a focus on subgroup-specific costs. Maturitas 2011;69(3):220-229.

[43] Di Lorenzo N, Antoniou SA, Batterham RL, et al. Clinical practice guidelines of the European Association for Endoscopic Surgery (EAES) on bariatric surgery: update 2020 endorsed by IFSO-EC. EASO and ESPCOP- Surg Endosc; 2020 [published online ahead of print, 2020 Apr 23].

[44] Thorell A, Hagström-Toft E. Treatment of diabetes prior to and after bariatric surgery. J Diabetes Sci Technol 2012;6(5):1226−32.

[45] Kosinski C, Jornayvaz FR. Effects of ketogenic diets on cardiovascular risk factors: evidence from animal and human studies. Nutrients 2017;9(5):517.

CHAPTER 5

Fluid therapy during bariatric surgery

Esther García-Villabona, Carmen Vallejo-Lantero
Department of Anesthesiology, University Hospital La Princesa, Madrid, Spain

Chapter outline

Fluid management approaches 63
    Preoperative period 64
    Intraoperative period 64
    Surgical factors affecting fluid therapy 65
    Goal-directed fluid therapy 66
Guiding parameters for administering fluids 67
    Monitoring of intravascular volume status 67
    Commonly used techniques in goal-directed fluid therapy 67
    Functional hemodynamic variables to guide GDFT 71
    What monitoring recommendations are there in bariatric surgery? 71
Conclusion 72
References 73

Fluid management approaches

Intravenous fluid therapy is an important and integrated treatment of patients undergoing surgery. Minimizing the risk of the intraoperative complications requires precise assessment of the patient's volume status. Estimation of intravascular volume is one of the most important clinical skills of the anesthesiologist.

The majority of perioperative patients experience a certain degree of preoperative hypovolemia. Hypovolemia can lead to vasoconstriction and inadequate perfusion with decreased oxygen delivery to organs and peripheral tissues causing organ dysfunction.

On the other hand, fluid overload can lead to interstitial edema and local inflammation and likely impair the regeneration of collagen, thus negatively affecting tissue healing and increasing the risk of wound dehiscence, wound infections, and anastomotic leakage. Therefore, it is imperative to manage each patient's fluid therapy in an individualized manner [1].

Preoperative period

There are some preoperative factors affecting bariatric patients that can complicate their management:

- Preoperative weight loss, including preparation by a rapid weight-loss diet, aims to facilitate laparoscopic bariatric surgery. However, this condition can expose patients to acute nutritional, electrolyte and fluid deficits.
- Obesity is associated with an increase in total and lean body mass; however, intracellular, extracellular, and absolute total body fluids are relatively reduced compared to those with normal weight.
- Although total blood volume is increased in obese patients, they have a reduced blood volume on a volume/weight basis compared with nonobese patients (50 mL/kg compared with 75 mL/kg).
- Cardiac involvement, including impaired relaxation and compliance of the left ventricle, is common in obesity of long duration.
- Traditionally, surgical patients have been required to fast for 8 h. This can potentially lead to preoperative hypovolemia. The resulting surgical stress can induce multiple endocrine responses, including the release of vasopressin (antidiuretic hormone). The reabsorptive actions of vasopressin on the collecting duct in the kidneys can cause water retention, which can, to some extent offset the hypovolemic effect of fasting [2].

Intraoperative period

Although fluid therapy is one of the main areas of anesthesia practice, there are no recognized, accessible guidelines for intraoperative fluid therapy in bariatric surgery. There are limited data for the optimal fluid regimen in morbidly obese patients.

Present fluid management paradigms are based on studies of liberal versus restrictive strategies in nonobese patients whereby fluid excess or "imbalance" resulted in worsened outcomes than maintaining "fluid balance." Both approaches (liberal vs. restrictive) have their own benefits and risks [3].

	Liberal (40 mL/kg)	Restrictive (15 mL/kg)
Benefits	✔ Rhabdomyolysis prevention ✔ ↓POSTOPERATIVE NAUSEA AND VOMITING	✔ GI function faster recovery ✔ Better wound healing ✔ Improvement in pulmonary function and tissue oxygenation ✔ ↓ HOSPITAL STAY
Risks	- Positive fluid balance - Weight gain - Congestive heart failure	- Risk of acute tubular necrosis - Rhabdomyolysis

The significance of the symbol "↓" in the table is "reduction", "decrease".

Fluid overload leads to a decrease in muscular oxygen tension. Due to surgical trauma, a systemic inflammatory response arises, which leads to a fluid shift to the extravascular space. Following a large fluid shift, generalized edema may occur, which decreases tissue oxygenation and impedes tissue healing. By contrast, hypovolemia leads to arterial and tissue hypoxia due to a decrease in cardiac output.

Patients with more liberal fluid management (40 mL/kg vs. 15 mL/kg total body weight) also produced significantly higher urine output in the operating room, in the postanesthesia care unit, and on postoperative days 0 and first [1].

On the other hand, surgical patients whose fluid balance was managed in the more restrictive fashion (15 mL/kg) demonstrated faster recovery of gastrointestinal function, better wound healing, and improvement in pulmonary function and tissue oxygenation. There were no differences in postoperative rhabdomyolysis following laparoscopic bariatric surgery compared to more liberal strategies (40 mL/kg). No differences in intraoperative urine output were noted when morbidly obese patients were randomized to intraoperative low (4 mL/kg/h) versus high (10 mL/kg/h) volumes of Ringer's lactate. In the bariatric setting, limiting intravenous fluids reduced the incidence of postoperative pulmonary dysfunction and hypoxia, and shortened hospital stay [1].

Surgical factors affecting fluid therapy

Most of the bariatric interventions are performed with a laparoscopic approach. Laparoscopy requires abdominal insufflation of CO_2 for intraabdominal pressures up to 15 mmHg. As long as the intraabdominal pressure elevates, venous stasis increases, intraoperative portal venous blood flow, intraoperative urinary output, and respiratory compliance are reduced, airway pressure increases, and cardiac function is impaired. Intraoperative management to minimize adverse effects of pneumoperitoneum includes appropriate ventilator support to avoid hypercapnia and acidosis, and optimization of intravascular volume to minimize effects of elevated intraabdominal pressure on renal and cardiac functions.

Reverse Trendelenburg position in the presence of pneumoperitoneum represents another challenge for the intraoperative assessment of fluid balance. Under general anesthesia, this position is associated with a gravity-induced shift of blood volume to the lower part of the body, which frequently results in a significant decrease of cardiac output and blood pressure (Fig. 5.1).

Apart from direct effects of the laparoscopy, morbidly obese patients that would undergo surgical procedure are also at risk of muscle injury, which, in turn, may result in rhabdomyolysis (RML), serious electrolyte disturbance, cardiac arrhythmias, and acute renal failure. In bariatric surgery rates of 5%—77% were reported (defined by elevation of serum creatine kinase of 1000 IU/L). Of those with RML, the overall incidence of renal failure was 14% and mortality 3%. Risk factors for RML identified in a meta-analysis were male sex, body mass index (BMI) (52 kg/m^2), and operation time [4].

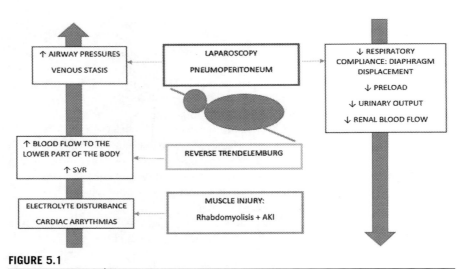

FIGURE 5.1

Physiological changes during bariatric surgery.

Although aggressive fluid replacement is the mainstay for the management of rhabdomyolysis, it is still contradictory whether or not liberal perioperative fluid therapy will prevent this complication. No difference was reported in the incidence of RML between bariatric surgery patients receiving either liberal or restrictive crystalloid fluid therapy. Administration of each liter of extra fluid added on the given fluids intraoperatively was reported to increase the risk of postoperative symptoms (16%) and complications (32%) [3].

Goal-directed fluid therapy

It is well established that both hypovolemia and hypervolemia are associated with postoperative morbidity. Goal-directed fluid therapy (GDFT) is based on the optimization of tissue perfusion by rational fluid management, guided by hemodynamic parameters. These algorithms are designed to avoid excessive fluid infusion and to maximize cardiac output by measuring hemodynamic parameters [5].

The historical method of predicting fluid losses is based on fasting duration and insensible losses that may occur during surgery. In addition, fluid administration was titrated based on static parameters such as urine output, heart rate (HR), and blood pressure (BP). The theory of GDFT encourages clinicians to manage fluid/volume administration based on objective goals of hemodynamic parameters that are evidence based.

GDFT encompasses a technique involving intensive monitoring to assess fluid responsiveness and aggressive management of intraoperative hemodynamics. Fluid responsiveness is defined as an ability of the heart to increase stroke volume in response to volume expansion [6].

Numerous meta-analyses showed outstanding benefits of GDFT over standard fluid therapies in terms of reducing morbidity and mortality rates in high-risk surgeries. Furthermore, administration of GDFT protocols were reported to decrease length of hospital stay, incidence of respiratory failure, acute renal failure, and surgical site infections, and reduce postoperative morbidity such as nausea and vomiting [5].

Guiding parameters for administering fluids
Monitoring of intravascular volume status

The purpose of monitoring intravascular volume status is to guide fluid administration to maintain adequate tissue perfusion. Reduced tissue perfusion can be associated with hypovolemia (hemorrhage) or hypervolemia (i.e., a patient with severe myocardial dysfunction and compensatory fluid retention). Volume status assessment can be achieved with continuous intraoperative monitoring of factors such as HR, BP, end-tidal CO_2, central venous pressure (CVP), urine output, stroke volume (SV), cardiac output (CO), and their derivatives. Classic static hemodynamic indicators (such as HR, BP, urine output, or CVP) are not the best indicators to estimate the patient's hydration status and they are poor predictor markers of fluid therapy response [6].

GDFT is defined as the monitoring of hemodynamic parameters and rational fluid administration based on information obtained to optimize tissue perfusion. The hemodynamic parameters used are stroke volume (SV) and CO, or dynamic volume response parameters such as pulse pressure variation (PPV) and stroke volume variation (SVV). According to the parameters measured, GDFT algorithms are designed to maximize the cardiac output while avoiding fluid excess [7].

Thus, some invasive, minimally invasive, and noninvasive hemodynamic monitors are used to assess volume status and predict fluid responsiveness in various surgical procedures.

Accurate intraoperative determination of intravascular volume status remains challenging because of some intraoperative conditions like the following: cardiovascular responses to anesthetic drugs, the variable surgical volume losses (that are often difficult to quantify), the presence of preoperative hypovolemia or an unknown preoperative volume status, as well as the manifestations of the normal physiological responses to surgery.

Additionally, not all patients who are fluid responders require volume expansion. The decision to administer fluid should be supported by an apparent need for hemodynamic improvement in the context of a volume deficit and by the lack of associated risk [6].

Commonly used techniques in goal-directed fluid therapy

There are now many different monitoring systems available, and physicians may feel somewhat confused by the multiple possibilities. These systems can be easily listed in order of invasiveness, from the highly invasive pulmonary artery catheter (PAC) to the completely noninvasive bioimpedance/bioreactance technique and the transthoracic echo-Doppler.

Advances in minimally and noninvasive monitoring technologies should be considered as an effort to decrease the degree of invasiveness and a possibility of increasing its frequency of application, especially in the operating room.

These techniques provide information of systemic flow and cardiac performance as well as intravascular fluid status. Classifying them according to how accurate (closeness of measured values to the "true" value, expressed as the bias) or precise (variability of values due to random errors of measurement) they are, is more difficult, in part because of the lack of a perfect "gold" standard for comparison.

Most devices have been evaluated by comparing their results with those obtained by intermittent thermodilution from the PAC as the reference, although this technique has its own limitations and may not represent the best choice of comparator [8].

- Pulmonary artery catheterization

The PAC, enabling pulmonary artery thermodilution, is certainly the most invasive CO-monitoring tool. The intermittent thermodilution technique, in which boluses of ice-cold fluid are injected into the right atrium via PAC, and the change in temperature detected in the blood of the pulmonary artery is used to calculate cardiac output, is still widely considered as the standard method of reference. Adaptation of the PAC to incorporate a thermal filament or thermal coil that warms blood in the superior vena cava and measures changes in blood temperature at the PAC tip using a thermistor, provides a continuous measure of the trend in cardiac output, with the displayed values representing an average of the values over the previous 10 min.

Although the PAC can now be largely replaced by less invasive hemodynamic monitoring techniques in many cases, in some complex clinical situations (e.g., cardiac surgery, organ transplant surgery, and surgery associated with major fluid shifts or high risk of respiratory failure or in patients with compromised right ventricle function), the PAC still represents a valuable tool when used by physicians adequately trained to correctly interpret and apply the data provided [8].

- Transesophageal echocardiography

Echocardiography allows measurement of cardiac output using standard two-dimensional imaging or, more commonly, Doppler-based methods. The main interest in echocardiography in general is that it can be used not only for the measurement of cardiac output but also for the additional assessment of cardiac function. Echocardiography is particularly useful as a diagnostic tool because it allows the visualization of cardiac chambers, valves, and pericardium.

Transesophageal echocardiography can measure SV, CO, and CVP, and thus it can be used intraoperatively to provide parameters for GDFT. The less invasive transthoracic echocardiography can be used preoperatively and postoperatively; however, it is often not possible to use transthoracic echocardiography during the intraoperative period.

However, echocardiography instruments and expertise may not be easily available everywhere; it requires formation and qualification.

- **Arterial waveform analysis-based techniques**

Pulse wave analysis derives CO/SV from continuous pressure waveform measurement via an arterial line. Characteristics of the arterial pressure waveform are determined by the interaction between cardiac action and vascular compliance, aortic impedance as well as peripheral arterial resistance. For adequate CO/SV measurement, some features and limitations need to be considered:

1. Optimal arterial waveform signal is a prerequisite, that is, damping or increased tubing resonance has to be eliminated or at least reduced.
2. Severe arrhythmias and the use of an intraaortic balloon pump impede adequate performance of pulse wave analysis.
3. Rapid changes of vascular resistance may limit reliable CO/SV measurements. This can be especially a problem for the uncalibrated devices. By contrast, calibrated devices require frequent recalibration for accurate CO estimation under these conditions.
4. Severe atherosclerosis may preclude the insertion of an arterial catheter or reliable measurements (e.g., subclavian stenosis and signal detection via radial arterial line).

Different calibrated and uncalibrated devices are currently available [9].

➢ **PiCCO$_2$ and LiDCO** are based on the same pulse pressure algorithm (PulseCO) and track SV continuously. The PiCCO$_2$ system requires a dedicated thermistor-tipped catheter that is typically placed in the femoral artery, to assess SV on a beat-to-beat basis. The PiCCO algorithm assumes that the area under the systolic part of the pressure curve corresponds with SV. A calibration is required, and it is performed using intermittent transpulmonary thermodilution via a central venous line.

➢ The LiDCOplus requires calibration by the transpulmonary lithium indicator dilution technique, which can be performed via a peripheral venous line. By contrast, the LiDCOrapid does not require calibration because CO estimation relies on hemodynamic nomograms.

➢ **FloTrac/Vigileo/EV1000** requires a proprietary transducer (the FloTrac), which is attached to a standard radial or femoral arterial catheter and connected to the Vigileo monitor. The FloTrac/Vigileosystem does not require calibration. To assess CO, the standard deviation of pulse pressure sampled during a time window of 20 s is correlated with "normal" SV based on patient's demographic data (age, gender, height, and weight) and a built-in database containing information regarding CO assessed by PAC in a variety of clinical scenarios. Impedance is also derived from these data whereas vascular compliance and resistance are determined using arterial waveform analysis. Another CO monitoring device based on pulse pressure analysis is the EV 1000 platform (with the Volume View catheter), which is also calibrated by transpulmonary thermodilution.

➢ Special mention deserves a completely noninvasive pulse pressure analysis devices (**Clearsight** and **CNAP**), which monitor pulse pressure using photoelectric plethysmography in combination with a volume-clamp technique (i.e., an inflatable finger cuff system). They are the only devices that provide continuous information on oxygen delivery via incorporated pulse oximetry [10]. With the finger cuff and a pressure transducer mounted on the forearm (and a noninvasive arterial pressure cuff for calibration), this technology offers the ability to continuously (beat to beat) measure blood pressure and PPV. The basic principles of calculating SV/CO in both systems are generally based on the pulse contour method, which are described in detail before.

- **Esophageal Doppler**

Esophageal Doppler devices measure blood flow in the descending aorta and derive CO by multiplying the cross-sectional area of the aorta by blood flow velocity. The aortic diameter is obtained from nomograms or by direct measurement using M-mode echocardiography.

There are several important limitations for the use of esophageal Doppler devices [11]:

1. Doppler devices assume a fixed partition between flow to the cephalic vessels and to the descending aorta. This may be a valid assumption in healthy volunteers; however, the relationship may change in patients with comorbidities and under conditions of hemodynamic instability.
2. Doppler probes are smaller than the conventional transesophageal echocardiography probes. Therefore, probe position may change unintentionally and continuous monitoring is restricted.
3. The device is operator dependent and studies have shown that roughly 12 insertions are required to obtain accurate measurements with an acceptable intra and interobserver variability.
4. Aortic cross-sectional area is not constant but rather dynamic in any individual patient. Therefore, the use of nomograms may result in less accurate measurements.

- **Bioimpedance-based technologies**
    ➢ **Thoracic Electrical Bioimpedance (TEB):** TEB determines the change of impedance via delivering a low amplitude high frequency electrical current across the thorax. The TEB electrodes are placed on the upper and lower thorax. TEB parameters are based on changes in the thoracic electrical conductivity to changes in the thoracic aortic blood flow during the cardiac cycle. TEB is an alternative technique to measure SV, CO, and cardiac index (CI).

> **Electrical Bioreactance-based Technology:** Electric bioreactance (EB) analysis is also based on alterations in frequency of electrical resistivity across the thorax. EB is significantly less susceptible to interference from chest wall movement, lung edema, and pleural effusion. EB measures CO centrally. When an alternative current is applied to the thorax, the pulsatile blood flow in the large thoracic arteries induces phase shifts or time delays between the measured thoracic voltage and the applied alternative current. By continuously measuring these phase shifts, EB can determine SV and other derivative parameters such as CO, CI, systolic volume index, and systemic vascular resistance index [10].

Functional hemodynamic variables to guide GDFT

GDFT protocols were recently developed to avoid excessive fluid loading and improve postoperative patient outcomes. Various hemodynamic parameters are utilized to guide these protocols. Ventilation-induced plethysmographic wave form variations were shown to be directly associated with intravascular volume [7].

Compared to standard fluid protocols, GDFT protocols were reported to allow for less fluid infusion intraoperatively, and shorten the length of hospital stay, reduce the incidence of surgical site infections, and accelerate the restoration of bowel movements and perfusion [8].

Dynamic parameters such as PPV and SVV, derived from arterial waveform analysis, have been suggested as the most reliable indicators of fluid responsiveness in mechanically ventilated patients as long as sinus rhythm is maintained. A recent study by Jain and Dutta demonstrated the value of SVV in the bariatric population. PPV or SVV values greater than 13% indicate fluid responsiveness, while patients with PPV below 9% should be considered nonresponders. Twenty-five percent of the patients with PPV value between 9% and 13% represent the so-called "gray zone" when fluid responsiveness cannot be reliably predicted [12].

Dynamic parameters were reported to have lower accuracy in predicting fluid responsiveness when used in patients with low pulmonary compliance, or when high tidal volume (>8 mL/kg) was administered. For increased elastic resistance of chest wall and decreased respiratory compliance in obesity, some studies reported clinical benefits of lung-protective ventilation by using low tidal volumes. As the use of lung-protective ventilation may interfere with dynamic parameters in predicting fluid responsiveness in bariatric patients, we did not include those patients with low pulmonary compliance [8].

What monitoring recommendations are there in bariatric surgery?

Plethysmographic waveform variation (PWV) obtained from the pulse oximeter is a completely noninvasive dynamic parameter, which can also be used to assess fluid responsiveness as described by Pizov et al. Its noninvasive nature, minimal additional cost, and practically universal availability represent a major benefit for its use [7]. However, compared to arterial waveform analysis, the authors found some delay in detecting hypovolemia. In other words, PWV may be useful at levels of more profound hypovolemia.

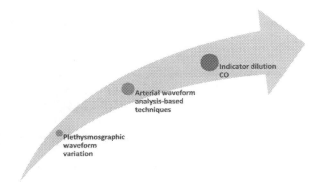

FIGURE 5.2

Recommendations for monitoring in bariatric surgery depending on the patient's risk.

There are other new technologies for noninvasive assessment of the cardiac output, PPV and SVV (Nexfin). It uses a finger cuff for assessment of blood pressure and derived variables. Early results from intraoperative use in a bariatric population suggest that this technology may be comparable to invasive PPV [8].

As we have explained earlier, there are some devices that are capable to calculate vascular tone and cardiac output by analyzing the waveform derived from the arterial line. Along with the SVV, they provide continuous CO and central venous oxygen saturation if connected to a central venous line. The additional parameters provided by this technology can be used in bariatric patients with significant cardiac comorbidities.

Pulse-contour analysis-based techniques are a comprehensive modality for perioperative cardiovascular assessment as they provide not only real-time measurement of PPV, SVV, and CO, but also useful newer parameters, such as global end diastolic index, intrathoracic blood volume, and extravascular lung water index. This technology can be used in patients with certain conditions (e.g., significant arrhythmia) that limit the use of PPV or in high-risk patients with morbid obesity undergoing high-risk surgical procedures. Due to the high cost and invasiveness, these devices are often reserved for the sickest patients undergoing major surgical interventions (Fig. 5.2).

Conclusion

Decisions regarding fluid therapy are among the most challenging and important tasks that clinicians face on a daily basis. Perioperative fluid management and accurate assessment of volume status in morbidly obese patients are a challenge. Reasons for this include physiological differences, the presence of multiple comorbidities (and associated polypharmacy), preoperative preparation (rapid weight loss diet), inaccuracies associated with the use of noninvasive monitoring, and higher incidence of rhabdomyolysis postoperatively [5].

When making decisions for intraoperative fluid management in patients with morbid obesity, clinicians should consider the following:

1. Optimal perioperative fluid management is an important component of the enhanced recovery after surgery pathways, and it can reduce postoperative complications.
2. Regardless of monitoring technique, it is important for the clinician to effectively plan and implement preoperative and intraoperative fluid goals.
3. Excess crystalloid fluid should be avoided.
4. In some low-risk patients undergoing low-risk surgery, a "zero-balance" approach is encouraged.
5. For most patients undergoing major surgery, GDFT is recommended.
6. In high-risk patients with morbid obesity undergoing high-risk surgical procedures, consider the use of advanced, invasive monitoring.

References

[1] Ogunnaike BO, Jones SB, Jones DB, et al. Anesthetic considerations for bariatric surgery. Anesth Analg 2002;95:1793—805.
[2] Poso T, Kesek D, Aroch R, et al. Morbid obesity and optimization of preoperative fiuid therapy. Obes Surg 2013;23:1799—805.
[3] Bundgaard-Nielsen M, Secher NH, Kehlet H. 'Liberal' vs. 'restrictive' perioperative fiuid therapy—a critical assessment of the evidence. Acta Anaesthesiol Scand 2009; 53:843—51.
[4] Chakravartty S, Sarma DR, Patel AG. Rhabdomyolysis in bariatric surgery: a systematic review. Obes Surg 2013;23:1333—40.
[5] Thorell A, MacCormick AD, Awad S, et al. Guidelines for perioperative care in bariatric surgery: enhanced recovery after surgery (ERAS) society recommendations. World J Surg 2016;40(9):2065—83.
[6] Kalantari K, Chang JN, Ronco C, et al. Assessment of intravascular volume status and volume responsiveness in critically ill patients. Kidney Int 2013;83:1017—28.
[7] Demirel I, Bolat E, Altun AY, et al. Efficacy of goal-directed fluid therapy via pleth variability Index during laparoscopic roux-en-Y gastric bypass surgery in morbidly obese patients. Obes Surg 2018;28:358—63.
[8] Vincent JL, Rhodes A, Perel A, et al. Clinical review: update on hemodynamic monitoring — a consensus of 16. Crit Care 2011;15:229.
[9] Hofer CK, Cecconi M, Marx G, et al. Minimally invasive haemodynamic monitoring. Eur J Anaesthesiol 2009;26:996—1002.
[10] Li MQ, Yang LQ, Zhou L, et al. Non-invasive cardiac output measurement: where are we now? J Anesth Perioper Med 2018;5:221—7.
[11] Renner J, Grunewald M, Bein B. Monitoring high-risk patients: minimally invasive and non-invasive possibilities. Best Pract Res Clin Anaesthesiol 2016;30:201—16.
[12] Michard F, Chemla D, Teboul JL. Applicability of pulse pressure variation: how many shades of grey? Crit Care 2015;19:144.

CHAPTER 6

Bariatric surgery options

Jaime Ruiz-Tovar[1,2], Lorea Zubiaga[3]
[1]Bariatric Surgery Unit, Garcilaso Clinic, Madrid, Spain; [2]Department of Surgery, University Alfonso X, Madrid, Spain; [3]Lille University, Institut National de la Santé et de la Recherche Médicale (INSERM)-U1190, EGID, CHU Lille, Lille, France

Chapter outline
Introduction 75
Restrictive procedures 76
Mixed procedures 78
Malabsorptive procedures 80
Conclusion 84
Acknowledgments 84
References 85

Introduction

Obesity is actually considered as the 21st century epidemy. It represents an important health problem in developed and even in developing countries, as it reduces life expectancy and quality of life, mostly associated with the development of obesity-related comorbidities and consequently cardiovascular risk factors. Obesity is associated with type 2 diabetes mellitus (T2D), hypertension, dyslipidemia, respiratory diseases, psychosocial disorders, and some types of neoplasms [1].

Bariatric surgery has shown to be the best therapeutic option for severely obese patients (BMI $\geq$ 35 kg/m^2) with obesity-related comorbidities and for morbidly obese patients (BMI $\geq$ 40 kg/m^2).[1] The different bariatric techniques show different features, related to the ponderal effect, postoperative complications evolution of comorbidities, and nutritional sequelae. Actually, a customized treatment must be selected for each patient, considering their characteristics [2]. Notwithstanding, the surgeons' preferences often influence the final selection of the technique to perform.

Globally, bariatric procedures can be divided into three groups [2]:

- Restrictive procedures (adjustable gastric banding, sleeve gastrectomy): Imply a functional or anatomic decrease of the gastric volume, and consequently reduce the food intake.

- Malabsorptive procedures (biliopancreatic diversion, duodenal switch, one-anastomosis gastric bypass, single anastomosis duodenum-ileal switch, etc.): These procedures include changes in the small bowel anatomy, bypassing part of the length of the intestine and consequently reducing the absorption of the nutrients.
- Mixed procedures (Roux-en-Y gastric bypass): It is a combination of restrictive and malabsorptive techniques, associating a reduction of the gastric volume with a partial bypass of the small bowel.

All types of procedures present advantages and disadvantages. Malabsorptive procedures appear to be more effective, in terms of weight loss and remission of comorbidities, and with a longer durability of the results. However, they associate greater nutritional deficiencies. On the other hand, restrictive procedures are at lower risk of developing nutritional sequelae, but present poorer outcomes and long-term weight regain and comorbidities recurrence. Thus, as previously mentioned, a careful selection of the most appropriate technique for each subject must be done.

Restrictive procedures

- **Adjustable gastric banding:**

Adjustable gastric banding (AGB) was the most frequently bariatric procedure in the last 2 decades of the 20th century, based on its simplicity and low risk of complications. The absence of visceral resections or anatomic changes and the reversibility were the keys to the growth of this approach.

AGB, as most bariatric procedures actually, is laparoscopically performed. The technique consists of the placement of an adjustable silicone band around the upper part of the stomach. The silicone band is filled with normal saline, injected through a special device located in the abdominal wall, and thereby the pass from the upper to the lower part of the stomach is narrowed. Consequently, the AGB artificially creates a small gastric pouch above the band and the size of the opening between the pouch and the rest of the stomach can be adjusted, according to the filling of the silicone band; the greater the filling of the band, the greater will be the restrictive effect. During the postoperative course, depending on the ponderal evolution or appearance of gastrointestinal symptoms (nausea or vomits, gastroesophageal reflux disease, etc.), the band can be adjusted in the outpatient clinic (Fig. 6.1) [3].

The benefit of the band is mostly restriction and satiety, resulting in a reduction of calorie consumption. The mean percentage of excess weight loss (EWL) at 1 year after surgery ranges from 16% to 50%. EWL obtains maximum levels 1—2 years after surgery, then remained stable between years 2 and 3, and tends to decrease after 4—5 years. The rates of complete remission of comorbidities are also one of the lowest of all bariatric techniques [4,5].

Late complications, such as band erosion, band slippage, gastroesophageal reflux, esophageal dilatation, and port infections, and the trend toward long-term weight regain in patients with noncompliance of dietary measures, were the most important factors to the decline in the use of AGB worldwide [6,7].

Restrictive procedures

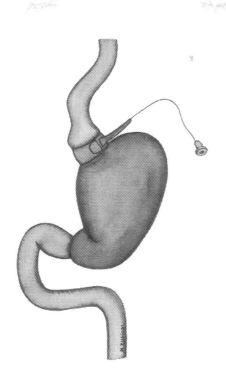

FIGURE 6.1

Adjustable gastric banding.

- **Sleeve gastrectomy:**

Sleeve gastrectomy (SG) was initially developed as the first step from a Duodenal Switch in superobese patients with high surgical risk to undergo the complete duodenal switch. The excellent results obtained in some patients, who did not require the second step of the duodenal switch, lead to the development of SG as independent bariatric approach [8]. Since 2014, the SG is the most performed procedure in the world representing more than 50% of all primary bariatric interventions [7]. The fear of nutritional consequences has led to the exponential growth of SG. With this technique, the nutritional deficiencies are less frequent, but it has other disadvantages, such as the appearance of de novo acid gastro-esophageal reflux disease and mid- and long-term weight regain [9].

SG consists of the resection of 80% of the total volume of the stomach. The greater curvature of the stomach is resected vertically, leaving a remaining long, tubular conduit (Fig. 6.2) [10].

Despite the pure restrictive mechanism that seems to be the basis of weight loss with this procedure, a certain metabolic effect has been also reported. The reduction of the ghrelin levels has been described as the most important hormonal effect of SG. The ghrelin is secreted mostly on the gastric fundus, which is removed during the SG. Ghrelin is an orexigenic hormone involved in appetite stimulation, and the reduced levels after surgery lead to a decrease in appetite feeling [11]. The hormonal

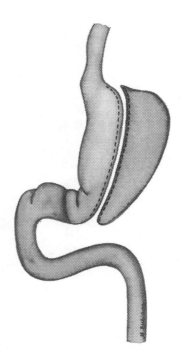

FIGURE 6.2

Sleeve gastrectomy.

effect of SG seems to be greater in the first 3 years after surgery and then the ponderal outcome depends mainly on lifestyle changes. Therefore, a weight regain after this period is increasingly described [9]. The mean EWL at 1 year after surgery ranges from 26% to 74.3%. This is maintained up to 3 years after surgery, but then a weight regain is observed. The European Accreditation Council for Bariatric Surgery reports means EWL 5 years after SG of around 20% [12].

The complete remission rate of T2D at 5 years after surgery overcomes in many cases 80%, but the long-term remission rate of dyslipidemia was below 30%. The main improvement of SG on the lipid profile is the significant increase of HDL cholesterol and a moderate decrease of triglycerides, whereas total cholesterol and LDL-cholesterol levels remain unaltered [13].

Mixed procedures

- **Roux-en-Y gastric bypass:**

Until 2014, the Roux-en-Y gastric bypass (RYGB) was considered the gold standard procedure by many bariatric surgeons, as it is a safe procedure with low complications and mortality, and obtains very good midterm ponderal results and remission of comorbidities. However, long-term results show a weight regain, with over 30% of the patients presenting a BMI >35 kg/m² and with less than 20% of the subjects nutritionally intact [14]. RYGB may also develop nutritional deficiencies, as a certain part of the small bowel is bypassed, impairing a correct absorption of all nutrients. RYGB patients are at risk of developing anemia, neuropathies, and osteoporosis [15].

The surgical technique of RYGB includes two parts: the first phase consists of the performance of a small gastric pouch of around 30 cm³. The second phase includes the division of the small intestine into three limbs: a first segment distal to the ligament of Treitz that represents the biliary limb, a second segment (alimentary limb) that is anastomosed to the gastric pouch, and a third segment (common limb), where the biliary and alimentary limbs are connected, so that the biliopancreatic secretion and the alimentary bolus contact in this limb, allowing the digestion and absorption of the nutrients (Fig. 6.3) [16,17].

The RYGB is considered as a mixed procedure. The small gastric pouch is a restrictive component, reducing the amount of food intake. The separation between the alimentary bolus and the digestive enzymes from the biliary limb represents the malabsorptive component of the technique. The exclusion of the duodenum and proximal jejunum determines many of the metabolic effects of RYGB. Undigested nutrients in the distal intestine stimulate the secretion of glucagon-like peptide 1 (GLP-1), which provokes satiety and decrease of insulin resistance [18].

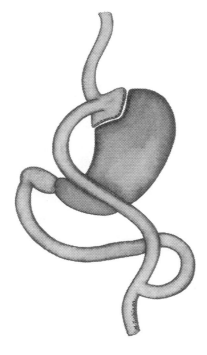

FIGURE 6.3

Roux-en-Y gastric bypass.

After RYGB, the mean EWL 1 year after surgery ranges from 41.4% to 82.8%, and the weight lost is maintained up to 5 years [4]. The complete remission rate of T2D ranges from 65% to 75% at 5 years, while the remission rate of dyslipidemia ranges from 79% to 100% at 5 years postoperatively [12,19].

Malabsorptive procedures
- **Biliopancreatic diversion (BPD)/duodenal switch (DS):**

The BPD, described by Scopinaro, consists of a subtotal gastrectomy and a distal gastroileostomy, creating a 50-cm-long common channel. Some years later, the horizontal subtotal gastrectomy was changed by an SG, to reduce the tension produced by raising the ileum to the supramesocolic area. This new variant was called DS. In the DS, the duodenum is divided just distal to the pylorus. A segment of the distal ileum is then divided at 250 cm proximal to the ileo-cecal valve and raised and anastomosed to the duodenum in a Roux-en-Y configuration. The other anastomosis (ileo-ileostomy) is performed at 100 cm proximal to the ileo-cecal valve to complete the operation (Figs. 6.4 and 6.5) [20].

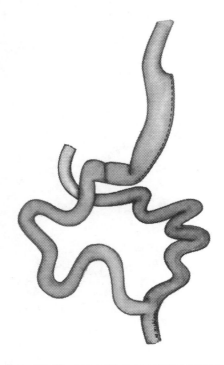

FIGURE 6.4

Duodenal switch.

Malabsorptive procedures 81

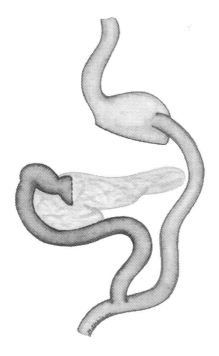

FIGURE 6.5

Biliopancreatic diversion (Scopinaro technique).

BPD/DS together represent less than 2% of the total number of surgeries performed worldwide. The technical complexity, the higher rates of complications, and the important deficiencies of macro and micronutrients are the reasons for the reduction in the number of these procedures. However, in all the surveys and in the different meta-analyses carried out so far, these procedures continue to have the best long-term results, in terms of weight loss and remission of comorbidities [7].

In both techniques, the gastric resection implies a certain restrictive effect. However, the effects of deriving large portions of the intestine that does not absorb are much more transcendent for the results. However, nutritional deficits also increase, forcing a strict follow-up throughout life.

In all malabsorptive techniques, and even in the RYGB with a malabsorptive component, the ideal measure of the different limbs remains unclear. There is enough evidence to support the measurement of the total bowel length, as there is high variability in the intestinal length between subjects and establishing fixed measurements may lead to severe nutritional deficiencies. Diverse groups defend that percentages, according to the total bowel length, should be considered rather than fixed measurements, always taking into account that the common limb is the determining factor in the degree of aggressiveness of the derivative techniques [21].

EWL after BPD/DS ranges from 72% to 96% after more than 10 years of follow-up. In addition, over 80% of patients lose more than 50% of their initial excess weight, and less than 1% lose less than 25% of their initial excess weight, confirming that these techniques are the ones obtaining greatest weight loss and maintained during long-term follow-up. Complete remission of T2D is obtained in over 85% of the cases and remission of dyslipidemia in over 90% [22–24].

- **One-anastomosis gastric bypass**:

One-anastomosis gastric bypass (OAGB) has shown an exponential growth during the last decade, mainly based on their excellent long-term results, its technical ease, and low complications rate. Actually, it represents the third most frequently performed bariatric procedure worldwide, after sleeve gastrectomy and RYGB [25].

OAGB consists of a long vertical gastrectomy and a unique gastro-enteral anastomosis. This technique was developed to simplify the RYGB to only one anastomosis. However, with the pass of time, it has been observed that both techniques are completely different. OAGB is more malabsorptive than RYGB, as the unique biliary limb in the OAGB is not able to have any absorption, whereas there is certain evidence that the alimentary limb in the RYGB may be able to absorb some nutrients (Fig. 6.6) [25].

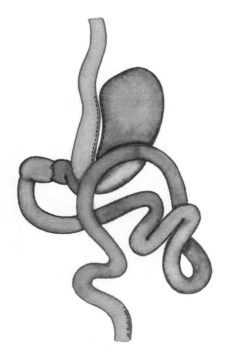

FIGURE 6.6

One-anastomosis gastric bypass (OAGB).

In 2018, the International Federation for Surgery of Obesity (IFSO) published a position statement, referring to OAGB [26]. In this statement, they decided to include all the bariatric procedures with a single gastroenteric anastomosis under the acronyms OAGB, abolishing the term "mini-gastric bypass (MGB)." This is a big problem as very different techniques are now denominated as OAGB, with the corresponding problem in future comparative studies. The OAGB developed by Carbajo has important differences with the "classical MGB" as described by Rutledge. Carbajo's technique includes a longer pouch of 20 cm, a calibrated 2.5-cm-long gastroenterotomy, and the measurement of the total bowel length, in contrast to a shorter gastric pouch, a 5-cm-wide anastomosis, and the measurement of only the biliopancreatic limb in the previously denominated MGB. The first modifications are focused on reducing the biliary reflux and the latter on decreasing the risk of malnutrition, which are the two main drawbacks of this technique. The absence of the alimentary limb triggered the alarm about the feared biliary reflux, which forced the abandonment of Billroth II long term ago. However, diverse studies could not demonstrate a higher incidence of gastric cancer after OAGB [25].

In comparison to RYGB, the OAGB reduces the risk of leakage, stenosis, or anastomotic ulcers. In addition, there is no need for dissection of the mesenterium and this reduces the risk of internal hernias. Moreover, the absence of the alimentary limb reduces the risk of complications derived from the loop foot [25].

A recently published study of our group determined that weight loss and remission of comorbidities were significantly higher after OAGB than after RYGB. We obtained 5-years EWL of 97.9%, and remissions rate of T2D and dyslipidemia of 95.7% and 100%, respectively [13].

- **Single-anastomosis duodeno-ileal switch**

Single-anastomosis duodeno-ileal switch (SADI-S) is a modification of the DS, in which after sleeve gastrectomy, the duodenum is anastomosed to an ileal loop in a Billroth-II fashion. In contrast to the OAGB, the SADIS refers to a pylorus sparing technique gastrectomy accompanied by a proximal duodenal-ileal end-to-side bypass (Fig. 6.7) [27].

As previously mentioned, the common limb is the determining factor in the degree of aggressiveness of the derivative techniques [21]. Thus, in the SADIS, the small bowel is measured from the ileocecal valve proximally. In the evolution of SADIS, surgeons have adopted a longer efferent limb as a result of late nutritional deficiencies [28].

SADIS bears the complications of a combined restrictive and malabsorptive procedure. Postoperative staple line leak, anastomosis leak, bleeding, hernia, infection and abscess formation, ileus, bowel obstruction, and diarrhea are among the reported early postoperative complications, being diarrhea the most common one [29].

SADIS achieves a long-term EWL ranging from 72% to 95% and obtains T2D remission in around 75% and dyslipidemia resolution in over 60% of the cases. However, there are still few studies reporting long-term results [30].

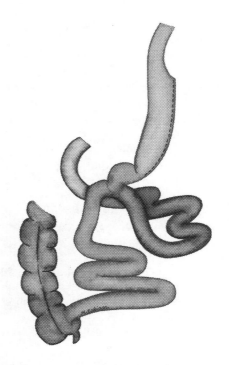

FIGURE 6.7

Single-Anastomosis duodeno ileal bypass (SADIS).

Conclusion

There is no universally accepted gold-standard bariatric technique, and the election of the procedure must be based on the individual characteristics of the patient, the experience of the surgeon, and the decision of the patient once he has received all the necessary information.

Globally, restrictive procedures are technically more simple and associated with lower morbidity and mortality rates, and few nutritional deficiencies, but they obtained poorer outcomes and with long-term weight regain. RYGB, as a mixed procedure, obtains better weight loss results and remission of comorbidities, than restrictive approaches, but it is also associated with long-term weight regain. Malabsorptive approaches are the most effective techniques to achieve significant and maintained weight loss and remission of comorbidities, but are associated with increased risk of severe nutritional deficiencies.

Acknowledgments

To Maite Zubiaga, for the performance of graphical illustrations.

References

[1] Salas-Salvado J, Rubio MA, Barbany M, Moreno B, Grupo Colaborativo de la SEEDO. SEEDO 2007 Consensus for the evaluation of overweight and obesity and the establishment of therapeutic intervention criteria. Med Clin 2007;128(5):184—96.

[2] Colquitt JL, Pickett K, Loveman E, Frampton GK. Surgery for weight loss in adults. Cochrane Database Syst Rev 2014;8:CD003641.

[3] Dixon JB, O'Brien PE, Playfair J, Chapman L, Schachter LM, Skinner S, et al. Adjustable gastric banding and conventional therapy for type 2 diabetes: a randomized controlled trial. J Am Med Assoc 2008;299(3):316—23.

[4] Panagiotou OA, Markozannes G, Kowalski R, Gazula A, Di M, Bond DS, et al. Short- and long-term outcomes after bariatric surgery in the medicare population. Rockville (MD): Agency for Healthcare Research and Quality (US); January 7, 2018.

[5] Loy JJ, Youn HA, Schwack B, Kurian MS, Fielding GA, Ren-Fielding CJ. Safety and efficacy of laparoscopic adjustable gastric banding in patients aged seventy and older. Surg Obes Relat Dis 2014;10(2):284—9.

[6] Kindel T, Martin E, Hungness E, Nagle A. High failure rate of the laparoscopic-adjustable gastric band as a primary bariatric procedure. Surg Obes Relat Dis 2014;10(6):1070—5.

[7] Angrisani L, Santonicola A, Iovino P, Vitiello A, Higa K, Himpens J, et al. IFSO worldwide survey 2016: primary, endoluminal, and revisional procedures. Obes Surg 2018;28(12):3783—94.

[8] Deitel M, Crosby RD, Gagner M. The first international consensus summit for sleeve gastrectomy (SG), New York City, October 25—27, 2007. Obes Surg 2008;18(5):487—96.

[9] Felsenreich DM, Langer FB, Prager G. Weight loss and resolution of comorbidities after sleeve gastrectomy: a review of long-term results. Scand J Surg 2019;108(1):3—9.

[10] Hutter MM, Schirmer BD, Jones DB, Ko CY, Cohen ME, Merkow RP, et al. First report from the American College of Surgeons Bariatric Surgery Center Network: laparoscopic sleeve gastrectomy has morbidity and effectiveness positioned between the band and the bypass. Ann Surg 2011;254(3):410—20.

[11] Keogh JB, Turner KM, McDonald F, Toouli J, Clifton PM. Remission of diabetes in patients with long-standing type 2 diabetes following placement of adjustable gastric band: a retrospective case control study. Diabetes Obes Metabol 2013;15(4):383—5.

[12] European accreditation council for bariatric surgery database. Available from: www.eac-bs.com. [accessed 02 08 2020].

[13] Ruiz-Tovar J, Carbajo MA, Jimenez JM, Castro MJ, Gonzalez G, Ortiz-de-Solorzano J, et al. Long-term follow-up after sleeve gastrectomy versus roux-en-Y gastric bypass versus one-anastomosis gastric bypass: a prospective randomized comparative study of weight loss and remission of comorbidities. Surg Endosc 2019;33(2):401—10.

[14] Higa K, Ho T, Tercero F, Yunus T, Boone KB. Laparoscopic roux-en-Y gastric bypass: 10-year follow-up. Surg Obes Relat Dis 2011;7(4):516—25.

[15] Kim J, Brethauer S. ASMBS Clinical Issues Committee; American Society for Metabolic and Bariatric Surgery Clinical Issues Committee, position statement. Metabolic bone changes after bariatric surgery. Surg Obes Relat Dis 2015;11(2):406—11.

[16] Rodriguez-Carmona Y, Lopez-Alavez FJ, Gonzalez-Garay AG, Solís-Galicia C, Meléndez G, Serralde-Zúñiga AE. Bone mineral density after bariatric surgery. A systematic review. Int J Surg 2014;12(9):976—82.

[17] Nguyen NT, Varela JE. Bariatric surgery for obesity and metabolic disorders: state of the art. Nat Rev Gastroenterol Hepatol 2017;14(3):160—9.

[18] Stefater MA, Wilson-Perez HE, Chambers AP, Sandoval DA, Seeley RJ. All bariatric surgeries are not created equal: insights from mechanistic comparisons. Endocr Rev 2012;33(4):595—622.

[19] Lee SK, Heo Y, Park JM, Kim YJ, Kim SM, Park do J, et al. Roux-en-Y gastric bypass vs. Sleeve gastrectomy vs. Gastric banding: the first multicenter retrospective comparative cohort study in obese Korean patients. Yonsei Med J 2016;57(4):956—62.

[20] Dapri G, Cadiere GB, Himpens J. Superobese and super-superobese patients: 2-step laparoscopic duodenal switch. Surg Obes Relat Dis 2011;7(6):703—8.

[21] Murad Jr AJ, Cohen RV, de Godoy EP, Scheibe CL, Campelo GP, Ramos AC, et al. A prospective single-arm trial of modified long biliopancreatic and short alimentary limbs roux-en-Y gastric bypass in type 2 diabetes patients with mild obesity. Obes Surg 2018;28(3):599—605.

[22] Michaud A, Marchand GB, Nadeau M, Lebel S, Hould FS, Marceau S, et al. Biliopancreatic diversion with duodenal switch in the elderly: long-term results of a matched-control study. Obes Surg 2016;26(2):350—60.

[23] Baltasar A, Bou R, Bengochea M, Serra C, Ferri L, Pérez N, et al. Four decades of bariatric surgery in a community hospital of Spain. Nutr Hosp 2017;34(4):980—8.

[24] Bolckmans R, Himpens J. Long-term (>10 yrs) outcome of the laparoscopic biliopancreatic diversion with duodenal switch. Ann Surg 2016;264(6):1029—37.

[25] Carbajo MA, Luque de Leon E, Jimenez JM, Ortiz-de-Solórzano J, Pérez-Miranda M, Castro-Alija MJ. Laparoscopic one-anastomosis gastric bypass: technique, results and long-term follow-up in 1200 patients. Obes Surg 2017;27:1153—67.

[26] De Luca M, Tie T, Ooi G, Higa K, Himpens J, Carbajo MA, et al. Mini gastric bypass-one anastomosis gastric bypass (MGB-OAGB)-IFSO position statement. Obes Surg 2018;28:1188—206.

[27] Sanchez-Pernaute A, Rubio Herrera MA, Perez-Aguirre E, García Pérez JC, Cabrerizo L, Díez Valladares L, et al. Proximal duodenal-ileal end-to-side bypass with sleeve gastrectomy: proposed technique. Obes Surg 2007;17(12):1614—8.

[28] Sanchez-Pernaute A, Herrera MA, Perez-Aguirre ME, Talavera P, Cabrerizo L, Matía P, et al. Single anastomosis duodeno-ileal bypass with sleeve gastrectomy (SADIS). One to three-year follow-up. Obes Surg 2010;20(12):1720—6.

[29] Sanchez-Pernaute A, Rubio MA, Perez Aguirre E, Barabash A, Cabrerizo L, Torres A. Singleanastomosis duodenoileal bypass with sleeve gastrectomy: metabolic improvement and weight loss in first 100 patients. Surg Obes Relat Dis 2013;9(5):731—5.

[30] Shoar S, Poliakin L, Rubinstein R, Saber AA. Single anastomosis duodeno-ileal switch (SADIS): a systematic review of efficacy and safety. Obes Surg 2018;28:104—13.

CHAPTER 7

Postoperative complications: indications and access routes for enteral and parenteral nutrition

E. Martín Garcia-Almenta, E. Martin Antona, O. Cano-Valderrama, A.J. Torres García
Department of Surgery, Hospital Clínico Universitario San Carlos, Madrid, Spain

Chapter outline

Early postoperative complications	89
Indications and access routes	89
Parenteral access route	91
Central venous catheters	91
Peripheral inserted central catheter	92
Enteral nutrition routes	92
Leaks	92
Remnant gastrostomy	93
Naso-jejunal tubes	94
Jejunostomies	94
Late postoperative complications	95
References	97

Adiposity-based chronic disease is the primary noninfectious epidemic disease of this century. The excessive accumulation of adipose tissue accompanied by chronic, systemic inflammation is associated with the development of more than a 100 conditions (hypertension, type 2 diabetes, cardiovascular disease, dyslipidemia, sleep apnea, orthopedic conditions, or some types of cancer). According to the last estimations of the World Health Organization, more than 2.1 billion adults are considered to be overweight or obese, of whom 1.5 billion are overweight, and 640 million are obese. On this basis, about 25 million people have the classical NIH criteria for bariatric surgery (BS) [1].

The most recent IFSO Worldwide Survey reported that 634,897 bariatric operations were performed worldwide in 2016 [2]. The most common primary surgical bariatric/metabolic procedure was sleeve gastrectomy (SG), followed by Roux-en-Y gastric bypass (GB) and one-anastomosis gastric bypass (OAGB). The following chapter will discuss several proposed techniques for the surgical management of morbid obesity. These operations can be divided into restrictive, mixt and malabsorptive procedures that are designed to reduce caloric intake by modifying the gastrointestinal tract.

The published studies demonstrate that these procedures are safe and well tolerated. They also demonstrate that, during the last years, they have decreased their mortality and morbidity rates. The Obesity Division of the "Asociación Española de Cirujanos" (Spanish Association of Surgeons, AEC) in collaboration with the "Sociedad Española de Cirugía de la Obesidad" (Spanish Society of Obesity Surgery, SECO) [3] has proposed identifying the key points that define the quality of bariatric surgery. Based on the published literature, the mortality rate should be below 0.5% and the general morbidity rate below 10%. In addition, leak rate should be below 4% and internal hernias below 3%. Recent publications of the Longitudinal Assessment of Bariatric Surgery Consortium data or the Bariatric Outcome Longitudinal Database, among others, confirm that the mortality rate is below 0.5%. This is an acceptable rate, considering that long-term mortality in nonoperated morbid obese patients is higher than 6%.

The most frequent cause of death after bariatric surgery was multiple organ failure due to sepsis (33%), followed by cardiac pathologies (28%) and pulmonary embolism (17%). Abdominal sepsis, primarily when associated with anastomotic leakage, continues to be a challenge in this type of patients. Mortality is variable and depends on the experience of the surgical group, which reinforces the importance of the learning curve. In the postoperative period, we refer to early morbidity (<30 days: pulmonary embolism, leaks, and hemorrhages) or late morbidity (>30 days: marginal ulcers, stenosis, and internal hernias).

In 2007, Kumpf [4] surveyed 467 members of the American Society for Parenteral and Enteral Nutrition (ASPEN) regarding nutrition support practices after complications from bariatric surgery. Sixty percent of respondents reported being consulted on 1—10 patients requiring nutrition support in the past year, and 20% of respondents were consulted on more than 10 cases per year. Anastomotic leak or fistula was the most common reason for nutrition support (49%), followed by chronic nausea and vomiting (27%) and severe malabsorption/diarrhea (19%).

There is a lack of published data on nutrition support in complicated bariatric surgical patients, and most of the recommendations are based on expert opinions [5]. The 2013 Clinical Practice Guidelines for the Perioperative Nutritional, Metabolic, and Nonsurgical Support of the Bariatric Surgery Patient [6] and most recent clinical practice guidelines of the European Association for Endoscopic Surgery [7] do not specifically address nutrition support goals for complicated bariatric patients. The first one refers readers to previous published clinical practice guidelines from other organizations. The ASPEN Clinical Guidelines Nutrition Support of Hospitalized Adult Patients with Obesity were published in 2013 with recommendations for both critically ill and nonintensive care unit (ICU) patients.

Early postoperative complications

Currently, the overall early morbidity rate is below 7% in centers with more extensive experience. The complication rate was influenced by the surgical technique, with a higher rate of major complications in GBP (2.5%—3.6%) compared to the SG (2.2%—2.4%).

Early surgical complications can be divided into two entities: septic complications, mainly fistula and anastomotic leak, and nonseptic complications, mostly due to hemorrhage.

Management of complicated BS patient is based on a combined approach including surgical and/or endoscopic procedures and medical care, largely depending on the nature and severity of the complication. The severity of the clinical features at the time of diagnosis is the most important factor guiding the treatment strategy.

General surgical management corresponds to the conventional rules of septic surgery including identification of the infectious source, collection of microbiological samples, peritoneal lavage and possibly drainage depending on the intensity and source of contamination, and elimination/control of the source of infection. In the presence of bleeding, surgery is required to identify the source of bleeding and to control blood loss. During the initial surgical or endoscopic management of complicated BS patient is also mandatory to evaluate the necessity/adequacy of placing an access route for feeding/enteral nutrition.

Medical management is based on supportive ICU care of organ dysfunctions, prophylactic or curative anticoagulation if required, nutritional support, and appropriate antiinfective therapy.

Indications and access routes

Due to the importance of nutritional support for complicated BS patients, it is important to clarify its aims: avoidance of overfeeding and its harmful effects (e.g., increased CO_2 production, which may increase respiratory effort; promotion of lip genesis causing hepatic dysfunction and also insulin resistance), preservation of lean body mass, and promotion of healing.

Obese patients may be malnourished despite having increased energy stores in the form of fat. Regardless of the body weight of the individual, the presence of malnutrition increases the risk of morbidity and mortality, especially in a stressful situation as postoperative complication. It is essential to meet nutritional needs and avoid the consequences of malnutrition. Taking an expectant position, assuming that patients can consume their energy reserves, would be inappropriate.

To prevent or delay the development of malnutrition, nutritional support should be introduced in obese patients as soon as in normal-weight individuals. Whenever possible, feeding is preferred by oral or enteral route because it is cheaper and more physiological and because it presents less serious complications than the parenteral route.

Nutritional support is poorly investigated in these patients. Traditionally, the route of feeding for patients after bariatric surgery that experiences complications would be parenteral nutrition (PN), providing complete gut rest allowing anastomotic leaks to heal. Most authors report placement of a feeding tube into the gastric remnant or at the jejunum to continue enteral nutrition below the anastomotic leak.

If possible, an oral diet or enteral nutrition should be initiated within the first 24–48 h of admission to the critical care area when the hemodynamic stability has been achieved. According to the approach of the ASPEN, if the patient cannot ingest at least 50% of his requirements by enteral route within more than 7–10 days, especially in the presence of a situation of metabolic stress, enteral nutrition (EN) should be supplemented with PN. The 2019 European Society of parenteral and enteral nutrition (ESPEN) guideline on clinical nutrition in the intensive care unit [8] establishes that every critically ill patient staying for more than 48 h in the ICU should be considered at risk for malnutrition. If oral intake is not possible, early EN (within 48 h) patients should be performed/initiated rather than early PN. In case of contraindications to oral and EN, PN should be implemented within 3–7 days. Early and progressive PN can be provided instead of no nutrition in case of contraindications for EN in severely malnourished patients. To avoid overfeeding, early full EN and PN shall not be used in critically ill patients but shall be prescribed within 3–7 days.

To establish an adequate nutrition therapy plan is crucial to know the characteristics of the postoperative complication, the gut resting time, and the anatomical changes in the upper gastrointestinal tract after each bariatric procedure. The type of postoperative complication plays an essential role in this decision; an anastomotic leak will not be managed like a hemorrhage or pulmonary embolism (Table 7.1).

Table 7.1 Summary of the most frequent bariatric complication in sleeve gastrectomy and Roux-Y gastric bypass and the expected delay of normal oral intake.

	Expected delay for adequate oral feeding	Prevalence in sleeve gastrectomy (%)	Prevalence in Roux-Y GBP (%)
Leak	++++	0–3.9	0.2–6.8
Hemorrhage (nonassociated to multiple organ failure)	+	0%–9	0.4–9
Pulmonary embolism	−	0.9	
Stenosis	++	0.1–3.9	9–10
Marginal ulcer	+	−	0.8–7.6

Source: F. Sabench et al. Quality criteria in bariatric surgery: consensus review and recommendations of the Spanish Association of Surgeons and the Spanish Society of Bariatric Surgery. Cir Esp 2017; 95 (1): 4–16. https://doi.org/10.1016/j.cireng.2016.09.015.

Table 7.2 Enteral feeding access routes.

Enteral access routes	Example
Gastric	Gastrostomy placed in gastric remnant (techniques without gastric resection as Roux-Y GBP, not in one-anastomoses GBP with GJ** leaks)
Jejunal	Surgical jejunostomy (evaluate the technical challenge and complications due to morbid obese patient's characteristic)
Jejunal	Naso-jejunal tube (placed through the anastomosis and distal to the leak or stenosis)

*, gastric bypass; **GJ, gastrojejunal.

Besides, the anatomical changes secondary to the bariatric procedure performed have a significant value to decide the access route for enteral nutrition (Table 7.2).

To estimate patient nutritional needs, resting energy expenditure (EE) is best assessed by indirect calorimetric (IC). If not available, energy intake can be guided by adjusted body weight (BW) and protein delivery by urinary nitrogen losses or lean body mass determination (using CT or other tools), according to the ESPEN guidelines. Several existing predictive scores, such as the Mifflin-St Jeor (MSJ) and the Harris—Benedict equations, can be applied if IC is not available in the case of complicated bariatric patients. However, it is important to consider that these scores are not specifically validated for postbariatric patients and IC is recommended in the first place.

PN is not in opposition to EN but can be used as an additional therapy as soon as a close monitoring of the medical nutrition therapy (MNT) is assured. However, the enlarged fatty liver that is commonly present in obese patients can complicate PN provision.

Parenteral access route

Whenever the parenteral route is chosen for delivery of nutrients, the type of intravenous access device, the catheter design, and its site of insertion must be determined [9]. Many nontunneled central venous catheters (CVCs), as well as peripherally inserted central catheters (PICCs) are suitable for in-patient PN.

Central venous catheters

The most appropriate site for central venous access will take into account many factors, including the patient's conditions and the relative risk of infective and noninfective complications associated with each site. Ultrasound-guided venipuncture is strongly recommended for access to all central veins. For parenteral nutrition, the ideal position of the catheter tip is between the lower third of the superior cava vein and the upper third of the right atrium; this should preferably be checked during the procedure. Catheter-related bloodstream infection is an important, and still too common, complication of parenteral nutrition. The risk of infection can be reduced by adopting cost-effective, evidence-based interventions such as proper education and specific training of the staff, an adequate hand washing policy, proper choices of the type of device and the site of insertion, use of maximal barrier protection during insertion, use of chlorhexidine as antiseptic before insertion and for disinfecting the exit site thereafter, appropriate policies for the dressing of the exit site, routine changes of administration sets, and removal of central lines as soon as they are no longer necessary. Most noninfective complications of central venous access devices can also be prevented by appropriate, standardized protocols for line insertion and maintenance. The use of the femoral vein for PN is relatively contraindicated, as this is associated with a high risk of contamination at the exit site at the groin, and a high risk of venous thrombosis.

Peripheral inserted central catheter
Some evidence suggests that PICC use may be preferable because associated with fewer mechanical complications at insertion, lower costs of insertion, and a lower rate of infection. Although this last issue is under debate, it is accepted that placement in the ante cubital fossa or the midarm carries the important advantage of removing the exit site of the catheter further away from endotracheal, oral and nasal secretions. In placement of PICCs, percutaneous cannulation of the basilic vein or the brachial vein in the midarm, utilizing ultrasound guidance and the microintroducer technique, is the preferred option.

Enteral nutrition routes
To evaluate the necessity/adequacy of placing an access route for feeding/enteral nutrition becomes mandatory during the initial surgical or endocopic BS complications management. Nowadays, endoscopy plays a main role in the management of postoperative complications (stenting, endo-vacuum therapy, endoluminal drainage, stenosis dilatation ...) and also giving an access route to enteral nutrition.

To establish an adequate enteral nutrition route is crucial to know the anatomical changes in the upper gastrointestinal tract in each bariatric procedure. Its knowledge will guide the right route for enteral feeding.

Leaks
Leaks or fistula deserve a special mention for indications of route enteral access. Despite the decreased incidence over time, gastrointestinal leak remains a significant cause of overall morbidity and mortality after primary stapled bariatric procedures. In 2015, the American Society for Metabolic and Bariatric Surgery [10] published a position statement to provide evidence-based findings on the prevention, detection, and management of GI leaks after GB and SG, but may also apply to leaks occurring after stapled biliopancreatic diversion (BPD) and BPD with duodenal switch (DS) procedures. However, the mention of handling the MNT is anecdotal, note that

Early postoperative complications

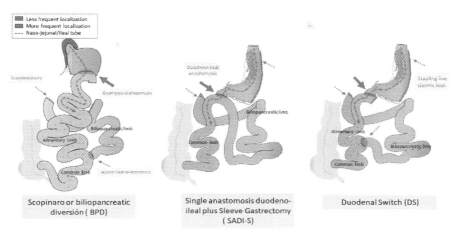

FIGURE 7.1

Malabsorptive procedures: leaks localization and EN routes.

the stenting of SG leaks may allow patients to support their own nutritional needs with oral feeding during the healing process, potentially decreasing the overall duration of treatment.

Traditionally, the route of feeding in-patients after bariatric surgery that experience complications would be PN, providing complete gut rest allowing anastomotic leaks to heal. Nevertheless, some authors report placement of a feeding tube into the gastric remnant or at the jejunum to continue enteral nutrition below the anastomotic leak. The anatomical recognition of leak localization guides the election for enteral feeding (Figs. 7.1–7.3).

Remnant gastrostomy

In critically ill patients, the standard gastric approach is recommended for enteral nutrition, but this is not available for the vast majority of complicated BS patients in whom gastric volume has been significantly reduced or harbors the complication. Just in case of nongastric resection procedure, as in GBP, the excluded gastric portion (remnant) could be used through a gastrostomy placed by laparoscopy or percutaneously by radiology (no accessible by endoscopy). In case that a surgical approach to a Roux-Y gastrojejunal (GJ) leak is performed, it is strongly recommended to insert a gastrostomy tube in the gastric remnant during the surgery. If conservative management is chosen, it could be placed percutaneously. We should be careful with the one anastomosis techniques that could change some of the routes used for enteral nutrition. For example, in an OAGBP GJ leak, the remnant gastrostomy is not indicated because it would not exclude this anastomosis.

Naso-jejunal tubes

As we have already mention, endoscopy plays a main role in treatment of leaks, through different options as stents, endo-vacuum therapy, endoluminal drainage, septotomy, and distal stenosis balloon dilatation. Giving an access route to enteral nutrition by placing a naso-jejunal tube below the leak is another option of endoscopic treatment. When the gastric remnant is not available or is not a safe option (organ interposition, high risk of bleeding …), it is recommended to place a nutrition tube at the jejunum in SG, OAGBP, or Roux-Y GBP, and at proximal ileum in DS, BPV, or SADI-s, preferably under endoscopy control (Figs. 7.1 and 7.3). In malabsorptive procedures, the length of the limb below to anastomotic leak (alimentary limb and/or common limb) has not enough absorptive surface to cover/support all the EN needed to cover the nutritional requirements, especially in a sepsis complication, and has to be associated to PN (Fig. 7.2). An untreatable diarrhea forces to stop enteral nutrition administration.

Jejunostomies

The most frequent complications of jejunostomies are tube dislodgment, aspiration events, and occlusion. Moreover, a distinctly uncommon but critical consequence of the use of jejunostomy tubes is the development of small bowel ischemia and necrosis during the immediate postoperative period [11]. Placing and maintaining of surgical jejunostomy suppose a challenge in morbid obese patients due to increase in abdominal fat (visceral and subcutaneous) [12].

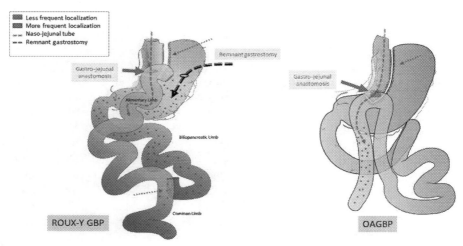

FIGURE 7.2

Leaks localization and EN routes in GBP and OAGBP.

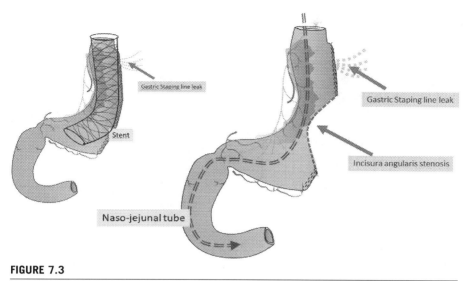

FIGURE 7.3

Sleeve gastrectomy complications.

Late postoperative complications

When a bariatric patient presents with nutritional problems, associated or not to digestive symptoms as diarrhea or vomits, we have to dismiss/rule out an anatomical/organic complications (i.e., stenosis, internal hernia, band erosion, etc.), eating disorders or maladaptation to a malabsorptive procedure.

- Stenosis: stenosis is a complication associated to different procedures. First of all, we will analyze SG. Stenosis after SG is uncommon, with an estimated incidence of 0.7%−5%. However, it is a common cause of revisional bariatric surgery. Some authors, as Shnell et al., have reported satisfactory results after sleeve gastrectomy with stents or balloon dilatation [13]. When conservative treatment fails, surgical approach is indicated. In this case, conversion to Roux-Y gastric bypass (the most common option) and seromyotomy are available options. Incidence of stenosis in a gastrojejunal anastomosis after gastric bypass has been reported to be as high as 12%. This complication usually presents late in the postoperative course (after 30 days). Endoscopic dilatation is usually useful, although several sessions are usually needed.
- Marginal ulcer: marginal ulcer incidence after gastric bypass varies according to the published series from 0.6% to 25%. Physiopathology of early (before postoperative day 30) and late (after postoperative day 30) marginal ulcer seems to be different, although there are some factors that are not properly understood. Some

of these factors are suture material, pouch shape, size of the anastomosis, *H. Pylori* infection, treatment with NSAIDs, tobacco use, and demographic factors. Spaniolas et al. studied 35,000 patients who underwent gastric bypass, and they concluded that the accumulated risk of marginal ulcer was 11.4% at 8 years, being tobacco use the most important risk factor [14]. Using the MBSAQIP database with 44,379 patients, Clapp et al. observed in 2019 that marginal ulcer incidence was 0.35%. Most of the marginal ulcers were late complications and were related to body mass index and development of deep vein thrombosis and/or pulmonary embolism [15]. Finally, Sverden et al. analyzed a cohort of 20,924 patients who underwent gastric bypass, and they observed that diabetes and previous peptic ulcer were both risk factors for marginal ulcer [16]. Endoscopy is usually the best treatment for marginal ulcer bleeding, although surgery is sometimes needed. Prophylaxis with pump proton inhibitors is effective, with an odds ratio of 0.5.

- Internal hernia: internal hernia is related to those procedures that create mesenteric defects such as the Petersen's space or the mesenteric opening after Roux-Y gastric bypass. Internal hernia incidence has decreased from 10% to 0.2% as the surgical technique has evolved (prophylactic closure of both defects and no section of the alimentary limb mesentery) [10]. Internal hernia is usually seen late in the postoperative course, at least 2 years after the surgery when the patient has lost enough weight.
- Eating disorders: patients submitted to BS have a higher prevalence of eating disorders than the general population. Binge-eating disorder is the most common disorder in patients submitted to BS, with a 10% prevalence. This disorder is not an absolute contraindication to undergo surgery. Picking and nibbling disorder is defined as repetitive and unplanned intake between meals. It can be seen in up to 30% of the patients. It is common that this disorder is seen in patients with anorexia or binge-eating disorder, but it is not associated with other psychopathologies. When this disorder is seen before the procedure, weight lost can be decreased. Night-eating disorder can be seen in 20% of the patients submitted to bariatric surgery, usually associated to binge-eating disorder. Night-eating disorder is not a parasomnia, as the patient is aware of the intake. It is not a contraindication for surgery, although it must be taken into account to assess and manage anxiety, depression, and substance abuse after the procedure. Nearly 65% of the patients who have weight regaining after BS have an eating disorder. Treatment of these disorders is usually based on cognitive behavior therapy [17].
- Malnutrition: it is very uncommon after restrictive procedures, but it is seldom seen after malabsorptive procedures such as gastric bypass, biliopancreatic diversion, or SADI-S. Exclusion of the proximal small bowel causes malabsorption of minerals, trace elements, vitamins, calcium, magnesium, iron, intrinsic factor, and vitamin B12. This malabsorption can cause anemia, osteopenia, osteomalacia, hypoproteinemia with generalized edema, Wernicke encephalopathy, diarrhea, cholelithiasis, renal lithiasis, and other disorders. To avoid these complications, long-term nutritional follow-up is needed [18].

Table of Recommendations:

Recommendation
Management of complicated BS patient is based on a combined approach including surgical and/or endoscopic procedures and medical care.
The severity of the clinical features at the time of diagnosis is the most important factor guiding the treatment strategy.
Nutritional medical therapy plays a crucial role in the medical management of complicated bariatric patients
Not all the postoperative bariatric complications need the same nutritional support
The obese patients may be malnourished despite having increased energy stores in the form of fat
To estimate patient nutritional needs, resting energy expenditure (EE) is best assessed by indirect calorimetry (IC). If not available, energy intake can be guided by adjusted body weight (BW) and protein delivery by urinary nitrogen losses or lean body mass determination (using CT or other tools),
If oral intake is not possible, early EN (within 48 h) patients should be performed/initiated rather than early PN.
In case of contraindications to oral and EN, PN should be implemented within 3—7 days.
Early and progressive PN can be provided instead of no nutrition in case of contraindications for EN in severely malnourished patients.
To avoid overfeeding, early full EN and PN shall not be used in critically ill patients but shall be prescribed within 3—7 days.
To establish an adequate nutrition medical therapy is crucial to know the characteristics of postoperative complication and the anatomical changes in upper gastrointestinal after each bariatric procedure
Non-tunneled central venous catheters (CVCs), as well as peripherally inserted central catheters (PICCs) are suitable for in-patient PN.
Ultrasound-guided venipuncture is strongly recommended for access to all central veins
Some evidence suggests that PICC use may be preferable because associated with fewer mechanical complications at insertion, lower costs of insertion, and a lower rate of infection
To establish an enteral nutrition route is crucial to know anatomical changes in upper gastrointestinal of each bariatric procedure. Its knowledge will guide the right route for enteral feeding.

References

[1] Himpens J. Fourth IFSO global registry report 2018. Prepared by published by Dendrite Clinical Systems Ltd. The Hub, Station Road, Henley-on-Thames, Oxfordshire RG9 1AY, United Kingdom. ISBN:978-0-9929942-7-3.

[2] Angrisani L. IFSO worldwide survey 2016: primary, endoluminal, and revisional procedures. Obes Surg December 2018;28(12):3783—94. https://doi.org/10.1007/s11695-018-3450-2.

[3] Sabench F, et al. Quality criteria in bariatric surgery: consensus review and recommendations of the Spanish Association of Surgeons and the Spanish Society of Bariatric Surgery. Cir Esp 2017;95(1):4—16. https://doi.org/10.1016/j.cireng.2016.09.015.

[4] Kumpf VJ, Slocum K, Binkley J, Jensen G. Complications after bariatric surgery: survey evaluating impact on the practice of specialized nutrition support. Nutr Clin Pract 2007;22(6):673—8.

[5] Kopp Lugli A. Medical nutrition therapy in critically ill patients treated on intensive and intermediate care units: a literature review. J Clin Med 2019;8:1395. https://doi.org/10.3390/jcm8091395.

[6] Mechanick JI, Youdim A, Jones DB, et al. Clinical practice guidelines for the perioperative nutritional, metabolic, and nonsurgical support of the bariatric surgery patient—2013 update: cosponsored by American Association of Clinical Endocrinologists, the Obesity Society, and American Society for Metabolic & Bariatric Surgery. Obesity 2013;21(Suppl. 1):S1—27.

[7] Di Lorenzo N, Antoniou SA, Batterham RL, et al. Clinical practice guidelines of the European Association for Endoscopic Surgery (EAES) on bariatric surgery: update 2020 endorsed by IFSO-EC, EASO and ESPCOP. Surg Endosc; 2020. https://doi.org/10.1007/s00464-020-07555-y.

[8] Singer P, et al. ESPEN guideline on clinical nutrition in the intensive care unit. Clin Nutr 2019;38:48—79.

[9] Pittiruti M, et al. ESPEN guidelines on parenteral nutrition: central venous catheters (access, care, diagnosis and therapy of complications). Clin Nutr 2009;28:365—77.

[10] Kim J, et al. ASMBS position statement on prevention, detection, and treatment of gastrointestinal leak after gastric bypass and sleeve gastrectomy, including the roles of imaging, surgical exploration, and nonoperative management. Obes Relat Dis 2015;11(4):739—48. https://doi.org/10.1016/j.soard.2015.05.001.

[11] Waitzberg D, Plopper C, Terra R. Access routes for nutritional therapy. World J Surg 2000;24:1468—76. https://doi.org/10.1007/s002680010264.

[12] Montravers P, et al. Diagnosis and management of the postoperative surgical and medical complications of bariatric surgery. Anaesth Crit Care Pain Med 2015;34:45—52.

[13] Shnell M, et al. Ballon dilatation for symptomatic gastric sleeve stricture. Gastroinest Endosc 2014;79:521—4.

[14] Spaniolas K, et al. Association of long-term anastomotic ulceration after Roux-en-Y gastric bypass with tobacco smoking. JAMA Surg 2018;153:862—4.

[15] Clapp, et al. Evaluation of the rate of marginal ulcer formation after bariatric surgery using the MBSAQIP Database. Surg Endosc 2019;33:1890—7.

[16] Sverden, et al. Risk factors for marginal ulcer after gastric bypass surgery for obesity: a population-based cohort study. Ann Surg 2016;263:733—7.

[17] Brode, et al. Problematic eating behaviors and eating disorders associated with bariatric surgery. Psychiatr Clin N Am 2019;42:287—97.

[18] Handzlik-Orlik, et al. Nutrition management of the post—bariatric surgery patient. Nutr Clin Pract 2015;30:383—92.

CHAPTER 8

Nutritional treatment in the critically-ill complicated patient

María Asunción Acosta Mérida[1], Pablo B. Pedrianes Martín[2], Gema M. Hernanz Rodríguez[3]

[1]*Esophagogastric, Endocrinometabolic and Obesity Surgery Division, Hospital Universitario de Gran Canaria "Dr. Negrin", Professor at the University of Las Palmas de Gran Canaria, Las Palmas de Gran Canaria, Canary Islands, Spain;* [2]*Department of Endocrinology and Nutrition, Hospital Universitario de Gran Canaria "Dr. Negrin", Las Palmas de Gran Canaria, Canary Islands, Spain;* [3]*Department of Anesthesiology and Critical Care Medicine, Hospital Universitario de Gran Canaria "Dr. Negrin", Las Palmas de Gran Canaria, Canary Islands, Spain*

Chapter outline

Introduction	99
Calculation of nutritional requirements	100
Calculations based on body weight	101
Protein needs	102
Low-calorie high-protein diets	102
Micronutrient supplementation	104
Complications of artificial feeding	104
Hyperglycemia	104
Hyperlipidemia	106
Considerations for support treatment in the critical obese patient	106
Respiratory system	106
Cardiovascular system	107
Kidney injury	108
Pharmacotherapy	109
Key points	110
References	110

Introduction

The incidence of obesity has increased steadily in the last decades, and intensive care units (ICUs) have also experienced an increment of the obese population [1], accounting for about 20% of their patients [2]. Despite the central role of nutrition in the development of obesity, there exists considerable uncertainty about the optimal nutritional support for obese patients with critical conditions. Estimation of caloric and protein needs in the critically ill obese patient may contrast with the requirements of subjects with normal BMI. Moreover, accompanying metabolic syndrome usually demands a more intense monitoring of hyperglycemia and other metabolic alterations, such as hyperlipidemia.

Apart from resuscitation and specific management of the acute situation that has led the patient to the ICU unit, a bariatric patient with a postsurgery complication most likely will require nutritional support, considering their stay in the ICU unit will take several days (ESPEN recommends initiation if ICU stay is > 48 h [3]) and the acute injury increases metabolic demands. If we chose any general nutritional screening test, such as the malnutrition universal screening tool [4], these patients would easily match the criteria of "acute disease or likeliness of not receiving food for 5 days" and be regarded as "in high risk of malnutrition." If we use the new Global Leadership Initiative on Malnutrition criteria [5], we could demonstrate inflammation related to acute disease (e.g., measuring PCR) and reduced muscular mass with bioimpedance (BIA), TC or phase angle. Bioimpedance is not appropriate in this setting, because edema affects its reliability and volume management is paramount in critical patients. Besides, an overestimation of fat-free body mass by BIA has been described in a recent review in subjects with BMI >35 kg/m^2, where scaling errors augmented with higher BMI [6]. CT scans are commonly performed on ICU patients and several studies have demonstrated its utility in assessing body composition, mainly measuring muscular mass in lumbar L3 level [7]. In critically ill patients, CT even has prognostic value with a sensitivity of 70% and a specificity of 69.5% for diagnosing sarcopenia (cut off value 41.2 cm2/m2) in oncologic ICU patients. Sarcopenia was associated with higher 30-day mortality and more noninfectious complications [8]. Thus, nutritional support becomes almost mandatory in these patients (Fig. 8.1).

Interestingly, an "obesity paradox" has been reported regarding a lower mortality in obese patients with certain pathologies, contrary to what is observed in large cohort studies based on the general population [2]. This paradox is observed in different conditions, including sepsis and critical illness. Mechanisms underlying this phenomenon are not completely understood, but probably energy obtained from fat cells and variations in the secretion of immune mediators play a role. Pharmacologic implications may also be important, as relatively less fluid therapy and vasopressor drugs are administered to these patients and thus, less secondary events might be observed. However, these findings have been founded on body weight instead of on body composition, so qualitative discrepancies could be established if this topic was thoroughly investigated.

Calculation of nutritional requirements

Individual characteristics of patients undergoing bariatric surgery with complications differ greatly. Previous weight, lean body mass, type of complication, and medical treatment modify basal metabolism in a variable manner. Thus, it would be desirable to have an objective method of assessing metabolic demands in ICU patients. The European Society for Clinical Nutrition and Metabolism (ESPEN) recommends indirect calorimetry and urinary nitrogen balance as the best tools for this purpose [3]. Indirect calorimetry is regarded as the gold standard, given its correlation with direct calorimetry in several studies [9,10], but it is seldom available in the hospital setting.

The mathematic calculation is still an acceptable means of assessing energy expenditure, especially in the acute phase of the illness. The goal is to provide 65%−70% of the obtained total energy expenditure initially, with a margin of 2−3 kg weight loss per week considered safe. A reasonable justification is that, apart from reducing the proinflammatory signals from fat tissue, a moderate weight loss also serves the main indication of surgery: reduction of body fat excess. An alternative to indirect calorimetry is determining oxygen consumption through a pulmonary arterial catheter or carbon dioxide production attained from the ventilator [3]. From the third day on, 80%−100% of the caloric needs of the patients should be met. Several formulas have been described as useful for calculating metabolic rate in obese subjects (Harris-Benedict, Ireton-Jones, Mifflin-St Jeor, or Swinamer), but most lack appropriate precision [9]. Besides, resting energy expenditure tends to vary intrinsically in the obese ICU population [11].

A review of this topic by Patel and cols [12] stated that Penn State University equation might better predict the requirements of this kind of patients. Published data showed higher accuracy (76%) compared to other formulas, even in patients older than 60 years of age with BMI > 30 kg/m^2, when a modification was applied. American Society for Parenteral and Enteral Nutrition (ASPEN) had already recommended Penn State University formula in a previous publication on this topic [13]. Estimation of caloric needs in elderly patients and women is considered the most difficult to perform. On the other side, etiology of critical illness, fever or SOFA score (Sequential Organ Failure Assessment) do not seem to affect the prediction value of equations [14]. Thus, professionals treating these patients might use any formulas with which they are familiar, as all of them predict acceptably well basal energy expenditure [15].

Calculations based on body weight

Another approach for initiating nutritional support is basing calculations on body weight. Here, too, there exist notable differences in recommendations. ASPEN offers a choice between 11 and 14 kcal per actual body weight in patients with BMI 30−50 kg/m^2 or 22−25 kcal per ideal body weight when BMI >50 kg/m2 [12], whereas ESPEN opts for ideal body weight (0.9 × height (in cm)−100 (in males) or−106 (in females). The latter statement takes into account the differential metabolic rate of muscular tissue (13 kcal/kg/day) versus fat (4.5 kcal/kg/day) [16], which could involve a theoretical lower incidence of complications such as hyperglycemia or infection [17]. Adjusted body weight is not appropriate for performing calculations because it has not been adequately validated and even its very definition varies among studies [18].

Protein needs

Nitrogen balance provides a means of measuring protein turnover by comparing oral amino acid intake and its excretion. Urinary excretion is the main via nitrogen disposal, accounting for about 81% of the total. Adding a constant for cutaneous and fecal excretion, total nitrogen balance can be calculated [19].

Not every ICU unit performs nitrogen balance so, frequently, the calculation is the preferred method to determine protein quantity. It has long been established that obese critical patients require an elevated protein support, with doses lower than 2 g/kg/day being insufficient to maintain neutral nitrogen balance [20]. Hence, both ASPEN and ESPEN recommend protein infusion of 2–2.5 g/kg/day to ensure normal protein anabolism, independently of the caloric density of the nutrition formula [21,22]. Estimations based on biochemical parameters, such as albumin or prealbumin, are not useful in this clinical setting [23].

Notwithstanding, some considerations must be taken into account when tailoring diet for a bariatric patient: the primary objective is avoiding excessive feeding while administering enough calories and proteins to favor anabolism and reduce catabolic phenomena. Loss of fat is only an extrabenefit.

Low-calorie high-protein diets

Nutritional support based on low-calorie high-protein regimens is the most widely used approach for the obese critical patient. However, this strategy has not yet been completely validated. What seems better founded is the administration of high doses of protein in critical patients. An observational study performed by Weijs and colleagues in 886 ICU mechanically ventilated, overweight patients (mean BMI 26.6 kg/m^2) showed that reaching a minimum of 1.2 g/kg/day of protein reduced 28-day mortality by 50% [24]. Allingstrup and colleagues also encountered a positive effect of proteins and amino acids on mortality, independently of caloric provision [25]. Indirect calorimetry and urine urea were used to calculate patient needs, but only protein was associated with fewer deaths, even when other factors (SOFA score, APACHE score, and age) were considered. Several other studies demonstrated that increasing the amount of protein in nutritional support improves the outcome of ICU patients [26–28]. Notwithstanding, a reduction in other parameters, including mortality has not been found consistently in all clinical trials. Ferrie and colleagues published an upgrade in fatigue, forearm muscle thickness, and nitrogen balance, but not in mortality rate in 119 patients in ICU receiving parenteral nutrition with 1.2 g/kg proteins compared to [26–28] those receiving 0.8 g/kg [29]. The EAT-ICU study was a single-center, randomized trial where 203 mechanically ventilated patients were treated with either an early nutrition based on indirect calorimetry and 24-h urinary urea vs a standard 25 kcal/kg nutrition, mainly through enteral route. The intervention group was administered a median of 1877 kcal (vs. 1061) and 1.47 g/kg/day protein (vs. 0.5 g/kg/day). There were no differences in its primary objective, physical quality of life, 6 months after discharge [30].

Investigations exclusively on obese patients do not abound, but some evidence exists specifically for this population. Burge et al. examined the effects of using a low-calorie parenteral nutrition in hospitalized obese patients [31]. The control group was given 100% of resting metabolic energy expenditure (plus 1.31 g/kg/day of protein), whereas the intervention group just received 50% (plus 1.23 g/kg/day of protein). Nitrogen balance was similar, proving that hypocaloric parenteral nutrition suffices for balancing protein turnover. Findings in the same direction were published by Choban et al. Their results suggested that 30 obese hospitalized patients were able to maintain nitrogen balance as long as enough parenteral protein was administered (i.e., 2 g/kg/day) [20]. The amount of calories was unimportant. In fact, weight loss did not differ between the hypocaloric or control groups.

Dickerson et al. have widely explored this topic in a series of publications. In the first one, 13 patients were treated with hypocaloric, high-protein parenteral nutrition [32] with 51.5% of measured resting energy expenditure and 2.13 g/kg of ideal body weight/day of proteins. Authors claimed that protein anabolism and clinical efficacy were not different from usual parenteral nutrition. In 2002, they performed a retrospective study on 40 critically ill obese patients treated with enteral feeding [21]. The eucaloric arm was administered 20 kcal/kg of adjusted body weight/day, and the hypocaloric arm received <20 kcal/kg of adjusted body weight/day. All patients were provided at least 2 g/kg of ideal body weight/day of protein. The hypocaloric group had a shorter stay in ICU (18.6 ± 9.9 days vs. 28.5 ± 16.1 days, $P < .03$) and a shorter duration of antibiotic therapy (16.6 ± 11.7 days vs. 27.4 ± 17.3 days, $P < .03$), but control group received about 30 kcal/kg of adjusted body weight/day. Influence of age was investigated in a study of 74 obese trauma patients who were divided according to age into old (>60 years) or young (<60 years) [22]. All subjects were treated with a hypocaloric (<25 kcal/kg of ideal body weight/day), high-protein (>2 g/kg of ideal body weight/day) diet. Most received enteral nutrition (81%). Nutritional and clinical outcomes were comparable, although the oldest patients were treated more frequently with parenteral nutrition and showed a higher risk of azotemia.

Low-calorie nutrition support has not always been proven to be better than standard-calorie nutrition. Krishnan et al. developed a prospective cohort study in 187 subjects (not obligatorily obese) admitted to ICU for at least 96 h [33]. Energy intake (based on American College of Chest Physicians recommendations) was divided into tertiles, and mortality, spontaneous ventilation, and nosocomial sepsis were assessed. Patients in the higher tertile were more likely to be alive at discharge and on spontaneous ventilation than the ones in the lowest tertile. Villet et al. found adverse outcomes in a prospective observational study on 48 critically ill patients in whom negative cumulative energy balance increased complications, mainly infections [34].

Based on the mentioned evidence, an approach focused on moderate energy administration and high-protein support seems the best for obese critically ill patients and can be applied both for enteral and parenteral regimens. This kind of nutrition is contraindicated if the patient suffers from renal insufficiency without renal replacement therapy or hepatic encephalopathy, given both might worsen by high protein diets. If type 1 diabetes is present, additional care is advised to avoid ketoacidosis and hypoglycemia. There is little experience with low-calorie high-protein diets in severe immunodeficiencies.

Micronutrient supplementation

ESPEN recommends the addition of glutamine (0.3—0.5 g/kg/day) only in enteral nutrition of patients suffering burns of >20% of body surface area for 10—15 days and in trauma patients (0.2—0.3 g/kg/d) for the first 5 days [3]. It also gives clinicians the choice to used omega-3 enriched oral or parenteral emulsions. Trace elements and micronutrients should be provided daily in parenteral nutrition and supplements must be used when a deficiency is detected. ESPEN is against the use of high doses of antioxidants.

ASPEN does not support the use of immune-modulating formulas, save in brain injuries or in the surgical ICU, and gives no endorsement concerning omega-3 lipids or antioxidants due to lack of evidence [35]. Neither do they recommend the adjuvant initiation of probiotics. On the other hand, if a patient with antecedents of bariatric surgery is admitted to ICU, ASPEN endorses preventive supplementation with thiamine and search of other micronutrient deficiencies (vitamins, folate, and minerals) and the enrichment of diets if any is detected.

Complications of artificial feeding
Hyperglycemia

Hyperglycemia is a common complication of artificial nutrition due to the intravenous infusion of glucose and the metabolic stress associated with acute illness. The fat excess of obese subjects also contributes to insulin resistance, leading to hyperglycemia in a high proportion of these patients. The transcendence of hyperglycemia and plasma glucose variability is their relation to adverse clinical outcomes, including mortality [36]. Blood glucose measuring is recommended when the patient enters the ICU or when artificial nutrition is started and a minimum of every 4 h during the first 2 days of admission [3]. More frequent monitoring should be granted to unstable patients and, ideally, with arterial or venous samples. Capillary glycemic control is less reliable in the critical setting. Fig. 8.1 shows the proposed scheme for the management of nutritional support in critical obese patients.

Although the exact range of blood glucose levels is not definitely established, there is a general consensus that the goal is keeping values between 140 and 180 mg/dL, and the upper desired level should not exceed 180 mg/dL [3,35]. The main concern is avoiding hypoglycemia because although some trials offered promising results with lower blood glucose levels, especially in surgical patients

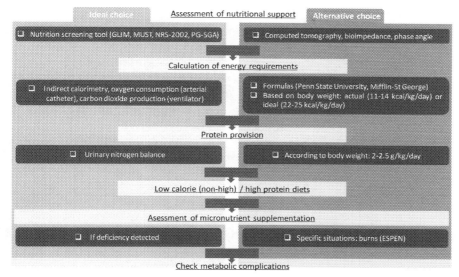

FIGURE 8.1

Scheme for management of nutritional support in critical obese patients.

(80—110 mg/dL) [37,38], these results were not confirmed in later publications. No diminished mortality could be demonstrated in the VISEP Trial despite the risk of severe hypoglycemia [39]. In fact, in the large NICE-Sugar Trial, where more than 6000 patients were included with a blood glucose target of 80—100 mg/dL, a tight glucose control group had higher mortality at 90 days (27.5% vs. 24.9%; $P = .02$) [40].

Treatment of choice for hyperglycemia in ICU is intravenous insulin, which must be adjusted to maintain blood glucose in the mentioned interval while reducing the risk of hypoglycemia. The amount of calories infused may influence insulin requirements, reducing both length (3.2 ± 2.7 vs. 8 ± 0.5 days) and dose (36.1 ± 47.1 UI vs. 61.1 ± 61 IU) [20]. A widely extended method for controlling hyperglycemia is starting intravenous insulin infusion at a minimum of 0.5 UI/h and then adjusting it in accordance with capillary glucose measurements every 1—2 h. An alternative could be to add insulin to parenteral nutrition, to provide both glucose and insulin simultaneously [41]. When enteral nutrition is the chosen support, subcutaneous insulin is also acceptable, with NPH showing the best results [42]. In our experience, subcutaneous regimens with once-daily basal insulin plus rapid-acting analogs every 4—6 h is a valid method for treating postsurgical patients.

There is no preference for specific diets for the nutritional support of diabetic patients, given the scarce evidence to prove a clinical benefit, although ESPEN remarks the possibility of improving glucose profiles and some economic advantage with enteral diabetes-specific preparations [3].

Hyperlipidemia

The quantity of lipids administered to obese patients has also been subject to investigation in the last decade. Fat tissue abounds in obese persons, who count on a larger deposit than nonobese patients when acute disease arises. This, together with the tendency to prescribe low-calorie diets, has limited lipid use in this population. This is more relevant during the first 48—72 h of admission in the ICU, when calorie restriction is recommended, except when long-chain omega-3 fatty acids are indicated (enteral nutrition in trauma and brain injury).

Some hints of lipid effects on the metabolism of obese patients can be identified in the literature. A small study on 13 obese adults who received both oral and intravenous infusion of lipids showed an increase in blood pressure and heart rate and an alteration in endothelial function [43]. A more recent retrospective analysis on 287 adults receiving parenteral nutrition studied the relationship between plasma triglycerides and BMI. Overweight and obese patients (BMI > 25 kg/m^2) showed higher triglyceride plasma concentrations despite the proportionally lower infusion of energy and lipids [44].

Considerations for support treatment in the critical obese patient

Respiratory system

Prevention of respiratory complications is the main goal in these patients [2], given the modifications that occur in pulmonary function in obesity: increased oxygen consumption and carbon dioxide production plus augmented respiratory labor and intraabdominal pressure [45]. Besides, obstructive apnea and hypoventilation-obesity syndromes are more frequent in this setting, with an incidence of 10%—20%, thus contributing to difficult management of the airway with increased atelectasis, respiratory complications, and longer need for mechanical ventilation [46]. All the described changes in pulmonary function provoke a rise in respiratory minute-volume which, added to an exaggerated caloric support, may cause a worsening of hypercapnia, especially when calories exceed more than 1.3 times the predicted energetic expenditure. This justifies an extravigilance in the caloric density of the nutrition given to patients with mechanical ventilation and obstructive chronic pulmonary disease or hypoventilation-obesity syndrome [47]. Table 8.1 shows the reference values for nutritional support and resuscitation in obese critical patients.

Obesity is an independent risk factor for intubation and ventilation with a facial mask. High Mallampati score, limited oral opening, presence of obstructive apnea syndrome, reduced cervical mobility, coma, and severe hypoxemia are associated with difficult intubation in the obese patient [48]. To limit desaturation during intubation maneuvers, preoxygenation must be optimized. The best results have been obtained by preoxygenating these patients for 5 min in a seating position with noninvasive mechanical ventilation (such as BIPAP), compared to the standard bag-mask ventilation [49].

Adult distress respiratory syndrome (ADRS), one of the complications with the highest morbidity and mortality in the critical patient has a greater incidence in obese subjects. Zhi et al. [50] performed a systematic review and meta-analysis with the combined data of 16 studies that examined the influence of obesity in ADRS and acute lung injury. Obesity was associated with a higher incidence of both conditions compared to patients with normal weight (OR 1.57, 95%CI 1.3−1.9), but with a lower mortality (OR 0.88, 95% CI 0.78−1), thus concurring with the above-mentioned obesity paradox.

Obese patients should be ventilated according to modern mechanical ventilation standards, with low volume flow rates (6 mL/kg) adjusted to body weight: 0.9 × height (in cm)−100 (males) or −106 (females), plateau pressure inferior to 30 cm H_2O, driving pressure lower than 14 cm H_2O, FiO_2 to maintain saturation between 92% and 95%, respiratory frequency appropriate for preserving normocapnia, Positive end-expiratory pressure (PEEP) values above 10 cm H_2O and alveolar recruitment maneuvers. Pirrone et al. observed that PEEP used in obese patients is commonly inadequate for minimizing atelectasis and optimizing ventilation (11.6 ± 2.9 cm H_2O) [51]. A careful titration of PEEP improves pulmonary volumes, respiratory elastance, and oxygenation while reducing its complications, so better results have been reported with elevated PEEP [52]. On the other hand, driving pressure is not useful in the evaluation of severity and prognosis of the obese patient with ADRS. Assessment of transpulmonary pressure through esophageal pressure monitoring is recommended to avoid lung collapse and loss of recruiting [53].

Prone decubitus is an elective ventilatory therapy in the obese patient with ADRS and must be considered in moderate and severe hypoxemia after alveolar recruiting maneuvers and optimization of ventilatory parameters. It has been proven as an efficient and safe technique in persons with BMI >35 kg/m^2, where it reaches a significant elevated PaO_2/FiO_2 compared to nonobese subjects [54]. When prone decubitus is contraindicated or if hypoxemia is refractory, some authors have used venovenous extracorporeal membrane oxygenation with good results [55].

For extubation, it is advisable to count on CPAP or noninvasive ventilation gear to reduce respiratory labor and oxygenation, especially if certain previous comorbidities are present, such as hypoventilation-obesity syndrome, domiciliary noninvasive ventilation, and heart conditions. The role of new devices, like high-flow nasal cannulas, remains to be elucidated.

Cardiovascular system

Obesity produces an increase in blood volume and cardiac output that leads to ventricular hypertrophy. Diastolic dysfunction is the earliest manifestation, but in time ventricular dilatation develops as part of the obesity myocardiopathy, which involves a higher risk of heart failure and fluid retention [2,47]. Atrial fibrillation is also a common complication and the possibility of pulmonary hypertension due to increased left atrium pressure, vasoconstriction secondary to hypoventilation, and chronic thromboembolism should be considered. Metabolic syndrome may affect vascular system too, as seen in hypertension with augmented afterload, dyslipidemia, or ischemic myocardiopathy [56].

Hemodynamic monitoring of the obese patient is mandatory, but the measurement of arterial pressure by oscillometry is less precise than in nonobese patients [57]. Pulse analysis devices have not proven to be reliable either in obese patient [58]. Hence, invasive arterial monitoring is the first choice for unstable obese patients, as well as through Swan-Ganz catheters. Transthoracic echocardiography gives limited information because of the bad acoustic window, so usually transesophagic echocardiography is required.

Resuscitation with fluid therapy must take into account both the increased blood volume and the risk of liquid overload and heart failure. Few investigations on resuscitation include obese patients and even the "surviving sepsis campaign" did not mention this subpopulation. Studies by Nelson et al. and Adams et al. on trauma and sepsis, respectively, demonstrate that obese patients receive less fluids in relation to their body weight and usually have longer septic shocks and demand more vasoactive drugs [59,60]. When fluid therapy is based on ideal body weight, metabolic acidosis is usually longer [61]. In a retrospective cohort of septic patients, better results were seen when adjusted body weight was used, instead of real or ideal weight [62]. Adjustment of vasoactive drugs in the obese septic patient seems to be more accurate when founded on clinical effects rather than employing doses founded on body weight [63].

Presently, more studies regarding resuscitation in the obese critical patient are necessary, but for the time being it would be reasonable to proceed with even more caution than in nonobese patients (Table 8.1).

Kidney injury

Obesity has been recognized as an etiologic factor in the development and progression of chronic kidney injury, a condition known as obesity-related nephropathy [64]. Association between BMI and kidney injury is multifactorial and proposed mechanisms include a rise in intraglomerular pressure, higher sodium reabsorption, and increased metabolic demands. Insulin resistance, type 2 diabetes mellitus, and hypertension also contribute to renal damage, which commonly ends up in glomerulomegalia and focal or segmental sclerosis. In the critical setting, obesity is a risk factor for acute kidney injury (AKI), which incidence increases with BMI in a lineal correlation [65]. Endocrine alterations related to excessive fat tissue could be transcendental too, although specific details are lacking.

However, AKI is submitted to the obesity paradox, given its lower mortality when compared to nonobese subjects. Possible explanations comprise higher plasmatic levels of beneficial inflammatory markers and a buffer effect of fat tissue on uremic toxins [66]. Obesity represents as well an issue for diagnosis and therapy of AKI. Utilizing bodyweight for applying oliguria criteria leads to false-positive diagnosis. On the other hand, it is not clear if adjusted, real, or ideal body-weight should be used in renal replacement therapies based on dosification with mL/kg/h.

Table 8.1 Reference values for nutritional support and resuscitation in obese critical patients.

Nutritional support	
Calories administered	Initial 48 h 65%−70%, after 72 h 80%−100%
Calculation of calories	11−14 kcal per actual body weight if BMI 30−50 kg/m^2, 22−25 kcal per ideal body weight if BMI >50 kg/m^2
Protein needs	2−2.25 g/kg/day
Lipid administration	Maximum 1 g/kg of ideal body weight/day (adjust according to low-calorie high-protein diet and presence of hyperlipidemia)
Glucose administration	3−5 g/kg of ideal body weight/day (adjust according to low-calorie high-protein diet and presence of hyperlipidemia)
Glutamin addition	0.3−0.5 g/kg/day in enteral nutrition for burn patients
Glycemic target	140−180 mg/dL
Resuscitation (mechanical ventilation)	
Volume flow rate	0.9 × height (in cm) − 100 (males) or − 106 (females)
Plateau pressure	<30 cm H$_2$O
Driving pressure	<14 cm H$_2$O
FiO$_2$	Keep saturation between 92% and 95%
PEEP	>10 cm H$_2$O

Pharmacotherapy

Obesity alters pharmacokinetics and pharmacodynamics. Hydrophilic drugs distribute in body fluids enriched in water, like interstitial fluid and muscles, whereas lipophilic drugs accumulate inside cells and in fat tissue. Higher volume of distribution (VOD) involves higher doses, while changes in drug clearance require modified intervals of administration.

Hydrophilic drugs suffer a slight increase in their VOD as a result of the augmented blood volume and fat-free mass. Lipophilic drugs undergo a climb of their VOD due to the accumulation of fat tissue. If weight-adjusted dosification is needed, the final dose might be difficult to assess. In general, adjusted body weight is preferable to ideal or real weight for calculations [67], although doses for over 100 kg are seldom required.

Other long-term comorbidities must be also taken into consideration, such as nonalcoholic fatty liver disease and peripheral vascular disease, as they alter pharmacokinetics. Predicting drug clearance for hydrophilic drugs with low VOD is troublesome if the patient requires renal replacement therapies or oxygenation by extracorporeal membrane oxygenation. Hypoalbuminemia transforms the clearance of drugs with high affinity for protein binding, like ceftriaxone or phenytoin; and also the VOD of hydrophilic drugs. The most desirable means of guiding optimal prescription is monitoring plasmatic concentration. This is routinely performed for antibiotics, such as vancomycin and amikacin [2].

Key points
- By default, consider all bariatric ICU patients as at risk of malnutrition
- Calculation of caloric needs with formulas is acceptable when direct measurements are not available (i.e., indirect calorimetry)
- Provide enough protein to minimize catabolism. In general, low-calorie high protein diets are chosen
- Search for micronutrient deficits and treat if detected
- Periodically check metabolic complications

References
[1] Schindler K, Themessl-Huber M, Hiesmayr M, Kosak S, Lainscak M, Laviano A, et al. To eat or not to eat? Indicators for reduced food intake in 91,245 patients hospitalized on nutrition days 2006-2014 in 56 countries worldwide: a descriptive analysis. Am J Clin Nutr 2016;104(5):1393−402.
[2] Schetz M, De Jong A, Deane AM, Druml W, Hemelaar P, Pelosi P, et al. Obesity in the critically ill: a narrative review. Intensive Care Med 2019;45(6):757−69.
[3] Singer P, Blaser AR, Berger MM, Alhazzani W, Calder PC, Casaer MP, et al. ESPEN guideline on clinical nutrition in the intensive care unit. Clin Nutr 2019;38(1):48−79.
[4] Stratton RJ, Hackston A, Longmore D, Dixon R, Price S, Stroud M, et al. Malnutrition in hospital outpatients and inpatients: prevalence, concurrent validity and ease of use of the 'malnutrition universal screening tool' ('MUST') for adults. Br J Nutr 2004;92(5):799−808.
[5] Cederholm T, Jensen GL, Correia M, Gonzalez MC, Fukushima R, Higashiguchi T, et al. GLIM criteria for the diagnosis of malnutrition - a consensus report from the global clinical nutrition community. Clin Nutr 2019;38(1):1−9.
[6] Johnson Stoklossa CA, Forhan M, Padwal RS, Gonzalez MC, Prado CM. Practical considerations for body composition assessment of adults with class II/III obesity using bioelectrical impedance analysis or dual-energy X-ray absorptiometry. Current Obes Rep. 2016;5(4):389−96.
[7] Mijan de la Torre A. El musculo, elemento clave para la supervivencia en el enfermo neoplasico. Nutr Hosp 2016;33(Suppl. 1):175.
[8] Toledo DO, Carvalho AM, Oliveira A, Toloi JM, Silva AC, Francisco de Mattos Farah J, et al. The use of computed tomography images as a prognostic marker in critically ill cancer patients. Clin Nutr ESPEN 2018;25:114−20.
[9] Frankenfield D, Hise M, Malone A, Russell M, Gradwell E, Compher C. Prediction of resting metabolic rate in critically ill adult patients: results of a systematic review of the evidence. J Am Diet Assoc 2007;107(9):1552−61.
[10] Daly JM, Heymsfield SB, Head CA, Harvey LP, Nixon DW, Katzeff H, et al. Human energy requirements: overestimation by widely used prediction equation. Am J Clin Nutr 1985;42(6):1170−4.

References

[11] Zauner A, Schneeweiss B, Kneidinger N, Lindner G, Zauner C. Weight-adjusted resting energy expenditure is not constant in critically ill patients. Intensive Care Med 2006; 32(3):428−34.

[12] Patel JJ, Rosenthal MD, Miller KR, Codner P, Kiraly L, Martindale RG. The critical care obesity paradox and implications for nutrition support. Curr Gastroenterol Rep 2016;18(9):45.

[13] Choban P, Dickerson R, Malone A, Worthington P, Compher C. A.S.P.E.N. Clinical guidelines: nutrition support of hospitalized adult patients with obesity. J Parenter Enter Nutr 2013;37(6):714−44.

[14] Frankenfield DC, Rowe WA, Smith JS, Cooney RN. Validation of several established equations for resting metabolic rate in obese and nonobese people. J Am Diet Assoc 2003;103(9):1152−9.

[15] Mogensen KM, Andrew BY, Corona JC, Robinson MK. Validation of the Society of Critical Care Medicine and American Society for Parenteral and Enteral Nutrition recommendations for caloric provision to critically ill obese patients: a pilot study. J Parenter Enter Nutr 2016;40(5):713−21.

[16] Wang Z, Heshka S, Gallagher D, Boozer CN, Kotler DP, Heymsfield SB. Resting energy expenditure-fat-free mass relationship: new insights provided by body composition modeling. Am J Physiol Endocrinol Metab. 2000;279(3):E539−45.

[17] McCowen KC, Friel C, Sternberg J, Chan S, Forse RA, Burke PA, et al. Hypocaloric total parenteral nutrition: effectiveness in prevention of hyperglycemia and infectious complications—a randomized clinical trial. Crit Care Med 2000;28(11):3606−11.

[18] McClave SA, Kushner R, Van Way 3rd CW, Cave M, DeLegge M, Dibaise J, et al. Nutrition therapy of the severely obese, critically ill patient: summation of conclusions and recommendations. J Parenter Enter Nutr 2011;35(5 Suppl. l):88s−96s.

[19] Kipnis V, Midthune D, Freedman LS, Bingham S, Schatzkin A, Subar A, et al. Empirical evidence of correlated biases in dietary assessment instruments and its implications. Am J Epidemiol 2001;153(4):394−403.

[20] Choban PS, Burge JC, Scales D, Flancbaum L. Hypoenergetic nutrition support in hospitalized obese patients: a simplified method for clinical application. Am J Clin Nutr 1997;66(3):546−50.

[21] Dickerson RN, Boschert KJ, Kudsk KA, Brown RO. Hypocaloric enteral tube feeding in critically ill obese patients. Nutrition 2002;18(3):241−6.

[22] Dickerson RN, Medling TL, Smith AC, Maish 3rd GO, Croce MA, Minard G, et al. Hypocaloric, high-protein nutrition therapy in older vs younger critically ill patients with obesity. J Parenter Enter Nutr 2013;37(3):342−51.

[23] Mesejo A, Sanchez Alvarez C, Arboleda Sanchez JA. Guidelines for specialized nutritional and metabolic support in the critically-ill patient: update. Consensus SEMICYUC-SENPE: obese patient. Nutr Hosp 2011;26(Suppl. 2):54−8.

[24] Weijs PJ, Stapel SN, de Groot SD, Driessen RH, de Jong E, Girbes AR, et al. Optimal protein and energy nutrition decreases mortality in mechanically ventilated, critically ill patients: a prospective observational cohort study. J Parenter Enter Nutr 2012;36(1):60−8.

[25] Allingstrup MJ, Esmailzadeh N, Wilkens Knudsen A, Espersen K, Hartvig Jensen T, Wiis J, et al. Provision of protein and energy in relation to measured requirements in intensive care patients. Clin Nutr 2012;31(4):462−8.

[26] Nicolo M, Heyland DK, Chittams J, Sammarco T, Compher C. Clinical outcomes related to protein delivery in a critically ill population: a multicenter, multinational observation study. J Parenter Enter Nutr 2016;40(1):45−51.

[27] Compher C, Chittams J, Sammarco T, Nicolo M, Heyland DK. Greater protein and energy intake may be associated with improved mortality in higher risk critically ill patients: a multicenter, multinational observational study. Crit Care Med 2017;45(2):156−63.

[28] Song JH, Lee HS, Kim SY, Kim EY, Jung JY, Kang YA, et al. The influence of protein provision in the early phase of intensive care on clinical outcomes for critically ill patients on mechanical ventilation. Asia Pac J Clin Nutr 2017;26(2):234−40.

[29] Ferrie S, Allman-Farinelli M, Daley M, Smith K. Protein requirements in the critically ill: a randomized controlled trial using parenteral nutrition. J Parenter Enter Nutr 2016; 40(6):795−805.

[30] Allingstrup MJ, Kondrup J, Wiis J, Claudius C, Pedersen UG, Hein-Rasmussen R, et al. Early goal-directed nutrition versus standard of care in adult intensive care patients: the single-centre, randomised, outcome assessor-blinded EAT-ICU trial. Intensive Care Med 2017;43(11):1637−47.

[31] Burge JC, Goon A, Choban PS, Flancbaum L. Efficacy of hypocaloric total parenteral nutrition in hospitalized obese patients: a prospective, double-blind randomized trial. J Parenter Enter Nutr 1994;18(3):203−7.

[32] Dickerson RN, Rosato EF, Mullen JL. Net protein anabolism with hypocaloric parenteral nutrition in obese stressed patients. Am J Clin Nutr 1986;44(6):747−55.

[33] Krishnan JA, Parce PB, Martinez A, Diette GB, Brower RG. Caloric intake in medical ICU patients: consistency of care with guidelines and relationship to clinical outcomes. Chest 2003;124(1):297−305.

[34] Villet S, Chiolero RL, Bollmann MD, Revelly JP, Cayeux RNM, Delarue J, et al. Negative impact of hypocaloric feeding and energy balance on clinical outcome in ICU patients. Clin Nutr 2005;24(4):502−9.

[35] McClave SA, Taylor BE, Martindale RG, Warren MM, Johnson DR, Braunschweig C, et al. Guidelines for the provision and assessment of nutrition support therapy in the adult critically ill patient: Society of Critical Care Medicine (SCCM) and American Society for Parenteral and Enteral Nutrition (A.S.P.E.N.). J Parenter Enter Nutr 2016; 40(2):159−211.

[36] Egi M, Bellomo R, Stachowski E, French CJ, Hart G. Variability of blood glucose concentration and short-term mortality in critically ill patients. Anesthesiology 2006; 105(2):244−52.

[37] Van den Berghe G, Wouters P, Weekers F, Verwaest C, Bruyninckx F, Schetz M, et al. Intensive insulin therapy in critically ill patients. N Engl J Med 2001;345(19):1359−67.

[38] Van den Berghe G, Wilmer A, Hermans G, Meersseman W, Wouters PJ, Milants I, et al. Intensive insulin therapy in the medical ICU. N Engl J Med 2006;354(5):449−61.

[39] Brunkhorst FM, Engel C, Bloos F, Meier-Hellmann A, Ragaller M, Weiler N, et al. Intensive insulin therapy and pentastarch resuscitation in severe sepsis. N Engl J Med 2008;358(2):125−39.

[40] Finfer S, Chittock DR, Su SY, Blair D, Foster D, Dhingra V, et al. Intensive versus conventional glucose control in critically ill patients. N Engl J Med 2009;360(13): 1283−97.

[41] Hakeam HA, Mulia HA, Azzam A, Amin T. Glargine insulin use versus continuous regular insulin in diabetic surgical noncritically ill patients receiving parenteral nutrition: randomized controlled study. Parenter Enter Nutr 2017;41(7):1110−8.

[42] Vercoza Viana M, Vercoza Viana L, Tavares AL, de Azevedo MJ. Insulin regimens to treat hyperglycemia in hospitalized patients on nutritional support: systematic review and meta-analyses. Ann Nutr Metab 2017;71(3−4):183−94.

[43] Gosmanov AR, Smiley DD, Robalino G, Siquiera J, Khan B, Le NA, et al. Effects of oral and intravenous fat load on blood pressure, endothelial function, sympathetic activity, and oxidative stress in obese healthy subjects. Am J Physiol Endocrinol Metab. 2010;299(6):E953—8.

[44] Frazee EN, Nystrom EM, McMahon MM, Williamson EE, Miles JM. Relationship between triglyceride tolerance, body mass index, and fat depots in hospitalized patients receiving parenteral nutrition. J Parenter Enter Nutr 2015;39(8):922—8.

[45] De Jong A, Chanques G, Jaber S. Mechanical ventilation in obese ICU patients: from intubation to extubation. Crit Care 2017;21(1):63.

[46] Bazurro S, Ball L, Pelosi P. Perioperative management of obese patient. Curr Opin Crit Care 2018;24(6):560—7.

[47] Dickerson RN. Metabolic support challenges with obesity during critical illness. Nutrition 2019;57:24—31.

[48] De Jong A, Molinari N, Pouzeratte Y, Verzilli D, Chanques G, Jung B, et al. Difficult intubation in obese patients: incidence, risk factors, and complications in the operating theatre and in intensive care units. Br J Anaesth 2015;114(2):297—306.

[49] Delay JM, Sebbane M, Jung B, Nocca D, Verzilli D, Pouzeratte Y, et al. The effectiveness of noninvasive positive pressure ventilation to enhance preoxygenation in morbidly obese patients: a randomized controlled study. Anesth Analg 2008;107(5):1707—13.

[50] Zhi G, Xin W, Ying W, Guohong X, Shuying L. "Obesity paradox" in acute respiratory distress syndrome: asystematic review and meta-analysis. PLoS One 2016;11(9): e0163677.

[51] Pirrone M, Fisher D, Chipman D, Imber DA, Corona J, Mietto C, et al. Recruitment maneuvers and positive end-expiratory pressure titration in morbidly obese ICU patients. Crit Care Med 2016;44(2):300—7.

[52] Bime C, Fiero M, Lu Z, Oren E, Berry CE, Parthasarathy S, et al. High positive end-expiratory pressure is associated with improved survival in obese patients with acute respiratory distress syndrome. Am J Med 2017;130(2):207—13.

[53] De Jong A, Cossic J, Verzilli D, Monet C, Carr J, Conseil M, et al. Impact of the driving pressure on mortality in obese and non-obese ARDS patients: a retrospective study of 362 cases. Intensive Care Med 2018;44(7):1106—14.

[54] De Jong A, Molinari N, Sebbane M, Prades A, Futier E, Jung B, et al. Feasibility and effectiveness of prone position in morbidly obese patients with ARDS: a case-control clinical study. Chest 2013;143(6):1554—61.

[55] Kon ZN, Dahi S, Evans CF, Byrnes KA, Bittle GJ, Wehman B, et al. Class III obesity is not a contraindication to venovenous extracorporeal membrane oxygenation support. Ann Thorac Surg 2015;100(5):1855—60.

[56] Piche ME, Poirier P, Lemieux I, Despres JP. Overview of epidemiology and contribution of obesity and body fat distribution to cardiovascular disease: an update. Prog Cardiovasc Diss 2018;61(2):103—13.

[57] Bur A, Hirschl MM, Herkner H, Oschatz E, Kofler J, Woisetschlager C, et al. Accuracy of oscillometric blood pressure measurement according to the relation between cuff size and upper-arm circumference in critically ill patients. Crit Care Med 2000;28(2): 371—6.

[58] Tejedor A, Rivas E, Rios J, Arismendi E, Martinez-Palli G, Delgado S, et al. Accuracy of Vigileo/Flotrac monitoring system in morbidly obese patients. J Crit Care 2015; 30(3):562—6.

[59] Nelson J, Billeter AT, Seifert B, Neuhaus V, Trentz O, Hofer CK, et al. Obese trauma patients are at increased risk of early hypovolemic shock: a retrospective cohort analysis of 1,084 severely injured patients. Crit Care 2012;16(3):R77.

[60] Adams C, Tucker C, Allen B, McRae A, Balazh J, Horst S, et al. Disparities in hemodynamic resuscitation of the obese critically ill septic shock patient. J Crit Care 2017; 37:219—23.

[61] Winfield RD, Delano MJ, Dixon DJ, Schierding WS, Cendan JC, Lottenberg L, et al. Differences in outcome between obese and nonobese patients following severe blunt trauma are not consistent with an early inflammatory genomic response. Crit Care Med 2010;38(1):51—8.

[62] Taylor SP, Karvetski CH, Templin MA, Heffner AC, Taylor BT. Initial fluid resuscitation following adjusted body weight dosing is associated with improved mortality in obese patients with suspected septic shock. J Crit Care 2018;43:7—12.

[63] Radosevich JJ, Patanwala AE, Erstad BL. Norepinephrine dosing in obese and nonobese patients with septic shock. Am J Crit Care 2016;25(1):27—32.

[64] Lu JL, Molnar MZ, Naseer A, Mikkelsen MK, Kalantar-Zadeh K, Kovesdy CP. Association of age and BMI with kidney function and mortality: a cohort study. Lancet Diabetes Endocrinol 2015;3(9):704—14.

[65] Druml W, Metnitz B, Schaden E, Bauer P, Metnitz PG. Impact of body mass on incidence and prognosis of acute kidney injury requiring renal replacement therapy. Intensive Care Med 2010;36(7):1221—8.

[66] Kovesdy CP, Furth SL, Zoccali C. Obesity and kidney disease: hidden consequences of the epidemic. Kidney diseases (Basel, Switzerland) 2017;3(1):33—41.

[67] Pai MP. Drug dosing based on weight and body surface area: mathematical assumptions and limitations in obese adults. Pharmacotherapy 2012;32(9):856—68.

CHAPTER 9

Nutritional recommendations after adjustable gastric banding

Amalia Paniagua Ruiz[1,2], Manuel Durán Poveda[3,4], Sonsoles Gutiérrez Medina[1]

[1]*Division of Endocrinology and Nutrition, Department of Medicine, Rey Juan Carlos University Hospital, Madrid, Spain;* [2]*Department of Medicine, Section of Endocrinology and Nutrition, Faculty of Health Sciences, Rey Juan Carlos University, Madrid, Spain;* [3]*Department of Surgery, Faculty of Health Sciences, Rey Juan Carlos University, Madrid, Spain;* [4]*Department of General Surgery, Rey Juan Carlos University Hospital, Madrid, Spain*

Chapter outline

Introduction	116
Postoperative nutritional stages	117
Stage 1 (immediately after surgery)	117
Stage 2 (days 2–9)	117
Stage 3 (days 10–14, depending on patient tolerance)	117
Stage 4 (4 weeks postop and beyond)	120
Calorie goals	121
Macronutrients	121
Protein	121
Carbohydrates	122
Fat	122
Micronutrients assessments and recommendations before and after bariatric surgery	122
Vitamin B1:	123
Assessment	123
Recommendation	123
Treatment	123
Vitamin B12 (cobalamin):	123
Assessment	123
Recommendation	123
Treatment	124
Folate (folic acid):	124
Assessment	124
Recommendation	124
Treatment	124

    Iron: 124
        Assessment 124
        Recommendation 124
        Treatment 124
    Vitamin D and calcium: 124
        Assessment 124
        Recommendation 125
        Treatment 125
    Vitamins A, E, and K: 125
        Assessment 125
        Recommendation 125
        Treatment 125
    Zinc: 126
        Assessment 126
        Recommendation 126
        Treatment 126
    Copper: 126
        Assessment 126
        Recommendation 126
        Treatment 127
Specific recommendations on LAGB and pregnancy 127
References 127

Introduction

Nowadays, adjustable gastric banding is mainly performed via laparoscopy. Among the advantages of the laparoscopic adjustable gastric band (LAGB) is the fact that it does not entail anatomic alterations, being removable and adjustable. Notably, this technique has the lowest early complications, shorter operative time, and shorter length of stay, when compared to laparoscopic gastric bypass, sleeve gastrectomy, and duodenal switch [1]. However, in the long term, it achieves less total body weight loss (TBWL), induces no metabolic effect, and reoperation rates can be high [2] due to complications such as high explant rate, erosion, slip, and prolapse. From a nutritional point of view, LAGB does not usually result in protein-calorie malnutrition and induces less micronutrient deficiencies.

For all these reasons, aftercare is critical for the success of this procedure, not only in terms of adjustment of the band and monitorization of the patients' symptoms [3], but also in terms of weight loss and nutritional success. Thus, nutritional management plays a vital role in these patients, to prevent malnutrition (which is rare) and gastrointestinal complications but also to enhance the amount of TBWL.

Briefly, preoperative care in these patients should always include evaluation of their ability to incorporate consequential changes in nutritional habits [4] (2019 AACE Guidelines, R31 Grade C, BEL. 3). All patients need to undergo a nutritional evaluation, including the micronutrient measurements described below. Enhanced recovery after bariatric surgery (ERABS) clinical pathways should be implemented. It includes continued oral nutrition with carbohydrates, including sips of clear liquids up to 2 h preoperatively [4].

Postoperative nutritional stages

Similarly, in postoperative care, patients should continue ERABS protocol [5] with an early return to oral intake to facilitate bowel function.

A multistage nutritional progressive program gets then started, for which consultation with a registered dietitian experienced with the postoperative specific LAGB diet is strongly recommended [4].

The phases described below are taken from the 2019 ASMBS clinical practice guidelines for the perioperative nutrition support of patients undergoing bariatric procedures [4] and from 2019 Tabesh M, Nutrition and Prescription of Supplements in Pre- and Post-bariatric Surgery Patients Practical Guideline [6]. Compared to the 2015 Academy of Nutrition and Dietetics Pocket Guide [7], the most current guides recommend faster progression (Table 9.1).

Stage 1 (immediately after surgery)

LAGB clear liquids (water, broth, plain gelatin) and ice chips.

Patients should be encouraged to begin fluid intake immediately after surgery, by slowly swallowing. Carbonated liquids or those with caffeine and sugar should not be used.

Stage 2 (days 2—9)

Clear liquids plus LAGB full liquids: low fat or skim milk; protein shakes; whey; whey isolate or soy protein powder; soy or almond milk, plain or Greek yogurt (although Consumption of plain yogurt with more than 25 g added sugar, should be limited); crystal light; broth; diluted natural fruit or vegetable juice; sugar-free jelly; smooth vegetable soup with no chunks, mixed with skim milk or water; sugar-free ice pops.

Patients should be encouraged to begin intake of high protein liquids. Recommended total fluid intake is 1500—1800 mL per day (50% of total intake, f.i.700—900 mL should be assigned to clear liquids, and full liquids could provide the rest). Liquids with more than 25 g sugar per servings and/or 2 g fat, should be limited.

Daily intake of protein supplement should be limited to 25—30 g per serving (100—200 cal; <10 g sugar; <15 g carbohydrates).

Patients should be encouraged to consume salty liquids only in moderation.

Carbonated liquids or those with caffeine and sugar should not be used.

Straw use should be limited.

Stage 3 (days 10—14, depending on patient tolerance)

LAGB clear liquids plus soft, pureed foods.

Having three to five small protein-rich meal increase satiety and prevent high-calorie intake.

Table 9.1 Dietary recommendations following bariatric procedure, focused on laparoscopic adjustable gastric band (LAGB).

Recommendations	UpToDate: postoperative nutritional management [8]	2008 ASMBS allied health nutritional guidelines [24]	Guidelines for perioperative care in bariatric surgery: ERAS society recommendations [5]	Academy of nutrition and dietetics pocket guide to bariatric surgery, 2nd ed [7]
Diet progression	Surgeon or institution-specific Stages 1 and 2: Hydration and liquids • Clear liquid diet (brief period) • Full liquids and possibly pureed foods—which includes liquid sources of protein and small amounts of carbohydrates (up to several weeks after surgery) Stage 3: Solid foods with an emphasis on protein sources, some carbohydrates, and fiber (~10–14 days after surgery) Stage 4: Micronutrient supplementation (when patient reaches a stable or maintenance weight) Long-term diet: • LAGB—generally resume a normal diet soon after surgery	Diet stage: Clear liquid (1–2 days after surgery) • Sugar-free or low sugar Full liquid (10–14 days after surgery) • Sugar-free or low sugar Pureed (10–14+ days) • Foods that have been blended or liquefied with adequate fluid Mechanically altered soft (>14 days after surgery) • Textured-modified • Require minimal chewing • Chopped, ground, mashed, flaked or pureed foods Regular textured (6–8 weeks after surgery) Purpose of nutrition care	Clear liquid meal regimen initiated a couple of hours postoperatively Balanced meal plan to include: • >5 servings of fruit and vegetables daily for optimal fiber consumption, colonic function, and phytochemical intake	Postoperative nutrition care of the bariatric patient has 2 distinct stages during the first year: • 0–3 months • 3 months–1 year Typically described in stages: • Diet stage 1: Clear liquid diet—very short-term; used in the hospital on post-operative days (POD) 1 and 2; liquids low in calories and sugar and free of caffeine, carbonation, and alcohol • Diet stage 2: Full liquid diet—started between POD 2 and POD 3; continues for ~14 days; clear liquids + full liquids that are low in sugar with up to 25–30 g protein per serving • Diet stage 3: Soft food texture progression—timing varies by type of surgery and duration depends on patient's response to foods; replace protein-containing full liquids with soft, semisolid protein sources (moist, soft, diced,

Table 9.1 Dietary recommendations following bariatric procedure, focused on laparoscopic adjustable gastric band (LAGB).—cont'd

Recommendations	UpToDate: postoperative nutritional management [8]	2008 ASMBS allied health nutritional guidelines [24]	Guidelines for perioperative care in bariatric surgery: ERAS society recommendations [5]	Academy of nutrition and dietetics pocket guide to bariatric surgery, 2nd ed [7]
		after surgical weight loss procedures: • Adequate energy and nutrients to support tissue healing after surgery and support preservation of lean body mass during extreme weight loss • Foods and beverages must minimize reflux, early satiety, and dumping syndrome while maximizing weight loss and weight maintenance		ground or pureed), 3–5 times/day, as tolerated • Diet stage 4: regular solid food diet
Fluids	Throughout all the diet stages, patients should be counseled to consume adequate fluid to prevent dehydration	N/A	>1.5 L daily	48–64 ounces (oz)/d • Women: 48 oz/d • Men: 64 oz/d • 50% goal should be met with clear liquids

From Mechanick J, Apovian C, Brethauer S et al. Clinical practice guidelines for the perioperative nutrition, metabolic, and nonsurgical support of patients undergoing bariatric procedures - 2019 Update: cosponsored by American Association of Clinical Endocrinologists/American College of Endocrinology, the Obesity Society, American Society for Metabolic & Bariatric Surgery, Obesity Medicine Association and American Society of Anesthesiologists. Endocrine Practice. 2019; 25(2):1–75.

Patients should spend at least 20 min eating their meals, chewing all food thoroughly.

Patients should be encouraged to stay well hydrated (at least 1500−1800 mL of liquids per day).

Patients should be encouraged not to drink water with or immediately after meal, recommending drinking it 15 min before or 30 min after meals to prevent gastrointestinal symptoms.

Carbonated liquids or those with caffeine and sugar should not be used.

Stage 4 (4 weeks postop and beyond)

Advanced diet based on the patient's tolerance.

Stop eating as soon as satiety is reached [8].

Patients should be encouraged to stay well hydrated (at least 1500−1800 mL of liquids per day).

New foods should be reintroduced separately to determine which ones are intolerable.

Patients should be encouraged not to drink water with or immediately after meal, again recommending drinking it 15 min before or 30 min after the meal.

Raw fruits and vegetables should be included slowly due to possible problems with the tolerance of their skin or texture. More than five servings of fruit and vegetables daily are recommended for optimal fiber consumption, colonic function, and phytochemical intake [5].

Intake of rice, bread, and pasta should be limited until patients can tolerate well protein-rich food, vegetables, and fruit.

Patients should be informed that as their experience of hunger increases in the following weeks, food intake should increase gradually (considering recommended daily calorie intake).

Patients should chew every meal for at least 20 min until it is smooth, making sure that the food is soft and moist enough to swallow without sticking.

Patients should be encouraged to include protein in every meal and snack.

Simple sugars should be limited to less than 10% of daily caloric intake.

Avoid/delay: concentrate sweets, carbonated beverages, fruit juice, high-saturated fat, fried foods, soft doughy bread/pasta/rice, tough or dry red meat, nuts, popcorn, other fibrous foods, caffeine, alcohol.

As recommended by the last AACE Guidelines [4], nutrition support (enteral nutrition [EN] or parenteral nutrition [PN]) should be considered in bariatric surgery patients at high nutritional risk; PN should be considered in those patients who are unable to meet needs using their gastrointestinal tract for at least 5−7 days with noncritical illness or 3−7 days with a critical illness. In patients with severe protein malnutrition and/or hypoalbuminemia, nonresponsive to oral or EN protein supplementation, PN should be considered. PN formulation for patients after bariatric procedures should be hypocaloric with relatively high nitrogen.

Calorie goals

One of the main concerns of patients undergoing LAGB is the weight regain. In the first week, calorie intake is usually equal to 500—800 kcal/day, which is gradually increased to 800—1000 kcal/day during 3—12 months. Regular nutritional follow-ups help patients to develop healthy eating habits that meet their nutritional needs instead of focusing on calorie intake [6]. Concentrated sweets should be eliminated after any bariatric procedure to reduce caloric intake [4].

Macronutrients
Protein

Previous studies showed that protein intake after bariatric surgery could not only enhance satiety but also alter long-term surgical outcomes in terms of weight and fat loss. Furthermore, postsurgery high protein diets play an important role in preserving the fat-free mass [9—11]. Kanerva et al. found that individuals who consumed more dietary protein and less fat lost more weight during 10 years after bariatric surgery [10]. Dagan et al. reported more loss of fat-free mass among those who consumed less than daily recommended protein intake after surgery [12].

Despite the effect of protein intake on body composition and its positive effects on blood glucose and triglyceride levels after surgery, it seems that bariatric patients face some problems in providing their daily protein needs. Previous studies found rates of low protein intake, especially among women and those who underwent restrictive bariatric surgery [13].

A minimal protein intake of 60 g/d and up to 1.5 g/kg ideal body weight per day should be adequate; higher amounts of protein intake—up to 2.1 g/kg ideal body weight per day—need to be assessed on individual bases and probably would not be recommended in LAGB [4]. Based on renal function, restriction of daily protein intake may be considered in patients with chronic kidney disease, especially in diabetics [14]. Furthermore, too much protein intake could affect daily consumption of other macronutrients and in the long run alter calcium homeostasis, producing liver function disorders, and influencing negatively the course of some cancers [15].

As some bariatric patients are exposed to protein deficiency with its complications, they are often advised to use protein supplements to achieve daily intake goals [16,17]. Today, a different type of protein supplement is available with the source of egg white, whey, casein, milk, and soy. All of the essential amino acids are found in these supplements [18]; although, in most cases, whey protein is recommended due to the high amounts of branched-chain amino acids that are needed in the rapid weight loss stage [19].

Carbohydrates

There is no definite recommendation for carbohydrates after bariatric surgery [11]. Previous studies found that 35%—48% of postsurgery energy needs come from carbohydrates [20,21]. However, for maintaining an optimal brain function, daily intake of carbohydrates should not be less than 50 g in the early postoperative, increasing to 130 g/day as the diet progresses [8]. Moizé et al. and Mechanick et al. suggested that after bariatric surgery, the calorie intake of carbohydrates should be limited to 45% of the total calorie intake [22,23]. According to Kanervaetal, limiting carbohydrate and fat intake and prioritizing the use of protein lead to a greater weight loss [10]. Patients should be instructed to decrease the intake of high-glycemic carbohydrates to less than 10% of the daily caloric intake to prevent nausea [8,10]. Eliminating refined sugars and processed carbohydrates and increasing the use of whole, fiber-rich carbohydrates is recommended. In addition, patients should be encouraged to use five servings of fruits and vegetables per day [19].

Fat

There are no data on LAGB, but some authors recommend that after bariatric surgery fat should represent 20%—35% of the daily caloric intake in the form of unsaturated fat [8].

Micronutrients assessments and recommendations before and after bariatric surgery

Current AACE Guidelines [4] in its 39th Recommendation stated that after consideration of preprocedure deficiency states, as well as risks and benefits in the early (<5 days) postprocedure period, patients with, or at risk for, demonstrable micronutrient insufficiencies or deficiencies must be treated with the respective micronutrient, which will be then adjusted based on recommendations for the late postprocedure period (Grade of Evidence A).

Minimal daily nutritional supplementation for patients with LAGB should always include these three medications: one adult multivitamin plus minerals (including iron, folic acid, and thiamine; which means half daily tablets recommended in the rest of surgical procedures) (Grade B), 1200—1500 mg/d of elemental calcium (in diet and as citrated supplement in divided doses), and at least 2000—3000 international units of vitamin D (titrated to therapeutic 25-dihydroxy vitamin D levels [>30 ng/mL]) (Grade B) [4]. Commercial products that are used for micronutrient supplementation need to be discussed with a healthcare professional familiar with dietary supplements, as many products are adulterated and/or mislabeled (Grade D) [4].

Rajabian Tabesh et al. prescribed the following recommendations [6]:

Vitamin B1:
Assessment
Routine screening is recommended in high-risk groups: patients with risk factors for thiamin deficiency, females, Blacks, patients not attending a nutritional clinic after surgery, patients with gastrointestinal symptoms (intractable nausea and vomiting, jejunal dilatation, megacolon, or constipation), patients with concomitant medical conditions such as cardiac failure (especially those receiving furosemide) (Grade B, BEL2), and patients with small bowel bacterial overgrowth (Grade C, BEL 3). If signs and symptoms or risk factors are present after surgery, thiamin status should be assessed at least during the first 6 months, then every 3—6 months until symptoms resolve (Grade B, BEL2).

Recommendation
All post-WLS patients should take at least 12 mg thiamin daily (grade C, BEL3) and preferably a 50 mg dose of thiamin from a B-complex supplement or multivitamin once daily (Grade D, BEL4).

Treatment
Practitioners should treat post-WLS patients with suspected thiamin deficiency before or in the absence of laboratory confirmation of deficiency and monitor and evaluate the resolution of signs and symptoms (Grade C, BEL3). Oral therapy consists of 100 mg 2—3 times daily until symptoms resolve (Grade D, BEL4). Intravenous therapy: 200 mg three times daily to 500 mg once or twice daily for 3—5 days, followed by 250 mg/day for 3—5 days or until symptoms resolve, then consider treatment with 100 mg/day orally, usually indefinitely or until risk factors have been resolved (Grade D, BEL4). Intramuscular therapy: 250 mg once daily for 3—5 days or 100—250 mg monthly (Grade C, BEL3). Simultaneous administration of magnesium, potassium, and phosphorus should be given to patients at risk for refeeding syndrome (Grade C, BEL3).

Vitamin B12 (cobalamin):
Assessment
There are no data about its deficiency after LAGB. Vitamin B12 deficiencies can occur due to food intolerances or restricted intake of protein and vitamin B12-containing foods. Although LAGB is not mentioned, frequent screening (every 3 months) is recommended in the first-year postbariatric surgery, and then at least annually or as clinically indicated for patients who chronically use medications that exacerbate the risk of B12 deficiency, such as nitrous oxide, neomycin, metformin, colchicine, proton-pump inhibitors, and antiepileptic medications. Serum B12 may not be adequate to identify B12 deficiency.

Recommendation
All post-WLS patients should take vitamin B12 supplementation (Grade B, BEL2). Orally by disintegrating tablet, sublingual, or liquid: 350—500 mcg. daily. Parenteral (IM or SQ): 1000 mg monthly.

Treatment
1000 mcg/day to achieve normal levels and then resume dosages recommended to maintain normal levels (Grade B, BEL2).

Folate (folic acid):
Assessment
As the estimated prevalence of folate deficiency after LAGB can be around 65% of the patients, routine screening is recommended (Grade B, BEL 2). Particular attention should be given to female patients of childbearing age. Poor dietary intake of folate-rich foods and suspected nonadherence with multivitamin may contribute to folate deficiency [4].

Recommendation
400—800 mcg oral folate daily from their multivitamins (Grade B, BEL2). Women of childbearing age should take 800—1000 mcg. oral folate daily (Grade B, BEL2).

Treatment
1000 mcg of folate daily to achieve normal levels and then resume the recommended dosage to maintain such levels (Grade B, BEL2). Folate supplementation above 1 mg/day is not recommended in post-WLS patients due to the potential masking of vitamin B12 deficiency. (Grade B, BEL2).

Iron:
Assessment
The prevalence of its deficiency 3 months—10 years post-AGB is 14% [4]. Iron deficiency can occur despite routine supplementation. Routine post-WLS screening of iron status is recommended within 3 months after surgery, then every 3—6 months until 12 months, and annually for all patients (Grade B, BEL2).

Recommendation
Low-risk patients (males and patients without a history of anemia) for post-WLS iron deficiency should receive at least 18 mg of iron from their multivitamins (Grade C, BEL3). Menstruating females should take at least 45—60 mg of elemental iron daily (cumulatively, including iron from all vitamin and mineral supplements) (Grade C, BEL3).

Treatment
Oral supplementation should be increased to provide 150—200 mg of elemental iron daily to amounts as high as 300 mg 2—3 times daily (Grade C, BEL3).

Vitamin D and calcium:
Assessment
The prevalence of deficiency reaches up to 100% of patients. The screening is recommended for all patients (Combination tests: Vit D, 25-OH, serum alkaline phosphatase, PTH, 24-h urinary calcium...) (Grade A, BEL 1).

Recommendation
All post-WLS patients should take calcium supplementation (Grade C, BEL3). The appropriate dose of daily calcium in LAGB is 1200—1500 mg/day. The recommended preventative dose of vitamin D in post-WLS patients should be based on serum vitamin levels: recommended vitamin D3 dose is 3000 IU daily until blood levels of 25(OH) D are greater than sufficient (30 ng/mL) (Grade D, BEL4).

Treatment
Vitamin D levels must be replenished if deficient or insufficient to normalize calcium (Grade C, BEL3). All post-WLS patients with vitamin D deficiency or insufficiency should be treated with the following doses: VitaminD3 at least 3000 IU/day and as high as 6000 IU/day, or 50,000 IU vitamin D2 1—3 times weekly (Grade A, BEL1). Vitamin D3 is recommended as a more potent treatment than vitamin D2 when comparing the frequency and amount needed for repletion. However, both forms can be efficacious, depending on the dosing regimen (Grade A, BEL1). The recommendations for repletion of calcium deficiency vary with the surgical procedure (Grade C, BEL3) being 1200—1500 mg/day calcium after LAGB.

Vitamins A, E, and K:
Assessment
As vitamins A, E, and K deficiencies are uncommon after LAGB, only symptomatic patients should be screened (Grade B, BEL2). It also seems reasonable to study Vitamin A levels in those patients with evidence of protein-calorie malnutrition.

Recommendation
Vitamin A 5000 IU/day; vitamin K 90—120 µg/day (Grade C, BEL3) and vitamin E 15 mg/day (Grade D, BEL4). Higher maintenance doses of fat-soluble vitamins may be required for post-WLS patients with a previous history of deficiency in vitamin A, E, or K (Grade D, BEL4). Special attention should be paid to post-WLS supplementation of vitamin A and K in pregnant women (Grade D, BEL3).

Treatment
Vitamin A
Deficiency without corneal changes: a dose of vitamin A 10,000—25,000 IU/day should be administered orally until clinical improvement is evident (1—2 weeks) (Grade D, BEL4). If corneal changes are present, a dose of vitamin A 50,000—100,000 IU should be administered IM for 3 days, followed by 50,000 IU/day IM for 2 weeks (Grade D, BEL4). Patients should also be evaluated for concurrent iron and copper deficiencies because these can impair the resolution of vitamin A deficiency (Grade D, BEL4).

Vitamin E
The optimal therapeutic dose of vitamin E in post-WLS patients has not been clearly defined. There is potential for antioxidant benefits of this vitamin to be achieved with

supplements of 100–400 IU/day. This recommendation is higher than the amount typically found in a multivitamin; thus, additional vitamin E supplementation may be required for repletion (Grade D, BEL4).

Vitamin K
For post-WLS patients with acute malabsorption, a parenteral dose of 10 mg vitamin K is recommended (Grade D, BEL4). For post-WLS patients with chronic malabsorption, the recommended dosage of vitamin K is either 1–2 mg/day orally or 1–2 mg/week parenterally (Grade D, BEL4).

Zinc:
Assessment
The prevalence of this deficiency seems high, representing up to 34% of patients post-AGB in some series [4]. Screening is not routinely recommended after LAGB but it should be evaluated in all post-WLS patients when the patient is symptomatic for iron deficiency anemia and screening results for iron deficiency anemia are negative (Grade C, BEL3). Post-WLS patients who have chronic diarrhea should be evaluated for zinc deficiency (Grade D, BEL4).

Recommendation
Multivitamin with minerals containing 100% of the recommended dietary allowance (RDA) (8–11 mg/day). To minimize the risk of copper deficiency in post-WLS patients, it is recommended that the supplementation protocol contains a ratio of 8–15 mg of supplemental zinc per 1 mg of copper (Grade C, BEL3).

Treatment
There is insufficient evidence to make a dose-related recommendation for repletion. The previous recommendation of 60 mg of elemental zinc orally twice a day needs to be reevaluated in light of emerging research that this dose may be inappropriate. Zinc status should be routinely monitored using consistent parameters throughout treatment (Grade C, BEL3).

Copper:
Assessment
Routine screening is not usually recommended after LAGB.

Recommendation
All post-WLS patients should take more than RDA copper as part of routine multivitamin and mineral supplementation, being 100% of the RDA (1 mg/day) after LAGB. In post-WLS patients, supplementation with 1 mg copper is recommended for every 8–15 mg of elemental zinc to prevent copper deficiency. In post-WLS patients, copper gluconate or sulfate is recommended (Grade C, BEL3).

Treatment
The recommended regimen for repletion of copper will vary with the severity of the deficiency:

- Mild-to-moderate deficiency (including low hematologic indices): Treat with 3–8 mg/day oral copper gluconate or sulfate until indices return to normal.
- Severe deficiency: 2–4 mg/day intravenous copper can be initiated for 6 days or until serum levels return to normal and neurologic symptoms resolve.

Once copper levels are normal: monitor these every 3 months (Grade C, BEL3).

Specific recommendations on LAGB and pregnancy
AACE 2019 Guidelines recommend pregnancy to be avoided preprocedure and for 12–18 months after procedure. Patients who become pregnant following bariatric procedure should have nutritional surveillance and laboratory screening for nutrient deficiencies every trimester, including iron, folate, vitamin B12, vitamin D, and calcium (no need for fat-soluble vitamins, zinc, and copper screening as LAGB is not a malabsorptive technique) (Grade D). They should have band adjustments as necessary for appropriate weight gain for fetal health (Grade B; BEL 2).

References
[1] Buchwald H, Avidor Y, Braunwald E, et al. Bariatric surgery: a systematic review and meta-analysis. J Am Med Assoc 2004;292(14):1724–37.
[2] Schouten R, Japink D, Meesters B, et al. Systematic literature review of reoperations after gastric banding: is a stepwise approach justified? Surg Obes Relat Dis 2011; 7(1):99–109.
[3] Weichman K, Ren C, Kurian M, et al. The effectiveness of adjustable gastric banding: a retrospective 6-year U.S. follow-up study. Surg Endosc 2011;25(2):397–403.
[4] Mechanick J, Apovian C, Brethauer S, et al. Clinical practice guidelines for the perioperative nutrition, metabolic, and nonsurgical support of patients undergoing bariatric procedures - 2019 update: cosponsored by American Association of Clinical Endocrinologists/American College of Endocrinology, The Obesity Society, American Society for Metabolic & Bariatric Surgery, Obesity Medicine Association and American Society of Anesthesiologists. Endocr Pract 2019;25(2):1–75.
[5] Thorell A, MacCormick AD, Awad S, et al. Guidelines for perioperative care in bariatric surgery: enhanced recovery after surgery (ERAS) society recommendations. World J Surg 2016;40:2065–83.
[6] Tabesh MR, Maleklou F, Ejtehadi F, et al. Nutrition, physical activity, and prescription of supplements in pre- and post-bariatric surgery patients: a practical guideline. Obes Surg 2019;29:3385–400.
[7] Cummings S, Isom KA, editors. Academy of Nutrition and Dietetics Pocket Guide to Bariatric Surgery. 2nd. ed. Chicago, IL: Academy of Nutrition and Dietetics; 2015.

[8] Kushner R, Cummings S, Herron DM. Bariatric surgery: postoperative nutritional management. In: J.A. Melin (ed.); UpToDate. Retrieved March 1, 2019.

[9] Steenackers N, Gesquiere I, Matthys C. The relevance of dietary protein after bariatric surgery: what do we know? Curr Opin Clin Nutr Metab Care 2018;21(1):58—63.

[10] Kanerva N, Larsson I, Peltonen M, et al. Changes in total energy intake and macronutrient composition after bariatric surgery predict long-term weight outcome: findings from the Swedish Obese Subjects (SOS) study. Am J Clin Nutr 2017;106(1):136—45.

[11] Faria SL, Kelly E, Faria OP. Energy expenditure and weight regain in patients submitted to Roux-en-Y gastric bypass. Obes Surg 2009;19(7):856—9.

[12] Dagan SS, Tovim TB, Keidar A, et al. Inadequate protein intake after laparoscopic sleeve gastrectomy surgery is associated with a greater fat free mass loss. Surg Obes Relat Dis 2017;13(1):101—9.

[13] Pattern of calorie and macronutrient intake after bariatric surgery in patient with obesity: a clinical trial. In: Tabesh M, editor. Obesity Surgery. 233 Spring St, New York: Springer; 2018.

[14] Beasley JM, Wylie-Rosett J. The role of dietary proteins among persons with diabetes. Curr Atheroscler Rep 2013;15(9):348.

[15] Delimaris I. Adverse effects associated with protein intake above the recommended dietary allowance for adults. ISRN Nutr 2013:126929.

[16] Schollenberger AE, Karschin J, Meile T, et al. Impact of protein supplementation after bariatric surgery: a randomized controlled double-blind pilot study. Nutrition 2016; 32(2):186—92.

[17] Gomes DL, Moehlecke M, Da Silva FBL, et al. Whey protein supplementation enhances body fat and weight loss in women long after bariatric surgery: a randomized controlled trial. Obes Surg 2017;27(2):424—31.

[18] Castellanos VH, Litchford MD, Campbell WW. Modular protein supplements and their application to long-term care. Nutr Clin Pract 2006;21(5):485—504.

[19] Tsai AG, Wadden TA. The evolution of very-low-calorie diets: an update and meta-analysis. Obesity 2006;14(8):1283—93.

[20] Sherf Dagan S, Goldenshluger A, Globus I, et al. Nutritional recommendations for adult bariatric surgery patients: clinical practice. Adv Nutr 2017;8(2):382—94.

[21] Sarwer DB, Wadden TA, Moore RH, et al. Preoperative eating behavior, postoperative dietary adherence, and weight loss after gastric bypass surgery. Surg Obes Relat Dis 2008;4(5):640—6.

[22] Alvarado R, Alami R, Hsu G, et al. The impact of preoperative weight loss in patients undergoing laparoscopic Roux-en-Y gastric bypass. Obes Surg 2005;15(9):1282—6.

[23] Moizé VL, Pi-Sunyer X, Mochari H, et al. Nutritional pyramid for post-gastric bypass patients. Obes Surg 2010;20(8):1133—41.

[24] Aills LL, Blankenship JJ, et al. Allied Health Sciences Section Ad Hoc Nutrition C. ASMBS allied health nutritional guidelines for the surgical weight loss patient. Surg Obes Relat Dis 2008;4(5 Suppl):S73—108.

CHAPTER 10

Nutritional recommendations after sleeve gastrectomy

Raquel Sánchez Santos[1], Alicia Molina López[2], Marta López Otero[1]

[1]*Department of Surgery, Complejo Hospitalario Universitario de Vigo, Vigo (Pontevedra), Spain;*
[2]*Department of Nutrition and Dietetics, Hospital Universitari Sant Joan de Reus; Reus (Tarragona), Spain*

Chapter outline

Sleeve gastrectomy: technique and patient selection	129
Recommendations in the immediate postoperative period	130
Nutritional recommendations in LSG at discharge	131
Nutritional recommendations in LSG in the follow-up	131
Complications and nutritional issues in LSG	135
Ulcers and upper gastrointestinal hemorrhage (0%−20%)	137
References	138

Sleeve gastrectomy: technique and patient selection

Laparoscopic sleeve gastrectomy (LSG) was initially proposed as a first-stage procedure to perform in higher risk patients, mostly superobese individuals, with a body mass index (BMI) of >60 kg/m^2. The goal was to achieve significant weight loss prior to the completion of more complex bariatric procedures in a second stage. Soon, it was noted that patients frequently lost so much weight that most of them did not undergo the second stage. Therefore, LSG was considered as a sole bariatric operation. Since then, it has been indicated as a multipurpose definitive treatment in patients with severe obesity (BMI 35−60 kg/m^2), and also it has been proposed for patients with moderate obesity (BMI <35 kg/m^2) as a restrictive procedure alone [1]. According to the published data by Welbourn et al. [2], the percentage of LSG increased from 0% in 2003 to 40% of procedures performed in bariatric surgery worldwide in 2015; but with great differences between world regions, in the Middle East, more than 80% of bariatric procedures are LSG compared to 25% in Europe.

There is a consensus for the accepted indications for LSG, including high risk patients, liver or renal transplantation, metabolic syndrome, inflammatory bowel disease, aged patients, lower BMI (30−35 kg/m^2) and also as a sole technique for almost every bariatric patient [3]. Because of this, we will have a big variety of patients who receive LSG and the preoperative nutritional status may be different for all of them.

The consensus regarding the contraindications is not so strong but many surgeons agree that LSG should be avoided in patients suffering from gastroesophageal reflux, Barret disease, or large hiatal hernias.

There are some technical issues that may influence the tolerance of oral intake. In most cases, a pneumoperitoneum is performed, and one to five trocars are placed in the upper abdomen. The sort vessels are cut from an area near the pylorus to the angle of His. An orogastric bougie is usually positioned, and a section performed with an endostapler removing the greater gastric curvature, leaving a tubular stomach. The first technical variation is the distance to the pylorus from the first stapling; some surgeons recommend starting at 2–3 cm and others at 6 cm; this will make a difference between some antrum remaining or not; and this may influence the emptying of the stomach [4]. The other significant technical variation is the size of the bougie that may vary from 34 to 60 F; this may influence the capacity of the remaining tubular stomach. We know that a wider bougie has been related to less weight loss in some studies but may also seem safer than stomachs that are too narrow [5]. From the patients' point of view, a narrow tubular stomach is more frequently associated with nausea and vomiting. For all these reasons, the technical variations must be considered when nutritional recommendations to the LSG patients are given.

Recommendations in the immediate postoperative period

LSG is a perfect fit for enhanced recovery after surgery (ERAS) programs. Obese patients are usually well committed to self-care after the whole process of preoperative education carried on by the multidisciplinary team; the operative time is usually short (less than an hour), and complications are not frequent if the surgery is performed by well-trained surgical teams. The ERAS protocol consists of goal-directed patient education, specific pre- and postoperative multimodal medication regimen, early ambulation, and early oral intake. If everything goes according to plan, the LSG patient could be discharged in the first or second postoperative day [6].

The same day of the surgery, the patient can try with small intakes of clear liquid diet (usually 4–6 h after surgery, if there are not contraindications in relation to intraoperative complications or anesthetic issues); and we must insist on early mobility (the patient should go to a comfortable chair, stand, and walk a few steps the same day of surgery). The ERAS protocol includes prophylaxis of nausea and vomiting and a reduction in the use of morphics to facilitate the early intake of liquids.

In the following day, we will recommend increasing the fluids in several intakes of 80–100 ml each; and we can add some soluble protein (10 g/8 h). we could also use some commercial preparations with proteins as OptiSource or similar.

If the patient can tolerate the oral intake with some soluble protein, the patient is capable to walk and stand; there are not any signs or symptoms that suggest any postoperative complications, there is a caregiver available at home and they do not live very far from the hospital; the patient could be discharged in the first or second postoperative day. It is crucial that the patient and the caregiver understand all the precautions, the warning signs indicating complications and the nutritional recommendations before being discharged. It is better to give all of this information before the operation and make a reminder at discharge.

Nutritional recommendations in LSG at discharge

Nutritional recommendations in the first month after an LSG follow two goals: first, we have to ensure enough intake of nutrients in a patient suffering from the stress of a surgery; second, we have to protect the suture line for an excessive pressure due to large amounts of food or liquids intake (Table 10.1).

Nutritional recommendations in LSG in the follow-up

From the month of surgery, if the patient has a good tolerance to solid foods, a balanced and varied diet is started, respecting an established volume.

In Table 10.2 are shown some general recommendations for good compliance with the dietary guideline during this period. The progression toward a balanced diet must be guided and follow specific guidelines regarding the distribution of macronutrients and the volume of food intake.

Table 10.1 Recommendations in the first month after LSG.

	Fist week	Second week	Third and fourth week
Type of food	Liquids[a]	Liquids ± pureed foods[b]	Soft solids[c] (emphasis on protein sources, some carbohydrates and fiber; well chewed) + liquids ± pureed foods
Volume in each meal	80–100 mL	150 mL	200 cc
Frequency of meals	7–8 per day	6–7 per day	5–6 per day
Total calories	600–800	800–1000	1000–1200

[a] **Liquids** soup, low fat milk, vegetables juice, yogurt, soy drink, commercial drinks (OptiSource); add soluble protein to complete daily needs (60 g protein/day).
[b] **Pureed food:** boiled fruit, boiled vegetables, chicken, turkey, ham, boiled egg, low fat cheese, white fish, omelet.
[c] **Soft solids:** boiled fruit, boiled vegetables, chicken, turkey, ham, boiled egg, low fat cheese, white fish, omelet, rice, pasta, squid, prawn, seafood.

Table 10.2 General recommendations for patients receiving LSG in the follow-up (excluding first month).

General recommendations for patients receiving LSG after the first month of follow-up
• Plan the menus. Never cook more food than you need, but in the case that there are some leftover, keep it in the fridge in nontransparent recipients.
• Choose high fiber foods like vegetables, whole grains, fruit … this can help to avoid constipation and contributes to satiety
• Cook food easily: on the grill, roasted, steaming, without sauces … never take fried foods. Cook imaginatively by making appetizing recipes with healthy foods
• To eat, use small plates to make the amount of food seem bigger
• Eat small but frequent meals (5–6/day). If you feel nauseous, stop eating for an hour and then eat the rest of the feed
• Chew well and eat slowly. Put the spoon or fork on the table after each bite. When you eat do not do another activity like reading or watching tv. Choose a different eating place than the one you use for other activities
• Drink plenty of fluids between meals but avoid taking food and beverages at the same time
• Reduce dietary fat with skim milk, lean meats, and low cooking oil
• Avoid the temptations: serve food on the plate and avoid leaving the platter on the table, do not stay in the kitchen while cooking; do not eat between meals; do not buy forbidden food or more food than necessary
• Do not skip meals, eat little if you are not hungry
• If you go to a party, choose soft drinks and low-calorie foods; plan ahead what you will eat at the party
• Avoid sugary drinks and alcohol; you can drink coffee, tea and infusions if your doctor has not prohibited them for another reason
• Tobacco use must be avoided after bariatric procedures given the increased risk of poor wound healing, anastomosis ulcer and overall impaired health

The patient will make five to six feedings a day, respecting a volume of about 200 mL in the main meals (lunch and dinner). They will make two or three small healthy snacks throughout the day depending on energy expenditure and the feeling of satiety. Meals should last at least 20–30 min.

The patient will follow the recommendations for a diet rich in protein foods, fresh vegetables and fruits, whole grains, low in fat, and simple sugars. This diet should provide more than 60 g/day of protein (or more than 1.5 g/kg ideal weight/day), as recommended by the latest guidelines [7]. In main meals, a contribution of 20–25 g of protein/intake is recommended in order to achieve daily recommendations. If persistent intolerance to protein foods appears, supplementation with a protein module should be considered.

In the main meals, the macronutrient food balance shown in Fig. 10.1 will be maintained, always using a dessert-sized dish. Priority will always be given to protein, so that if the patient feels prematurely full, they will be instructed to start eating the protein first.

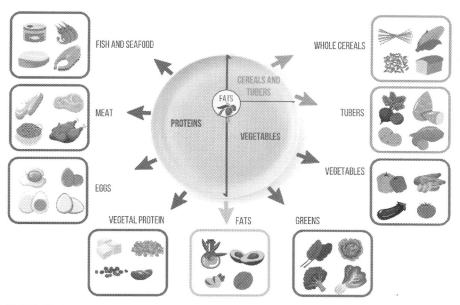

FIGURE 10.1

The balanced bariatric dish portions after surgery.

The intake of fresh vegetables and fruits is recommended, due to its fiber, vitamin, and mineral content, as well as the consumption of whole grains, which provide fiber and a greater feeling of satiety [8]. It is necessary to guarantee an intake of about 20 g/day of fiber, to avoid problems such as constipation.

The fats must be of quality, and extra virgin olive oil is recommended for cooking and other foods, such as nuts and avocado, to meet a minimum intake of 20 g/day of fat that guarantees the intake of essential fatty acids.

An adequate water intake of about 1500 mL/day should also be achieved to avoid dehydration. To fulfill this recommendation, infusions or tea, broths and flavored water with fresh frozen fruit can be added.

In addition, the vitamin and mineral supplementation established by endocrinology must be followed, which will perform control analyses to monitor possible deficits. The guideline to follow is specified in the corresponding chapter. Table 10.3 specifies how to introduce food during follow-up.

To follow all these guidelines, Fig. 10.2 shows some examples of main meals with the macronutrient distribution indicated above and the amount of protein/ intake.

Table 10.3 Food introduction guide.

	Highly recommended	Occasional consume	Not recommended
More than 6 weeks	Chicken, turkey, cooked ham White fish Eggs (not fried) Low fat dairy rich in calcium and vitamin D Green beans, carrot, chard spinach, onion, zucchini, leek, potato Boiled or baked fruit without sugar Toast bread Extra virgin olive oil Water, infusions, vegetable drinks Sugar free jelly	Salad Low-fat sausages Semi-fat cheeses Ripe raw fruit without skin Legumes Other vegetable oils Rice, pasta	Buns, cakes[a] Alcohol[a] Butter[a] Concentrated sweets[a] Carbonated beverages[a] High saturated fat, fried foods[a] Simple sugars[a] Tough dry red meat Fibrous vegetables Nuts
2 months	To incorporate: Rabbit, lean pork Blue fish, canned fish Cottage cheese and ricotta Fresh fruits	Seafood Tender or chopped beef Artichokes, asparagus, broccoli, cabbage and cauliflower Nuts Caffeine Soft doughy bread	Tough dry red meat Fruit juice (except orange and pineapple) Jams
3–6 months	To incorporate: Whole toast bread, whole cereals Salad Legumes	Caffeine Natural fruit juice Sugar free ice lollies	Homemade desserts, sauces, bechamel Prepared, ultraprocessed meals
Follow-up	Follow the pattern of the balanced Mediterranean diet, respecting the volume of the intakes (dessert dish). This pattern is characterized by: High consumption of plant-based foods Fat consumption less than 30% Olive oil main source of fat Moderate/high consumption of fish Moderate or low amounts of chicken and dairy products Low consumption of red meat and meat products Whole grain consumption Avoid sugary and carbonated drinks Avoid drinking alcohol Avoid consuming simple sugars Avoid consumption of pastries and ultraprocessed Other: Reduce the number of intakes to 3–4 from the year of surgery.		

[a] Not recommended at least in 6 months.

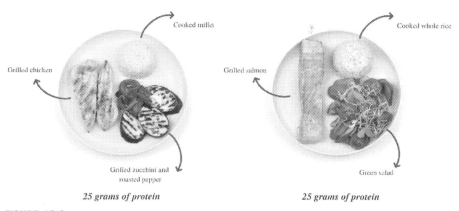

FIGURE 10.2

Examples of servings and amount of protein (dessert dish, 20 cm diameter).

It is recommended not to drink during meals, and avoid solid and liquid foods at the same time. To eat the dessert (preferably fresh fruit), patients should wait for 45–60 min. If a feeling of fullness appears, stop eating and continue later. If any food is not tolerated, eliminate it for a few days and then reintroduce it to test its tolerance.

Maintaining a balanced diet in the long term is essential to maintain the results of the surgery and achieve weight goals. Success does not only depend on surgery, dietary treatment and physical activity also play an especially important role. The acquisition of good eating habits and an active life will increase the quality of life of the patient.

Complications and nutritional issues in LSG

By resecting more than 60% of the stomach, patients undergoing an SG are at risk of *nutritional deficiencies*, firstly due to a decrease in oral intake and early satiety feeling, but also with a decrease in the levels of hydrochloric acid and extrinsic factor, secondary to the reduction in the number of parietal cells and with the consequent B12 deficiency and possible anemia.

Maintaining a well-controlled weight loss, especially after the first 12–18 months, reduces the risk of nutritional deficiencies as long as there are no pathological symptoms (persistent vomiting), the patient follows dietary instructions given and takes a standard multivitamin complex.

LSG has a long-term effect on significant improvement in the median values of triglycerides, low-density lipoproteins, and high-density lipoproteins, but not on total cholesterol levels according to published studies [9].

At 5-year follow-up, 50% of patients used vitamins regularly and 14% used them irregularly in a Stonian study [9]. The main daily intake of calcium, magnesium, phosphorus, and iron was less than the current recommendation in patients after LSG and RYGB in Moize et al. [10]. Despite the recommendation of universal supplementation, the prevalence of nutritional differences was comparable after LSG and RYGB; vitamin D, iron, and vitamin B12 were the most frequent deficiencies [9,11].

Other studies found that nutritional deficiencies are not more common after than before LSG when you consider the whole group of patients receiving LSG, but surely there are patients with more deficiencies before surgery that will be needing additional supplementation. Indeed, there is an interest of targeted supplementation in patients with deficiencies rather than systematic supplementation after LSG but this needs to be confirmed by randomized studies [11]. Nutritional deficiencies before surgery and difficulties in oral intake after surgery must be taken into consideration when the supplementation recommendations are adjusted to each patient. Patient with risk for micronutrient insufficiencies or deficiencies must be treated with the respective micronutrient and then adjusted based on recommendations for the late postprocedure period [12].

During the immediate postop period, nausea and vomiting are the main reasons for delaying oral nutrition in any bariatric procedure.

To avoid this situation, prevention is mandatory. There are several score systems (modified Apfel score) to know which patient has a higher risk to suffer from nausea and vomiting. Prophylaxis should start intraoperatively ensuring an adequate hydration, using opioid free anesthesia protocols and managing corticoids and antiemetics.

When a bariatric patient presents oral intolerance in the follow-up, it is not always related with an actual complication but usually associated with dietary transgressions.

After ruling out the diagnosis of food impaction, we can go back in oral feeding and restart with liquids and pureed food. It will be essential to closely monitor the evolution to ensure that hydration is correct, and malnutrition does not occur.

The following chart summarizes the main complications that can compromise the oral intake after a sleeve gastrectomy (Table 10.4).

Symptomatic stenosis (0.7%—4%) is a subacute/late complication. Usual symptoms include food intolerance and vomiting, and these may increase the risk of nutritional deficiencies [13].

The stenosis may be related to an inflammatory response in relation to a progressive twisting of the staple line or to an excessively narrow area. To prevent this, it is important to pull the front and back of the stomach balanced when sectioning. The

Table 10.4 Main LSG complications.

Stenosis	0.7%—4%
Leaks and fistulas	1%—3%
Ulcers and digestive hemorrhage	<1%

diameter of the probe is important; if it is too narrow it can associate stenosis more frequently, especially in the area of the incisura angularis.

The treatment of stenosis is complicated; endoscopic dilation is usually not effective, especially if it is long stenosis. In these cases, a reoperation and a gastric bypass may be necessary. In cases of mild stenosis, adequate fluid and nutrient intake must be ensured [14].

Leakage in the staple line (2%—3%) is potentially the most serious complication, representing the second leading cause of death in patients undergoing bariatric surgery (1.5%) [15].

Depending on the timing of appearance, we can classify fistulas in acute (<7 days), early (1—6 weeks), late (6—12 weeks), and chronic (>12 weeks) [16].

They usually appear in the upper third of the tube, near the angle of His, a poor vascularized area.

There are several factors that increase the risk of leakage, such as stenosis, high pressure inside the gastric tube, preoperative malnutrition or hemodynamic instability [17].

The treatment of this complication will depend on the clinical situation of the patient. In the event of instability and after diagnose confirmation by CT scan, urgent drainage of the collection or leakage is mandatory. Broad spectrum antibiotics and proton pump inhibitors will be administered, and the need for a diagnostic/therapeutic endoscopy will be assessed (placement of a self-expanding stent for 6—8 weeks, negative pressure vacuum therapies, endoscopic sutures, clips, biological glues, etc.).

At the acute moment of the fistula, the patient will not be able to take an oral diet for this reason, another alternative for nutrition must be ensured.

A central line/PICC line can be placed for parenteral nutrition and enteral nutrition can be administered through a naso-jejunal tube or by creating a laparoscopic feeding jejunostomy. In these cases, we will administer commercial hyperprotein formulas, which the patient could even manage after discharge if a longer supply of enteral nutrition is required.

Ulcers and upper gastrointestinal hemorrhage (0%—20%)

Hemorrhages are usually related with a bleeding point on the staple line. It can be endoluminal, producing hematemesis and melena, or extraluminal, resulting in a hemoperitoneum [16].

Bleeding does not normally produce hemodynamic instability, so it can be managed conservatively with close clinical surveillance, fluid therapy, and, occasionally, blood transfusions. However, the eventual appearance of a late leak has been described in patients with conservatively treated bleedings.

Ulcers are a cause of delayed bleeding in patients undergoing SG. The consumption of NSAIDs, tobacco or alcohol, advanced age or gastroesophageal reflux disease (GERD) are predisposing risk factors for its appearance.

To prevent this risk, it is advisable to perform the gastric sections using reinforced loads and tall enough staples, or even perform an invaginating suture over the staple line. In addition, it is recommended to move 1—2 cm away from the angle of His when performing the last shot of the gastroplasty.

Finally, the biggest long-term drawback to sleeve gastrectomy, according to the international series, is the onset of "de novo" GERD, found in up to 50% of patients.

If symptomatic GERD was found, in addition to maintaining the treatment with proton pump inhibitors, postural and dietary hygiene measures should be reviewed with the patient (avoiding decubitus after eating, avoiding large meals and consumption of liquids during the intake of food, avoiding gastric irritants such as caffeine, tobacco, alcohol, mint, or chocolate, etc.).

A systematic endoscopy is recommended every 5 years from the intervention for the screening of esophagitis, which would turn annual if Barret's disease was diagnosed. In the latter case, the option of a surgical revision converting the bariatric technique, usually to a gastric bypass, should at least be considered.

We can conclude that any postop morbidity puts at risk the patients' well-being, delays the weight loss results and resolution of comorbidities, and plays a negative role in a proper nutrition, requiring a deescalation in oral tolerance or even need long periods of enteral/parenteral nutrition without oral intake.

References

[1] Braghetto I, Csendes A, Lanzarini E, Papapietro K, Cárcamo C, Molina JC. Is laparoscopic sleeve gastrectomy an acceptable primary bariatric procedure in obese patients? Early and 5-year postoperative results. Surg Laparosc Endosc Percutan Tech 2012; 22(6):479—86.

[2] Welbourn R, Pournaras DJ, Dixon J, Higa K, Kinsman R, Ottosson J, et al. Bariatric surgery worldwide: baseline demographic description and one-year outcomes from the second IFSO global registry report 2013-2015. Obes Surg 2018;28(2):313—22. Springer US.

[3] Gagner M, Hutchinson C, Rosenthal R. Fifth International Consensus Conference: current status of sleeve gastrectomy. 2016. p. 750—6.

[4] Vives M, Molina A, Danús M, Rebenaque E, Blanco S, París M, et al. Analysis of gastric physiology after laparoscopic sleeve gastrectomy (LSG) with or without antral preservation in relation to metabolic response: a randomised study. Obes Surg 2017; 27(11):2836—44. Springer US.

[5] Sanchez-Santos R, Corcelles R, Vilallonga Puy R, Delgado Rivilla S, Ferrer JV, Foncillas Corvinos J, et al. Prognostic factors of weight loss after sleeve gastrectomy: multi centre study in Spain and Portugal. Cirugía Española 2017;95(3):135—42.

[6] Lam J, Suzuki T, Bernstein D, Zhao B, Maeda C, Pham T, et al. An ERAS protocol for bariatric surgery: is it safe to discharge on post-operative day 1? Surg Endosc 2019; 33(2):580—6. Springer US.

[7] Mechanick JI, Apovian C, Brethauer S, Timothy Garvey W, Joffe AM, Kim J, et al. Clinical practice guidelines for the perioperative nutrition, metabolic, and nonsurgical support of patients undergoing bariatric procedures — 2019 update: cosponsored by American association of clinical endocrinologists/American college of endocrinology. Obesity 2020;28(4):1.

References

[8] Parrott J, Frank L, Rabena R, Craggs-Dino L, Isom KA, Greiman L. American society for metabolic and bariatric surgery integrated health nutritional guidelines for the surgical weight loss patient 2016 update: micronutrients. Surg Obes Relat Dis 2017;13: 727−41.

[9] Kikkas EM, Sillakivi T, Suumann J, Kirsimägi Ü, Tikk T, Värk PR. Five-year Outcome of laparoscopic sleeve gastrectomy, resolution of comorbidities, and risk for Cumulative nutritional deficiencies. Scand J Surg 2019;108(1):10−6. SAGE Publications UK: London, England.

[10] Moizé V, Andreu A, Flores L, Torres F, Ibarzabal A, Delgado S, et al. Long-term dietary intake and nutritional deficiencies following sleeve gastrectomy or roux-en-Y gastric bypass in a mediterranean population. J Acad Nutr Diet 2013;113(3):400−10. Elsevier.

[11] Coupaye M, Sami O, Calabrese D, Flamant M, Ledoux S. Prevalence and determinants of nutritional deficiencies at mid-term after sleeve gastrectomy. Obes Surg 2020;30(6): 2165−72. Springer US.

[12] Mechanick JI, Apovian C, Brethauer S, Timothy Garvey W, Joffe AM, Kim J, et al. Clinical practice guidelines for the perioperative nutrition, metabolic, and nonsurgical support of patients undergoing bariatric procedures - 2019 update: cosponsored by American association of clinical endocrinologists/American college of endocrinology, the obesity society, American society for metabolic and bariatric surgery, obesity medicine association, and American society of anesthesiologists. Obesity 2020;28(4): O1−58. John Wiley & Sons, Ltd.

[13] Management of leakage and stenosis after sleeve gastrectomy. Surgery 2017;162(3): 652−61.

[14] Sanchez-Santos R, Corcelles Codina R, Vilallonga Puy R, Delgado Rivilla S, Ferrer Valls JV, Foncillas Corvinos J, et al. Prognostic factors for morbimortality in sleeve gastrectomy. The importance of the learning curve. A Spanish-Portuguese multicenter study. Obes Surg 2016:1−10. Springer US.

[15] Nedelcu M, Danan M, Noel P, Gagner M, Nedelcu A, Carandina S. Surgical management for chronic leak following sleeve gastrectomy: review of literature. Surg Obes Relat Dis 2019;15(10):1844−9.

[16] Souto-Rodríguez R, Alvarez-Sánchez M-V. Endoluminal solutions to bariatric surgery complications: a review with a focus on technical aspects and results. WJGE 2017;9(3): 105−23.

[17] Frattini F, Delpini R, Inversini D, Pappalardo V, Rausei S, Carcano G. Gastric leaks after sleeve gastrectomy: focus on pathogenetic factors. Surg Technol Int Surg Technol Int 2017;31:123−6.

CHAPTER 11

Nutritional recommendations after mixed procedures

Amador García Ruiz de Gordejuela[1], Alicia Molina López[2], Ramón Vilallonga Puy[1]

[1]*Bariatric Surgery Unit, Vall de Hebron University Hospital, Barcelona, Spain;* [2]*Department of Nutrition, Universitat Rovira i Virgili, Tarragona, Spain*

Chapter outline

Introduction	141
Recommendations in the immediate postoperative period	143
Clear liquid diet or tolerance phase	143
Complete liquid diet	143
Crushed diet	144
Soft diet	144
Balance diet	145
Long-term recommendations	146
Specific nutritional aspects in relation to gastric bypass	148
Nutritional complications in the gastric bypass patient	149
Food intolerance	149
Micronutrient deficiencies	150
Dumping syndrome	151
Hypoglycemias	152
Malnutrition	152
Supplementation in the gastric bypass patient	153
References	153

Introduction

Roux-n-Y gastric bypass is one of the most common bariatric procedures. For a long time, it has been considered as the gold standard in bariatric surgery. The procedure itself consists of a creation of a small pouch (20–50 mL) and an intestinal deviation based on a Roux-n-Y reconstruction. This procedure is considered as a mixed procedure as it combines both restriction and malabsorption [1] (Fig. 11.1).

There are several modifications of the procedures and there is no real consensus about how to construct it, especially in terms of limb length. Other variations described are the use of a ring in the pouch to add more restriction, and the size and construction of the gastroenteric anastomosis mainly.

CHAPTER 11 Nutritional recommendations after mixed procedures

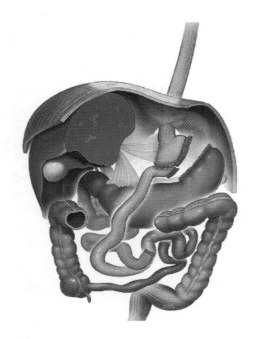

FIGURE 11.1

Roux-n-Y Gastric Bypass© Dr. Levent Efe, courtesy of IFSO.

The small pouch and the—usually—mild malabsorption are the keys to the general nutritional recommendations in these patients. The small pouch does not usually work as a normal stomach. There is just few amount of acid production in the pouch, and the size is usually too small to achieve a normal stomach digestion process.

This small pouch will determine that the patients must be instructed to eat slowly, after slow and proper chewing of the food in the mouth. They have to learn to eat small pieces several times a day (5—7 times per day). Some kinds of foods may be poorly tolerated. It usually may happen with pasta, rice, red meat, and some vegetables. These foods may be avoided and another sources of protein and long-chain carbohydrates should be recommended [2].

The ingested food will move quickly to the small bowel. Depending on the limb lengths used, it will be usually mild or distal jejunum. The Roux limb is constructed usually 80—180 cm, so after this tract, the food will be mixed with the biliary salts and the digestion of the fats will proceed. During the pass of the food for this Roux limb, only sugars and some proteins and amino acids will be absorbed.

The bowel derivation may cause some nutrient deficiencies. The bypass of the distal stomach, duodenum, and proximal jejunum is responsible for less absorption of iron, calcium, and some vitamins. Nutritional counseling should be addressed to include a diet that may redress these potential deficiencies. Patients should also be instructed to take some supplementation [3—5].

Nutritional care is the key to adequate long-term weight loss and prevention for weight regain. The objective of the postoperative diet is to meet the nutritional needs based on patients' tolerance. The exact calorie intake for every patient is calculated based on age, sex, and daily activity level, and always under the premise that negative energy balance is crucial for the first weeks and months after surgery [6,7].

Preoperatively, patients who are going to be submitted for gastric bypass require the same nutritional recommendations than the overall bariatric surgery patients [8]. In general, all bariatric patients are recommended for preoperative weight loss to avoid big left lobe livers, better respiratory compliance, and reduce postoperative complications. The amount of weight to be lost is not clearly determined. It was stated that at least 10% of preoperative weight should be lost, but there are some recent publications that reflect more complications in greater preoperative weight loss. The amount of weight to be lost and preoperative diet should be tailored to every single patient depending on their clinical and morphological characteristics.

Recommendations in the immediate postoperative period

Immediately after surgery, the goal of nutrition therapy focuses on preventing complications, side effects (nausea, diarrhea, vomiting, etc.), ensure adequate tolerance to diet and prevent deficiencies of micronutrients.

In the early stages, caloric intake is below 800 kcal/day, so adequate nutritional support is required from a specialized team to prevent situations such as protein and/or calorie malnutrition.

Once the patient is operated, the following steps and food progression are set:

Clear liquid diet or tolerance phase

It begins 24 h after surgery, or even before, with small intakes (30–50 mL approx.) of water, infusions, and if there is a good tolerance, nonacidic broths and juices (except orange and pineapple) are incorporated. This diet is limited to 2–3 days of hospital stay. It is recommended to proceed to the next phase without delay if the patient does not present symptoms of intolerance.

Complete liquid diet

- **Duration**: 7–14 days depending on the patient's degree of tolerance.
- **Volume**: 80–100 mL in each shot, fractioned and slowly.
- **Duration of each shot**: about 20–30 min.
- **Number of shots**: 7–8 per day.

The main objective of this diet is for the patient to gradually adapt to the capacity of his new gastric pouch and the consolidation of sutures. It is a dairy-based diet (milk, liquid yogurt) that is usually supplemented with the addition of a powdered protein module or with an enteral protein supplement (Optisource, Vegestart complet or Bi [1] Bificare). This diet contributes 600–800 kcal and must reach 60 g of protein/day. Avoid intake of caffeine for its diuretic effect and because it could interfere negatively in the absorption of iron. Carbonated beverages should also be removed during the initial stages. (Table 11.1)

Crushed diet

- **Duration:** 14 days (assess tolerance).
- **Volume:** a maximum of 150 mL.
- **Duration of each shot:** should be about 30 min.
- **Number of shots:** 5–6 per day.

The diet is composed of pureed foods and liquids. This phase will begin with liquid purees, and the consistency will be gradually increased depending on the patient's tolerance. This type of diet is generally more complete, as it includes a greater variety of foods. In the main meals, a complete puree consisting of vegetables, starch, and protein of animal origin will be prepared (the egg will be introduced first, then fish, and finally meat). This diet should provide a minimum of 60 g of protein per day or 1.5 g/kg ideal weight/day. (Table 11.2)

Soft diet

- **Duration:** 14 days (assess tolerance).
- **Volume:** about 150–200 mL approx.
- **Duration of each shot:** more than 30 min.
- **Number of shots:** 5–6 per day.

Table 11.1 Recommendations during the complete liquid phase.

Recommendations
• Maintain the duration established by your specialist and if you have any type of intolerance, contact your nutritionist.
• Respect the amounts and drink liquids in a fractional way as indicated.
• Avoid extreme temperatures (very cold or hot).
• Stop intakes if feeling fullness and retry later.
• Try to respect the instructions and eat all shots as indicated to reach the minimum daily target proteins. In case of not completing the indicated intakes, the administration of an enteral supplement should be considered.
• Avoid the use of reeds to drink liquids, since a lot of air could enter the digestive tract throughout the day, causing abdominal discomfort.
• Start the vitamin and mineral supplementation regimen.
• Complete the established instructions with other liquids such as water, infusions, or light broths to achieve adequate hydration.
• Do not make physical efforts.
• Do not lie down immediately after eating to avoid a possible reflux.
• Prioritize the use of medications in liquid form during the first weeks, following the instructions of your surgeon.

Table 11.2 Recommendations during the crushed phase.

Recommendations
• Start with liquid purees and progress consistency. • Ensure a correct protein intake. It is convenient to weigh protein foods the first few days to ensure the adequate portion in each intake. • Use small cutlery and eat slowly, without distractions. • Stop intake if you feel fullness or discomfort. • Ensure adequate hydration through fluid intake, separating at least 30 min from main meals. • Take the vitamin and mineral supplement. • Food example: hake puree, green beans, and potato.

In this phase, soft solid foods such as soft-boiled eggs or tortillas, cooked fruit, fresh cheese, yogurts, and cooked ham are introduced. Special importance is given to chewing food and the food environment so that the patient eats in a relaxed and leisurely way. It should monitor protein intake, which should be a minimum of 60 g of protein or day 1.5 g/kg ideal body weight/day. (Table 11.3)

Balance diet

Start: 1–2 months after surgery and will remain forever.
Volume: about 200 mL approx (dessert plate for main meals).
Duration of each: greater than 30 min.
Number of shots: 4–5 per day.

It begins when the patient has good tolerance to solids and can carry out a varied and balanced diet. You should follow a diet rich in protein, vegetables, and fruits, and low in fat and simple sugars. This diet should contribute 1000–1200 kcal per day and must ensure a supply of 60–120 g of protein per day. In the main meals, the protein contribution should reach 20–25 g per intake.

Nutritional education is essential at this stage to consolidate correct eating habits that guarantee a good weight evolution after surgery, and this guideline must be followed forever [9].

Table 11.3 Recommendations during the easily digestible phase.

Recommendations
• Start with soft foods and in very small portions. • In main meals prioritize protein intake and in case of early satiety leave the rest of the food. • Use small cutlery and dessert plate. • Ensure adequate hydration. • Take the vitamin and mineral supplement. • Start light physical activity to preserve lean mass. • Food example: French omelet, grilled zucchini, and cooked potato.

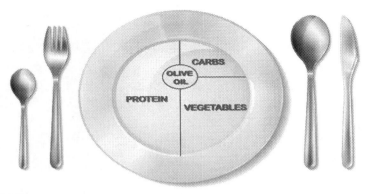

FIGURE 11.2

Balanced distribution of intake after surgery.

At mealtimes maintain a balanced diet macronutrient as shown in Fig. 11.2, using a dessert plate as reference. (Table 11.4)

Long-term recommendations

Once the initial period and the adaptation phases have been completed, the patient must consolidate good eating habits, which allow him to maintain the weight loss in the long term and guarantee good physical condition. Therefore, you will need to follow a guideline that enables you to meet your macronutrient and micronutrient requirements [3,6,10].

Table 11.4 Recommendations during the balanced diet phase.

Recommendations
• Respect the amounts of macronutrients. • In main meals prioritize protein intake, and in case of early satiety leave the rest of the food. • Use a dessert plate in main meals. • Chew food very well. • Try to keep structured schedules. • Maintain good oral hygiene. • Ensure adequate fiber intake from vegetables, whole grains, or fruit. • Ensure adequate hydration, separating liquids at least 30 min from food intake. • Avoid carbonated drinks and alcohol. • Maintain a diet low in fat and sugar. • Take the vitamin and mineral supplement. • Practice physical activity regularly and maintain an active lifestyle. • Food example: Grilled salmon, salad, and rice.

Aspects to consider maintaining food balance:

1. **Proteins:** It is the most important macronutrient after surgery, taking on special importance in those patients who have a poor tolerance to protein foods. The minimum recommendations are established at 1.5 g/kg of ideal weight/day, which in practice is equivalent to ingesting between 60 and 120 g of protein daily and represents more than 25% of the daily energy intake. It has been observed that around 37% of the patients who undergo gastric bypass fail to ingest the minimum amount of 60 g of protein per day. To achieve these recommendations, the patient must be provided with the appropriate tools. It is very important to educate them from the early stages of the cooking methods and recipes that make it easier to intake and tolerance of proteins.
2. **Carbohydrates:** There is no general recommendation on the percentage of this macronutrient after surgery, but a minimum intake of 130 g/day is recommended in most consensus documents. It will be particularly important to those foods with a lower glycemic load to minimize the occurrence of dumping syndrome. The intake of whole grains will be prioritized for its content in complex carbohydrates and fiber.
3. **Fats:** Fat intake should be around 20 g/day to guarantee the intake of essential fatty acids and the correct functioning of the gallbladder. Foods rich in fat should be avoided, not only because of possible intolerance but also because their excessive caloric weight slows down the weight loss curve. The intake of extra virgin olive oil and nuts will be prioritized, due to their contribution of monounsaturated and polyunsaturated fatty acids, respectively.
4. **Fiber**: Adequate fiber intake must be guaranteed, which should be around 20 g/day. The shortage of hydrochloric acid caused by the reduction of the gastric pouch does not allow the insoluble fiber of the cell walls of vegetables to be well digested and causes a feeling of gastric heaviness and flatulence. In contrast, soluble fiber contained in food is better tolerated.
5. **Alcohol:** Alcohol acts negatively on the body, adds empty calories, and prevents fats oxidation and, therefore, decrease the effectiveness of losing weight. After surgery, your intake regularly promotes the development of shortcomings of vitamins and minerals, as well as bone demineralization. The decrease of alcohol dehydrogenase enzyme contributes to acute poisoning following ethanol drinking. Therefore, it is important to avoid alcohol consumption after surgery.

These recommendations are designed to help the patient maintaining a balanced food intake, following the structure presented in the figure. Fig. 11.3 shows examples of balanced dishes complying with that structure.

Maintaining an adequate long-term regimen is essential to maintain the results of the surgery. There are different questionnaires to assess the food tolerance of patients undergoing bariatric surgery, such as the one presented by Suter et al., which assesses the degree of satisfaction with food, food tolerance to a specific food group, and the frequency of vomiting. This type of questionnaire is very easy to use in daily

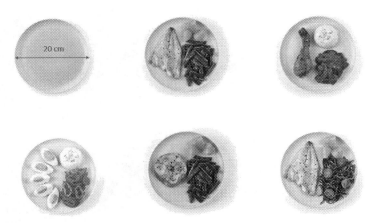

FIGURE 11.3

Examples of balanced macronutrient distribution.

clinical practice and provides information that may be relevant to the management of this type of patient. Early detection of food intolerances will help to provide the best nutritional support to our patients.

The success of surgery depends not only on the technique used. Dietary treatment is by large the main pillar to guarantee success at the long-term follow-up of the patient. The maintenance of weight loss will be responsible for remission or improvement of comorbidities and improvement of quality of life. This is the reason to maintain long-term follow-up of patients, trying to minimize the loss of patients during follow-up.

Another very important goal to achieve is the regular practice of physical activity, tailored to the characteristics of the patient. Before carrying out any type of activity, it is advisable to carry out an initial assessment by a qualified specialist. The exercise may be an adjunctive therapy to bariatric surgery, especially in patients with insufficient weight loss.

Specific nutritional aspects in relation to gastric bypass

Follow-up of these patients after bariatric surgery units is carried out in a coordinated and multidisciplinary way (surgeon, endocrine, dietitian-nutritionist, psychologist, etc.).

Regarding the frequency of consultations, they should be more frequent at the early stages. A monthly visit is necessary during the first 3 months. During these first visits, a control of the patient's food tolerance will be made during the food progression, modifying the diet according to the established diet plan. Weight loss will be monitored and the adherence to nutritional supplementation will be verified. It is important to insist on this aspect because often the good general condition of the patients makes them forget to take the prescribed supplements daily.

From the first 3 months, and until the end of the first year, if complications do not arise, a quarterly visit of the surgeon and the endocrinologist will be enough. Those visits have the objective to check weight loss, food tolerance, supplementation intake, as well as the evolution of the possible comorbidities that the patient presents. It is recommended to perform a blood test periodically. If the tolerance is correct, and the diet varied, subsequent reviews should verify that the patient maintains adherence to the initially proposed nutritional approach, to detect possible deviations from the established protocol.

From the first year and for the following 2 years, the patient must follow periodic visits every 6 months. After 3 years, if everything goes normally, an annual consultation will be enough.

Throughout the process, it will be the dietitian-nutritionist who will attend the patients the most frequently. They will make sure of the good nutrition, and the acquisition of good habits and lifestyles after the intervention [2,5,10]. Coordination with the rest of the professionals will allow an early referral to the rest of the team if it is needed.

The main societies recommend the evaluation of the results of the surgical treatment analyzing the evolution of weight, comorbidities, complications of surgery, quality of life, and eating habits.

Nutritional complications in the gastric bypass patient
Food intolerance

Food intolerance can be an important nutritional issue in gastric bypass patients. The main prevalence of this complication is in early postoperative time and related to stenosis of the gastrojejunal anastomosis. It has been described that anastomosis with a diameter lower than 1 cm will develop stenosis and food intolerance. In the mid- and long-term follow-up, food intolerance can be related to stenosis due to marginal ulcers or complications for banded pouches. In all cases, upper gastrointestinal series and endoscopy are the key to diagnosis.

Clinical manifestation is nausea and vomiting. In early postoperative time, patients can not move to different food textures and refer vomits and severe nausea. It is important to evaluate proper food patterns and discard potential food transgression, inadequate chewing, or excessive food volumes. In the late postoperative period, patients usually describe progressive difficulties to appropriate feeding. Sometimes they also refer to abdominal pain (ulcers).

The main nutritional concern in those patients is to keep appropriate protein ingestion and prevent nutritional deficiencies. During the diagnostic procedure, patients may be put on protein and vitamin supplementation, especially those in early postoperative time and with long-lasting vomiting. Those patients may also require hospital admission or enteral feeding through nasojejunal tube until the stenosis is solved. It is important to remember that those patients with chronic vomiting must be supplemented with B family vitamins, especially B1 to avoid neurological syndromes.

Micronutrient deficiencies

Micronutrient deficiency is a common issue after hypoabsorptive procedures. Gastric bypass induces usually mild hypoabsorption, and it is usually related to B1, B9, D, calcium, and iron. This micronutrient deficiency is variable from patient to patient depending on how the bypass is constructed (pouch size and limb lengths) and the patient adherence to surgical, endocrinologist, and nutritional surveillance.

Postoperative nutritional counseling is addressed to avoid or minimize those deficiencies, but always oral supplementation must be indicated [3,4,7].

There are several conditions and complications that may provoke those complications: vomiting, alcohol abuse, pharmacological interactions, etc. It is important to maintain a routine blood test check every 3—6 months during the first 2 years, and then every 6—12 months. This routine revision can prevent severe complications.

In women, iron and folate deficiencies should be closely monitored, especially in fertile age. Women may suffer for greater severity of anemia due to menstrual losses, and oral supplementation is usually needed. Folate deficiencies must be monitored and replaced in case of a desire for pregnancy.

Fertile women have no specific risks for childbearing. Routine postoperative monitoring is usually enough to develop an uneventful pregnancy.

Vitamin deficiency	Common manifestations	Recommended supplementation	Replacement
B1—Thiamine	Weakness, beri beri, Wernicke—Korsakoff encephalopathy	High-quality multivitamins are routinely recommended after bariatric procedures, irrespective of deficiencies, which are often recommended to be chewable or liquid	If hyperemesis, then 100 mg IV for 7 days, then 50 mg/d until thiamine in the normal range.
B9—Folate	Megaloblastic anemia, loss of appetite, weight loss	High-quality multivitamins are routinely recommended after bariatric procedures, irrespective of deficiencies, which are often recommended to be chewable or liquid	Total of 1200 ug/d of folic acid until RBC folate in the normal range, and then a multivitamin with at least 400 μg/d of folic acid
B12—Cobalamine	Macrocytic anemia. Guillain—Barré syndrome	Monthly intramuscular supplementation. Oral intake can be considered	1000 μg/mo IM, 1000 μg/wk sublingually, or 350—500 μg/d orally until B12 in the normal range

Vitamin deficiency	Common manifestations	Recommended supplementation	Replacement
D	Decreased bone mineralization, osteopenia, secondary hypoparathyroidism, hypocalcemia	2.000–3.000 IU of vitamin D (titrated to therapeutic 25-hydroxyvitamin D levels > 30 ng/mL).	Typical dose for mild deficiency of vit. D is 1000 IU/d after gastric bypass. For severe deficiency, a single dose of vit. D 50,000 IU/wk, then 3000 IU
Calcium	Decreased bone mineralization, osteopenia, secondary hypoparathyroidism	Calcium citrate 1500 mg/d, preferably with vitamin D	Calcium citrate 1200–1800 mg/d.
Iron	Microcytic anemia	18–60 mg total iron via multivitamins and additional supplements	For moderate deficiency, total elemental iron intake (including in a multivitamin) should be 50–100 mg/d. For severe deficiency, IV iron is sometimes required

Dumping syndrome

Dumping syndrome is a specific complication of gastric bypass related to the bypass of the pyloric emptying mechanism. It occurs in 70%–85% of the patients, and it is due to a quick deployment of the food into the bowel. It is presented as facial flushing, light-headedness, fatigue, reactive hypoglycemia, and postprandial diarrhea. These symptoms characteristically appear 10–30 min after eating It is common during the first 18 months postoperatively.

Early dumping has been classically related to hyperosmolarity of intestinal contents and increased fluid in the intestinal lumen, but more recently has been associated with the release of gut peptide due to food entering the bowel after bypassing the stomach.

Treatment includes nutritional counseling. Mostly, avoidance of food with a high glycemic index and avoid drinking fluid with meals. Patients are advised to chew thoroughly and eating slowly. Octreotide 15–30 min before surgery can be used in severe cases.

Hypoglycemias

It is rarely reported metabolic complication gastric bypass. It occurs after a meal along with biochemical detection of postprandial hyperinsulinemia and hypoglycemia. It should be suspected when postprandial neuroglycopenic symptoms like confusion, altered levels of consciousness, reduced cognition, weakness, fatigue, warm sensation, slurred speech, and visual disturbances; it occurs after bariatric surgery. A low blood glucose level must be screened and measured. Severe cases may develop hypoglycemia unawareness, loss of consciousness, seizures, coma, and even death.

The pathophysiological mechanism is unknown but may be related to the misregulation of GLP-1 after gastric bypass with overstimulation of insulin after glucose ingestion. Treatment begins with nutritional counseling. These include multiple small meals throughout the day to avoid large volume carbohydrate feeding. Meals should be high in fiber and protein, and low in simple, rapidly absorbable carbohydrates. Pharmacotherapy includes the use of acarbose, nifedipine, and GLP-1 receptor antagonists that have shown efficacy and promise for long-term treatment.

In severe cases, reversion surgical procedures to restitute food passage through the duodenum are the best choice.

Malnutrition

Malnutrition includes two different kinds of issues: protein malnutrition and energy malnutrition.

Protein malnutrition is not a common complication after gastric bypass. It can be more frequent in distal bypass cases or in patients with a poor compliance or even alcohol or substance abuse. It can also present in patients with chronic diarrhea, prolonged vomiting, or anorexia.

Protein malnutrition is usually presented as weakness, poor general aspect, peripheric edema and several blood test abnormalities, hair loss, etc, The main clinical sign is lean body mass loss. There is no physiological reserve of proteins, so in cases of deficient high-quality protein intake, the lean body mass in consumed, and this is an important part of weight loss.

There are different formulas to restore protein deficiency, and they need to evaluate the overall clinical status and patient condition. Nutritional advise is mandatory to look for high-quality protein foods. In severe cases, protein supplementations in different preparations can be used. More severe cases may need nasojejunal enteral feeding or even hospital admission and parenteral nutrition.

It is crucial to elucidate the cause that has triggered the protein malnutrition and correct it. Some cases of distal gastric bypass may require surgery for remodeling the limb lengths. In those cases, and before going to the operating room, it is important to improve the nutritional status to avoid surgical complications.

Energy malnutrition occurs in those situations in which the patient exceeds the expected weight loss, due to significant energy restriction as a consequence of the lack of appetite, the sensation of early satiety with a minimal intake of food, the elimination of some foods of the diet ruled by bad tolerance or inappetence, etc. This situation must be monitored and studied if it occurs as a consequence of an anatomical problem, such as gastrojejunal anastomosis stenosis (manual or mechanical) or due to an alteration in the patient's eating behavior. In the absence of anatomical problems, other possible causes must be studied, and the patient must be adequately treated to stop this type of malnutrition.

Supplementation in the gastric bypass patient

Patients submitted to gastric bypass will present some sequelae related to the pouch and the hypoabsorption induced by the distal stomach, duodenum, and proximal jejunum exclusion. The main deficiencies that may present related to this anatomical change have been presented through this chapter. Main bariatric surgery and endocrinological societies recommend routine supplementation in these patients [11].

Overall recommendations include:

- 1 bariatric dose of multivitamins plus minerals.
- 1.500 mg elemental calcium.
- 2.000–3.000 IU of vitamin D (titrated to therapeutic 25-hydroxyvitamin D levels > 30 ng/mL).
- 18–60 mg total iron via multivitamins and additional supplements.
- Vitamin B12 (parenterally, as sublingual, subcutaneous, or intramuscular preparations, or orally, if determined to be adequately absorbed).

Those recommendations may be adapted to patient preoperative and postoperative conditions. It is important to remark that morbid obesity patients may present vitamin D deficiencies before surgery, and fertile women are more prone to have anemia and iron deficiency. Finally, patients' conditions usually change during follow-up and other deficiencies may appear: vitamin A, copper, zinc, magnesium,etc. Routine blood test and clinical consultation are the keys to prevent complications.

References

1. Rubio Herrera M, Ballesteros Pomar M, Sánchez Pernaute A, Torres García J. Manual de obesidad mórbida. 2nd ed. Madrid: Editorial Panamericana; 2015.
2. Gil Hernández A, Fontana Gallego L, Sánchez de Medina F. Tratado de nutrición. Tomo V. 3rd ed. Madrid: Editorial Panamericana; 2017.
3. Parrott J, Frank L, Rabena R, Craggs-Dino L, Isom KA, Greiman L. American society for metabolic and bariatric surgery integrated health nutritional guidelines for the surgical weight loss patient 2016 update: micronutrients. Surg Obes Relat Dis 2017;13(5):727–41.
4. Obesity Algorithm®. ©2016-2017 Obesity Medicine Association.
5. Martin García-Almenta E, Ruiz-Tovar Polo J, Sánchez Santos R. Vía Clínica de Cirugía Bariátrica, 1. AEC, GERM, SECO, Funseco; 2017.

6. Tabesh MR, Maleklou F, Ejtehadi F, Alizadeh Z. Nutrition, physical activity, and prescription of supplements in pre- and post-bariatric surgery patients: a practical guideline. Obes Surg 2019;29(10):3385—400.
7. Vilallonga R, Pereira-Cunill J, Morales-Conde S, Alarcón I, Breton I, Domínguez-Adame E, et al. A Spanish Society joint SECO and SEEDO approach to the postoperative management of the patients undergoing surgery for obesity. Obes Surg 2019; 29(12):3842—53.
8. Gu L, Fu R, Chen P, Du N, Chen S, Mao D, et al. In terms of nutrition, the most suitable method for bariatric surgery: laparoscopic sleeve gastrectomy or Roux-en-Y gastric bypass? A systematic review and meta-analysis. Obes Surg 2020;30(5):2003—14.
9. Moizé VL, Pi-Sunyer X, Mochari H, Vidal J. Nutritional pyramid for post-gastric bypass patients. Obes Surg 2010;20(8):1133—41.
10. Moizé V, Andreu A, Flores L, Torres F, Ibarzabal A, Delgado S, et al. Long-term dietary intake and nutritional deficiencies following sleeve gastrectomy or Roux-en-Y gastric bypass in a mediterranean population. J Acad Nutr Diet 2013;113(3):400—10.
11. Backes CF, Lopes E, Tetelbom A, Heineck I. Medication and nutritional supplement use before and after bariatric surgery. Sao Paulo Med J 2016;134(6):491—500.

CHAPTER 12

Nutritional recommendations after hypoabsorptive procedures: OAGB, duodenal switch, SADI-S

Luciano Antozzi[1], Gisela Paola Latini[1], Joao Caetano Marchesini[2],
Tamires Precybelovicz[2], Andres Sánchez Pernaute[3], Miguel Ángel Rubio-Herrera[4]

[1]*Centro de Cirugías Especiales, Bahía Blanca, Buenos Aires, Argentina;* [2]*Clínica Doctor Caetano Marchesini, Curitiba, Brazil;* [3]*Hospital Clínico San Carlos, Madrid, Spain;* [4]*Endocrinology and Nutrition Department, Hospital Clinico San Carlos, Madrid, Spain*

Chapter outline

Introduction	156
Preoperative nutritional evaluation and supplementation	157
Micro/macronutrients	157
Bone health	157
Liver function	158
Preoperative eating behavior screening and weight loss	158
Postoperative diet and supplementation	159
Protein	160
Micronutrient supplementation recommendations	163
Thiamin—vitamin B1	163
Cobalamin—vitamin B12	163
Folate	165
Iron	165
Vitamin D and calcium	165
Vitamin A	165
Vitamin E	165
Vitamin K	166
Zinc	166
Copper	166
Bone health	166
Liver function	167
Gastrointestinal symptoms	167
Long-term follow up	168

Nutrition and Bariatric Surgery. https://doi.org/10.1016/B978-0-12-822922-4.00007-7
Copyright © 2021 Elsevier Inc. All rights reserved.

Chapter 12 Nutritional recommendations after hypoabsorptive procedures

Conclusions 169
References 169

Introduction

Bariatric/metabolic surgery is no longer considered only mechanically. Complex physiological changes, where gut signaling influences organs like the liver and brain, make profound changes in hunger, satiety, weight, glucose metabolism, and immune functions. Microbiota transformations and bile acids levels play a major role and justify that the effect of hypoabsorptive procedures (HAP) is not only related to the intestinal portion in contact with micronutrients, but with the excluded segment also. Hypoabsorptive techniques have significantly better weight loss and comorbidities resolution in the long term, but frequent nutritional deficiencies are still a significant concern [1]. Many of these can be avoided with proper multidisciplinary team (MDT) management.

The procedures considered in this chapter are One Anastomosis Gastric Bypass (OAGB), Biliopancreatic Diversion with Duodenal Switch (BPD/DS), and Single Anastomosis Duodenoileal Bypass with Sleeve Gastrectomy (SADI/S) as performed by the authors involved. The characteristics of each procedure are as follows (Table 12.1):

The length of intestinal segments has been a matter of debate and is still under constant research. BPD/DS is the most widely studied of the three HAP mentioned, and with a CL of 100 cm, it has the lowest contact of nutrients with endocrine secretions. OAGB has two variations, one with fixed lengths as described by Rutledge, and another one described by Carbajo that proposes a ratio taking into account total bowel length (TBL) and common limb. A CL/TBL ratio of 0.43 was found as the most accurate parameter to predict a 5-year postoperative BMI under 25 kg/m^2 with low protein or calorie malnutrition [2]. SADI/S most frequent CL is 250 cm, considering this as a length that ensures the greatest weight loss with fewer metabolic complications. Except for fat-soluble vitamins and vitamin B12 that are absorbed in the distal ileum,

Table 12.1 Hypoabsorptive procedures.

OAGB (Carbajo's technique)	BPD/DS	SADI/S
18–22 cm long, 36–40 Fr wide gastric pouch	50–60 Fr wide sleeve gastrectomy	50–60 Fr wide sleeve gastrectomy
~3 cm wide gastrointestinal anastomosis with an antireflux system	Wide duodenoileal anastomosis	Wide duodenoileal anastomosis
Single anastomosis configuration with the exclusion of 40%–60% of total bowel length	Roux-en Y configuration with 100 cm common limb (CL) and 250 cm alimentary limb (AL)	Single anastomosis configuration, 250 cm from the ileocecal valve

most vitamins and minerals are adequately absorbed along small bowel. The functional integrity and adaptation capacity of the CL are fundamental to avoid micronutrient deficiencies. The patient's age, a socioeconomic status that grants access to the designated diet, and patients' responsibility are key elements to avoid complications. Younger patients can maintain an adequate nutritional status, with a well-planned diet and a simple multivitamins/minerals complex. On the other hand, older patients or those who sabotage diets can find greater imbalances.

The nutritional status of patients in the preoperative period is frequently suboptimal. Evaluation, preoperative diet, and supplementation are of key importance. After surgery, reeducation is needed concerning diet progression, eating behaviors, and symptoms related to gastrointestinal adaptation. Finally, lifelong supplementation and lifestyle advice are necessary. This chapter abridges recommendations to attain long-term success and prevent complications in each part of this process.

Preoperative nutritional evaluation and supplementation

Candidates for bariatric surgery frequently have conditions that can aggravate after surgery. Bone health, liver function, fat-free mass depletion, and micronutrient/mineral levels should be screened before HAP are performed.

Micro/macronutrients

Chronic inflammation, improper diets, and low intake of fruits and vegetables may develop nutrient and vitamins decay in patients suffering from morbid obesity. These include low levels of ferritin, hemoglobin, vitamin B12, and vitamin D [3,4]. McKay et al. found that as BMI increased the serum concentration for vitamin D, folate, potassium, and magnesium decreased [5]. In Spain or Italy, vitamin D levels <30 ng/dL affect 80% of the population, being worse in obese patients due to adipose tissue accumulation [6]. They should be corrected before surgery, as the first postoperative months can aggravate a previously poor situation.

- Biochemical assessment: ferritin, folic acid, hemoglobin, blood potassium, magnesium, phosphorus, copper, iron, zinc, transferrin, transthyretin, vitamin A, B1, B2, B6, B12, D, E, and cobalamin.
- Recommendation: preoperative daily multivitamin supplementation because diet alone may not be sufficient.

Bone health

Sufficient levels of nutrients and hormones that are important for bone health, including vitamin D, calcium, albumin, and PTH, should be properly addressed before surgery with enough time to make corrections if necessary. Grace et al. reported that almost 90% of their patients considering bariatric surgery had an inadequate vitamin D status [7]. Deficiencies may be aggravated after HAP leading to osteomalacia and osteoporosis.

The utility of DEXA scans for bone mineral density before and after bariatric surgery is debated. Baseline DEXA scans should be considered in young postmenopausal women, men aged 50–69, and those with clinical risk factors for osteoporosis [8].

- Biochemical assessment: Measure serum calcium, albumin, PTH, and D3/25OHD levels. Treat any deficiencies before surgery (vitamin D, 28,000 IU of vitamin D3 per week for 8 weeks).
- Bone mass density assessment: DEXA scans are recommended for young postmenopausal women, men older than 50, and patients at risk of fracture.

Liver function

Non alcoholic fatty liver disease (NAFLD) is almost constant in morbidly obese patients. Body fat percentage, central adiposity, hyperinsulinemia, and insulin resistance are good predictors of liver dysfunction development. To evaluate liver disease, blood samples of function tests need to be performed. Most routine biochemical studies have a poor correlation with NAFLD. Common blood sample findings are mild-to-moderate ALT and/or AST elevation. AST/ALT index usually remains under 1 but it rises with fibrosis progression along with γ-glutamyl transferase (GGT). Albumin, prothrombin, or bilirubin alteration can indicate liver dysfunction or cirrhosis. Many imaging studies can detect hepatic steatosis, but none can distinguish NAFLD from NASH, this can only be done with liver biopsies. If there is a high suspicion of fibrosis, magnetic resonance (MR), MR spectrometry, MR elastography, transient elastography, or acoustic radiation force can be used. It is recommended to avoid HAP in cirrhotic patients since liver dysfunction may aggravate.

- Biochemical assessment: AST, ALT, AST/ALT index, GGT, blood glucose, albumin, prothrombin, INR, and bilirubin.
- Imaging studies: abdominal ultrasound is mandatory to detect fatty liver existence, and further studies can be performed when needed.

Preoperative eating behavior screening and weight loss

Eating behavior should be screened with a clinical interview to know the number and type of meals per day, liquid intake, and eating patterns like grazing, and binge eating. The patients should be properly informed about the significant effort and lifestyle change that any HAP involves. If the patient does not seem trustworthy regarding adherence to diet or follow-up, other procedures can be recommended.

Preoperative weight loss role can be controversial. The American Society for Metabolic and Bariatric Surgery (ASMBS) set it as a grade B recommendation because an increased risk of preoperative malnutrition and depleted free fat mass (FFM) could lead to complications. In contrast, a large-scale study showed that patients with preoperative weight loss >9.5% had a reduced rate of postoperative complications compared to patients with weight loss <0.5% [9]. Given that HAPs are usually indicated in higher BMI patients and can produce a significant rapid weight loss in the first months after surgery, we recommend the routine use of a controlled preoperative weight loss regimen.

Postoperative diet and supplementation

It has been proven that nutritional care not only prevents malnutrition and gastrointestinal complications but also decreases the risk of weight regain in morbidly obese patients. The objective of short-term postoperative diets is to meet the nutritional needs of the patients based on their tolerance to food texture [10].

Food intake should be started early after bariatric surgery. Diets are divided into three general categories before a regular ingestion is reached: clear liquid diets, full liquid diets, and soft diets. Despite there is no specific protocol, the use of locally validated ones based on tolerance to food texture, jointly established by surgeons and nutritionists, is strongly recommended [11].

Patients are instructed to begin with clear liquids at room temperature after surgery, increasing amounts gradually. Liquids with low calories are allowed, like water, light herbal tea, nonsugary drinks, juice, and coconut water. Carbonated liquids or those with caffeine and sugar should not be ingested. Patients should consume 150−200 mL of liquids every hour with at least four cups of water included. They should drink liquids in small portions, and as tolerated, add other liquid foods, such as low or no-fat milk, vegetable milk, broth without chunks, diluted natural fruit juice, and sugar-free ice pops. Protein shakes with 60−80 g of protein per day facilitate the adaptation to the new "gastric capacity" avoiding bloating, nausea, or vomiting. Advise small sips, without straw, 6−10 times per day to reach 600−800 kcal "Bariatric smoothies" can be prepared on the basis of milk, liquid yogurt, soy, oat, rice, or almond beverages, to which fruit, vegetables, or protein powder is added to reach nutritional recommendations. Usually, this stage lasts 2−4 weeks, depending on patient tolerance.

At 2−4 weeks after surgery, patients are advised to progress to a mashed or puréed diet. This diet ensures 800−1200 kcal, divided into six or eight servings. It is considered a transition diet that is achieved by chopping, grinding, mashing, flaking, or pureeing foods. Begin with smooth foods and slowly progress to less homogeneous mashed foods. Water ingestion remains primordial. Incorporate into the diet: ground or pureed low-fat meat, poultry and fish, egg, ham, low-fat cheese, cottage cheese, soft tofu, strained soups, well-cooked vegetables, canned fruit in water, and pureed fruits. Protein must be served first to ensure daily ingestion. Patients should be encouraged to consume 100−150 g per meal. In the last stage of this phase, servings that can be cut easily with a fork can be incorporated like scrambled, soft-boiled or omelet eggs, cooked ham, pudding, yogurt, fresh low-fat cheeses, and cooked fruit.

Special attention must be given to patients that hesitate to progress to solid foods postoperatively for fear of gaining weight, pain, nausea, or vomiting. Solid foods cause greater satiety and have an enhanced nutritional composition.

The final step advocates progression to a balanced solid, hypocaloric (1000–1500 kcal), Mediterranean diet with more than 90 g per day of protein. It usually takes the patients 8–12 weeks to attain the required tolerance. Reintroduce foods separately ascertaining which are intolerable, highlight adequate chewing, and encourage hydration (at least 1500–1800 mL of liquids per day). Promote water consumption 15 min before or 30 min after meals, but not during food ingestion. Dietetic counseling is mandatory during the first year, optional later [6,12,13].

Protein

A protein intake of 60–120 g or 1.5 g/kg of ideal body weight per day should be adequate; higher amounts of protein intake—up to 2.1 g/kg ideal body weight per day—need to be assessed on an individualized basis [14]. To achieve these recommendations, protein-rich food must be served first (animal sources, such as lean meat and fish or low-fat dairy products, and vegetable sources, such as legumes combined with cereals, tofu) and are preferred over food rich in carbohydrates or fats [15]. The main issue in practice is that protein-rich food is generally not well tolerated within the first weeks after surgery. Approximately 50% of patients cannot reach the minimum goal of 60 g. This is why, in the first stages of the diet, patients are advised to use protein supplements to achieve daily intake goals. In most cases, whey protein is recommended due to the high amounts of branched-chain amino acids that are needed in the rapid weight loss stage [16]. The exact calorie intake for better weight loss after bariatric surgery is not known yet and should be defined based on age, sex, and daily activity level. However, a negative energy balance is vital [17]. Protein malnutrition is the most severe macronutrient complication associated with HAP [18]. Protein deficiency can affect up to 30% of patients in the long term after BPD/DS [19]. The clinical manifestations of protein deficiency include hair loss, peripheral edema, poor wound healing, and loss of lean body mass. Bacterial overgrowth usually coexists. Treatment with enteral nutrition, supplementation, antibiotics, and dietary instruction is usually enough. Advanced cases may require surgical elongation of the CL.

Guidelines recommend that carbohydrates should be limited to 45% of the total calorie intake. Limiting carbohydrates to two servings per day of whole grains and cereals, and prioritizing the use of protein leads to a greater weight loss [20]. In addition, patients should be encouraged to use five servings of fruits and vegetables per day.

Recommendations for fat intake after bariatric surgery are like those for the general population, 20% of the total calorie intake. This goal should be thoroughly screened and should not exceed 30%–35% of daily kcal because high-fat diets lead to diarrhea based on the malabsorptive character of the procedures. Steatorrhea caused by fat malabsorption may lead to deficiencies in zinc, copper, magnesium, and fat-soluble vitamins (Table 12.2) [21].

Table 12.2 Diet progression.

Diet stage	Food	Recommendations
Stage 1: Clear liquid diet.	Water, light herbal tea, nonsugary drinks, juice, and coconut water 30 mL of liquids every 15 min.	Liquids should be ingested slowly, intercalated to advocate tolerance. The usage of straws should be limited. Carbonated liquids or those with caffeine and sugar should not be incorporated.
Stage 2: Full liquid diet.	Add to previous indications: low or no-fat milk, vegetable milk, whey, isolated whey, broth, diluted natural fruit or vegetable juice, sugar-free jelly, smooth vegetable soup with no chunks. 150–200 mL of liquids every hour.	Avoid carbonated liquids or those with caffeine and sugar. Start whey proteins. Add at least 800 mL of water.
Stage 3: Mashed, pureed, soft diet.	Well-cooked vegetables: potato, carrot, beetroot, zucchini, sweet potato, broccoli, corn, pumpkin, eggplant, strained soups, pureed of nonfibrous fruits, ground or pureed low-fat meat, poultry and fish, eggs, cottage cheese, low or no-fat yogurt 100–150 g.	Prioritize protein ingestion first at every meal. Encourage not to drink water with or immediately after a meal (15 min before or 30 min after meals is recommended) The use of protein powders should be continued. Sugar should not be used. Advice thorough chewing. At least 3–5 small meals per day. At least 1500–1800 mL of water per day.
Stage 4: Normal diet.	❏ Feed normally, according to tolerance. ❏ Total calories calculated based on physical activity, sex, and age, maintaining negative energy balance, distributed in 45% of carbohydrates, at least 90–120 g per day or 1.5g/kg. of ideal weight of protein and 20% of fat. ❏ Avoid simple carbohydrates: ice cream, cakes, cookies, soda, and alcohol. ❏ Two servings of carbohydrates in the day, one serving corresponds to 90 g of rice or pasta, 30 g of breakfast cereals, bread, and toast, 80 g of lentils, peas, beans, and 85 g of potatoes, sweet potatoes. ❏ 5 servings of fruits and vegetables per day. ❏ 3 servings of dairy products per day. ❏ Organize and plan 4 to 6 meals a day. ❏ Prioritize protein consumption and maintain protein supplements as required. ❏ Adjust chewing. ❏ Maintain good water intake.	

Table 12.3 Micronutrient supplementation.

Micronutrient	Preventative recommendations supplements	Repletion recommendations for micronutrient deficiency	Other considerations
Thiamin —Vitamin B1	50—100 mg/d.	Should be based on the route of administration and severity of symptoms: Oral therapy: 100 mg 2—3 times daily until symptoms resolve. IV therapy: 200 mg 3 times daily to 500 mg once or twice daily for 3—5 d, followed by 250 mg/d for 3—5 d or until symptoms resolve, then consider treatment with 100 mg/d orally, usually indefinitely or until risk factors have been resolved. IM therapy: 250 mg once daily for 3—5 d or 100—250 mg monthly.	Simultaneous administration of magnesium, potassium, and phosphorus should be given to patients at risk for refeeding syndrome.
Cobalamin —Vitamin B12	350—500 mcg/d.	Oral therapy: 1000 mcg/d. IV therapy: 5000 mg monthly.	Patients who chronically use medications that exacerbate the risk of B12 deficiency: nitrous oxide, neomycin, metformin, colchicine, proton pump inhibitors, and seizure medications.
Folate (Folic Acid)	400—800 mg/d.	Supplementation above 1000 mg/d is not recommended in patients because of the potential masking of vitamin B12 deficiency.	Women of childbearing age should take 800 —1000 mg oral folate daily.
Iron	Men: 18 mg. Women: 45—60 mg.	Oral therapy: 300 mg two to three times a day. IV therapy: If iron	Other studies recommend 200 mg/day for

Micronutrient supplementation recommendations

HAPs have always been associated with an increased risk of vitamins and other micronutrient deficiencies. Exclusion of jejunal contact with nutrients can result in poor iron, vitamin B12, and zinc absorption, whereas a short common channel affects the absorption of fat-soluble vitamins. Patients are advised to meticulously adhere to the use of multivitamins lifelong. The necessity of specific vitamin and mineral supplementation can be many times higher than other bariatric procedures. Multivitamin complexes designed for each surgical technique are ideal, but sometimes they are not available or patients cannot afford them. A wide variety of deficiencies can be found depending on the patient's age, supplementation indicated, CL length, and technique employed (Table 12.3). Biochemical assessment at regular periods is recommended (every 3—6 months within the first year, and every 6—12 afterward). Frequently vitamins and minerals results are slightly under normal values without any clinical impact; if this happens, there is no need for an obsessive supplementation.

Minimal daily nutritional supplementation for HAP is two multivitamins complex plus minerals in chewable form, containing iron, folic acid, thiamine, elemental calcium citrate, vitamin D, and vitamin B12. Despite preventive strategies, patients can experience clinical burden. It is worrisome that the number of patients receiving reimbursement for a nutritional supplement decreased significantly over time [22].

Thiamin—vitamin B1

Vitamin B deficiency can manifest at any stage, but this usually occurs within the first year after surgery. Clinical manifestations are paresthesia, muscle weakness, abnormal gait, and polyneuropathy. To avoid irreversible Wernicke—Korsakoff syndrome, patients must be under care [23]. There is an estimated deficiency frequency lower than 7.5% of patients after HAP [24,25]. Malnutrition, excessive and/or rapid weight loss, proton pump inhibitors, diuretics, persistent vomiting, bacterial overgrowth, and excessive ingestion of coffee, tea, raw fish, or alcohol are risk factors for thiamine deficiency. Patients should take 50 mg of thiamin from a B-complex supplement or multivitamin once or twice daily. In case of deficiency, the dose depends on the route of administration and severity of symptoms: oral 300 mg/d, intravenous 1000 mg/d, and intramuscular 250 mg/d [26].

Cobalamin—vitamin B12

Cobalamin deficiency can emerge secondary to the reduced mass of gastric parietal cells necessary for hydrolysis of vitamin B12 and conformation of the cobalamin-intrinsic factor complex. Restricted intake of protein and vitamin B12-containing foods, atrophic gastritis, PPI, and metformin use aggravate this situation. A frequency of 0%—29% has been described [27,28], usually lower than RYGB series [29]. Supplementation of vitamin B12 is based on the route of administration: orally by disintegrating tablet, sublingual, or liquid, 350—500 mg/d; nasal spray as suggested by the manufacturer; IV therapy: 1000 mg/month. Patients with B12 deficiency should take 1000 mg/d to achieve normal levels and then resume regular dosage [26].

Table 12.3 Micronutrient supplementation.—cont'd

Micronutrient	Preventative recommendations supplements	Repletion recommendations for micronutrient deficiency	Other considerations
		deficiency does not respond to oral therapy.	women and 100 mg/day for men.
Vitamin D	Vitamin D3: 3000—6000 UI/d.	Adequate vitamin D, calcium and parathormone.	Dose of 7.000 IU/day is suggested by other studies with patients undergoing BPD/DS.
Calcium	1800—2400 mg/d.	Adequate vitamin D, calcium and parathormone.	Other studies suggest 3000 mg/day. Carbonate: with meals. Citrate: with or without meals.
Vitamin A	10.000—25.000 UI/d.	Patients with corneal changes: 50.000—10.000 UI/d IM for 3 days, followed by 50.000 UI/d IM for 2 weeks.	50.000 IU/d is another suggestion for maintenance doses.
Vitamin E	15 mg/d.	Little reported deficiency.	There is potential for antioxidant benefits of vitamin E to be achieved with supplements of 100—400 IU/d.
Vitamin K	300 mcg/d.	—	—
Zinc	16—22 mg/d.	Multivitamin with minerals containing 200% of the RDA (16—22 mg/d).	Other studies suggest the need for 40—100 mg/d.
Copper	2 mg/d.	Multivitamin with minerals containing 200% of the RDA (2 mg/d).	Supplementation with 1 mg of copper is recommended for every 8—15 mg of elemental zinc to prevent copper deficiency. Copper gluconate or sulfate is recommended.

Folate
Poor dietary intake of folate-rich foods and nonadherence to multivitamins contributes to folate deficiency. After surgery, patients should take 400−800 mg folate daily from a multivitamin complex. Women of childbearing age should take 800−1000 mg of oral folate daily. All patients with folate deficiency should take an orally 1000 mg/d to achieve normal levels and then resume the recommended dosage to maintain normal levels. Folate supplementation above 1 g/d is not recommended in patients because of the potential masking of vitamin B12 deficiency [26].

Iron
Iron deficiency can occur despite routine supplementation. Patients at low risk (males and patients without a history of anemia) of iron deficiency should receive at least 18 mg of iron from their multivitamins. Menstruating females should take at least 45−60 mg of elemental iron daily (cumulatively, including iron from all vitamin and mineral supplements). However, other studies show elemental iron has to be introduced at a mean daily dose of 200 mg for menstruating females and 100 mg for men after biliopancreatic diversion [1,30]. If iron deficiency does not respond to oral therapy, the intravenous iron infusion should be administered [26].

Vitamin D and calcium
The recommended preventative dose of vitamin D is 3000 IU/d. Patients with vitamin D deficiency or insufficiency should be repleted with 6000 IU/d, or 50,000 IU vitamin D2 1−3 times weekly [26]. Cholecalciferol can be absorbed erratically after HAP and calcifediol conversion is altered in obesity [31]. Thus, 2000−3000 IU/d orally of calcifediol is more reliable. IM or subcutaneous administration may be necessary in severe deficiency with secondary hyperparathyroidism. The appropriate dose of daily calcium is 1800−2400 mg or 1−2 g as citrate, which is better absorbed in low gastric acid levels. When PTH levels remain high, monitoring of calcium and phosphorus, as well as oxalates in urine, are useful for appropriate management.

Vitamin A
Patients who have undergone HAP should be screened for vitamin A deficiency regardless of symptoms. Theoretically, retinol deficiency is very frequent, but vitamin A is transported by *Retinol Binding Protein* (RBP). Therefore, vitamin levels should be adjusted to RBP levels, reducing the incidence of the deficiency by half. For BPD/DS, ASMBS guidelines suggest 10.000 UI/d of vitamin A [26], but the findings of a recent study show that 50.000 UI/d are necessary to prevent deficiency [1]. In patients with vitamin A deficiency with corneal changes: a dose of vitamin A 50,000−100,000 IU should be administered IM for 3 days, followed by 50,000 IU/d IM for 2 weeks.

Vitamin E
Vitamin E deficiency is infrequent. The prevalence of deficiencies is 10% after 5 years of biliopancreatic diversion. ASMBS guidelines suggest 15 mg/d of

vitamin E [26]. There is potential for antioxidant benefits of vitamin E to be achieved with supplements of 100−400 IU/d. This is higher than the amount typically found in a multivitamin complex, thus additional vitamin E supplementation may be required [26].

Vitamin K

Vitamin K is found in leafy green vegetables, such as cabbage, spinach, turnip greens, kale, chard, mustard greens, parsley, romaine lettuce, and vegetables like Brussels sprouts, broccoli, cauliflower, and cabbage. The appropriate dose of vitamin K supplementation is 300 mcg/d [26]. High vitamin K deficiency rates are present in 60% of the patients with BPD/DS [30]. Therefore, for patients with acute malabsorption, a parenteral dose of 10 mg vitamin K is recommended. For patients with chronic malabsorption, the recommended dosage of vitamin K is either 1−2 mg/d orally or 1−2 mg/week parenterally.

Zinc

Zinc is absorbed in the duodenum and the first part of jejunum, exclusion of this area elevates the risk of deficiency. Despite low levels are frequently found, clinically relevant findings are unusual. Anyway, it should be monitored, and especially if patients have chronic diarrhea, hair loss, or dysgeusia. All patients should take zinc with multivitamins and minerals containing 200% of the RDA, 16−22 mg/d, some studies suggest 40 a 100 mg/d for the prevention of deficiency [30]. To minimize copper deficiency a ratio of 8−15 mg of Zn should be provided for each milligram of copper [32].

Copper[1]

Monitoring copper and ceruloplasmin is necessary to detect deficiencies at an early stage. Severe deficiency should be suspected when nonferropenic anemia or pancytopenia are found along with neuropathy or myeloneuropathy. All patients should take 2−3 mg/d [26]. This can be doubled or tripled in case of severe deficiency.

Bone health

Despite larger studies are needed to compare specific techniques, fracture risk is described as more frequent after procedures that affect absorption. After HAP, vitamin D is not properly absorbed, and mean serum 25OHD concentrations usually remain <30 ng/mL despite supplementation. Low calcium intake association justifies the hyperparathyroidism frequently found. Fracture patterns associated with obesity switches to the type found in osteoporosis, and this can start even 24/36 months after surgery [33,34]. Adequate protein intake minimizes muscle and bone loss [35].

---

[1] The ingestion of multivitamin complex must include Selenium.

- ❏ Biochemical assessment: calcium, albumin, PTH, 25OHD, and 24-h urinary calcium every 6 months for 2 years.
- ❏ DEXA 2 years after surgery, then once a year until the fifth year.
- ❏ Calcium citrate to achieve total daily calcium intake of 1800−2400 mg.
- ❏ Vitamin D3 3000 IU with titration to 25OHD level >30 ng/mL.
- ❏ BMI adjusted protein intake 45−75 g/d.
- ❏ Physical activity: aerobic and strength training at least two times/week. Mandatory during the weight-loss period.

Liver function

Rapid weight loss can affect liver function. A hypoabsorption too powerful can lead to not only a lack of regression of NAFLD, but progression or liver failure. It is prevalent to find biochemical markers alteration in the first 18 months after HAP. There are reports of increased de novo fibrosis after, but the development of cirrhosis or liver function alterations are infrequent in a controlled postoperative scenario. Weight loss should be thoroughly controlled along with biochemical status. If a preoperative cirrhosis is detected, many groups avoid HAP, but experts consensus has determined that HAP can be indicated even in Child A cirrhosis. This topic is of particular importance if a patient has a previous hepatic disease, as the procedure can be tailored according to the existence of this comorbidity. A longer common limb is safer in these cases.

- ❏ Biochemical assessment: AST, ALT, AST/ALT index, GGT, albumin, prothrombin, bilirubin.
- ❏ Longer common limb recommended if there is a diagnosis of preexisting hepatic conditions.
- ❏ Be alert and avoid rapid weight loss.

Gastrointestinal symptoms

All clinicians involved in the management of the postoperative course should be aware of the risk of early and repeated vomiting after surgery. Although infrequent, this can generate further complications. If upper GI swallow does not show any sign of surgical complications, the most frequent causes are functional or psychological. In these cases, prokinetics and antiemetics could be helpful. In some cases, these symptoms appear early in the first stages of diet progression and resolve without further treatment. Sustained dysphagia or vomits can suggest mechanical/functional obstruction secondary to twist or stenosis of the sleeve in SADI/S or BPD/DS. In OAGB, other causes like a twisted, small, or ulcered anastomosis should be suspected. This can generate intolerance even to liquids and diagnosis and treatment should not be delayed to avoid nutritional complications or dehydration.

Dumping syndrome and postprandial hypoglycemia are more common after RYGB but very unusual in HAP. Dumping syndrome refers to predominantly GI symptoms that occur early (30–60 min) after a meal, often precipitated by "inappropriate" foods. Postprandial hypoglycemia (PPH) refers to symptomatic hypoglycemia that is often provoked by high glycaemic foods or drinks, resulting 45–90 min after ingestion. Nutritional intervention is the mainstay of dumping and PPH syndromes (small, frequent, low carbohydrate meals). However, for hyperinsulinemic hypoglycemia, an urgent referral might be required to an endocrinologist for detailed investigations, such as a CT scan or selective arterial calcium stimulation test, to exclude other causes and to consider pharmacological management if dietary advice is insufficient to control the problem.

Usually bowel movement shifts after HAP, diarrhea is far more common than constipation. Two or three bowel movements per day are usual, but this is very variable. If diarrhea is present, treatment should focus on loperamide use, pH modification, increased water intake, and reduced dietary intake of fat, lactose, or fiber. Pancreatic enzymes replacement therapy for chronic diarrhea with an initial dose of 500 units/kg/meal is usually a very effective treatment during intestinal adaptation phase. After 30–90 days, it can be progressively discontinued. Besides bowel movement, flatulence can have serious effects on social life. This should be treated the same way as diarrhea. Bismuth subgallate 200 mg, two capsules per meal, has been beneficial for gastrointestinal and steatorrhea-like symptoms [36]. Bacterial overgrowth is suspected when diarrhea and flatulence associate with abdominal pain. In this case, stools should be examined for *Clostridium Difficile* and treatment established with Rifaximin/Ciprofloxacin for 14 days.

Long-term follow up

Despite within 18 months after surgery most changes and complications occur, bariatric surgery is a lifelong change and long-term follow-up adherence is advised. The information provided in this chapter is based on evidence and experience. Patients usually have a variable response to treatment, which makes systematic guidelines difficult to write. Therefore, patients have to be treated on an individual basis. A recommended short- and long-term screening schedule is described in Table 12.4, and it can be modified depending on patients' comorbidities and complications.

Laboratory testing	Preop	1 M	3 M	6M	9M	12M	18M	24M	36M	Yearly
Hemogram	X	X	X	X	X	X	X	X	X	X
Folic acid	X	—	—	—	—	X	X	X	X	X
Ferritin	X	—	—	—	—	X	X	X	X	X
Ionogram	X	X	—	—	—	X	X	X	X	X
Magnesium	—	—	—	—	—	X	X	X	X	X
Phosphorus	—	—	—	—	—	X	X	X	X	X
Copper	X	—	—	X	X	X	X	X	X	X

Laboratory testing	Preop	1 M	3 M	6M	9M	12M	18M	24M	36M	Yearly
Iron	X	—	—	—	—	X	X	X	X	X
Zinc	X	—	—	X	X	X	X	X	X	X
Transferrin	X	—	—	X	X	X	X	X	X	X
Transthyretin	X	—	—	X	X	X	X	X	X	X
Vitamin A	X	—	—	—	—	X	X	X	X	X
Vitamin B1	X	X	—	—	—	X	X	X	X	X
Vitamin B2	X	—	—	—	—	X	X	X	X	X
Vitamin B6	X	—	—	—	—	X	X	X	X	X
Vitamin B12	—	—	—	—	—	X	X	X	X	X
Vitamin D3/25OHD dicalciferol	X	—	—	X	X	X	X	X	X	X
Vitamin E	X	—	—	—	—	X		X	—	—
Cobalamin	X	—	—	—	—	X	X	X	X	X
Calcium	X	—	—	X	X	X	X	X	X	X
Glucose	X	X	—	—	—	X	X	X	X	X
Urinary calcium	—	—	—	—	—	X	X	X	X	X
Creatinin	X	X	—	—	—	X	X	X	X	X
PTH	X	—	—	X	X	X	X	X	X	X
INR	X	X	X	X	X	X	X	X	X	X
Total proteins/albumin	X	X	X	X	X	X	X	X	X	X
Hepatic profile	X	X	X	X	X	X	X	X	X	X

Conclusions

Hypoabsorptive procedures are described in the literature as the most effective bariatric therapies. It has also been widely demonstrated that they require proper surveillance to avoid complications. If the recommendations mentioned in this chapter can be fulfilled, the excellent clinical results over morbid obesity and associated comorbidities will widely outweigh complications.

References

[1] Nett P, Borbély Y, Kröll D. Micronutrient supplementation after biliopancreatic diversion with duodenal switch in the long term. Obes Surg 2016;26(10):2469−74.

[2] Ruiz-Tovar J, Carbajo MA, Jimenez JM, Luque-de-Leon E, Ortiz-de-Solorzano J, Castro MJ. Are there ideal small bowel limb lengths for one-anastomosis gastric bypass (OAGB) to obtain optimal weight loss and remission of comorbidities with minimal nutritional deficiencies? World J Surg 2020;44(3):855−62. https://doi.org/10.1007/s00268-019-05243-0.

[3] Ernst B, Thurnheer M, Schmid SM, Schultes B. Evidence for the necessity to systematically assess micronutrient status prior to bariatric surgery. Obes Surg 2009;19(1): 66–73.

[4] Lefebvre P, Letois F, Sultan A, Nocca D, Mura T, Galtier F. Nutrient deficiencies in patients with obesity considering bariatric surgery: a cross-sectional study. Surg Obes Relat Dis 2014;10:540–6.

[5] Mckay J, Ho S, Jane M, Pal S. Overweight and obese Australian adults and micronutrient deficiency. 2020. p. 1–13.

[6] Mechanick JI, Apovian C, Brethauer S, et al. Clinical practice guidelines for the perioperative nutrition, metabolic, and nonsurgical support of patients undergoing bariatric procedures – 2019 Update: Cosponsored by American Association of Clinical Endocrinologists/American College of Endocrinology, The Obesity Society, American Society for Metabolic & Bariatric Surgery, Obesity Medicine Association, and American Society of Anesthesiologists – executive summary. Endocr Pract 2019;25(12):1346-1359.

[7] Grace C, Vincent R, Aylwin SJ. High prevalence of vitamin D insufficiency in a United Kingdom urban morbidly obese population: implications for testing and treatment. Surg Obes Relat Dis 2014;10(2):355–60.

[8] Heber D, Greenway FI, Kaplan LM, Livingston E, Salvador J, Still C. Endocrine and Nutritional management of the post-bariatric surgery patient: an Endocrine Society clinical practice guideline. J Clin Endocrinol Metab 2010;95(11):4823–43.

[9] Anderin C, Gustafsson UO, Heijbel N, Thorell A. Weight loss before bariatric surgery and postoperative complications: data from the Scandinavian obesity registry (SOReg). Ann Surg 2014. https://doi.org/10.1097/SLA.0000000000000839.

[10] Dagan SS, Goldenshluger A, Globus I, Schweiger C, Kessler Y, Sandbank GK, Ben-Porat T, Sinai T. Nutritional recommendations for adult bariatric surgery patients: clinical practice. Adv Nutr: Int Rev J 2017;8(2):382–94.

[11] Thibault R, Huber O, Azagury DE, Pichard C. Twelve key nutritional issues in bariatric surgery. Clin Nutr 2016;35(1):12–7.

[12] Aills L, Blankenship J, Buffington C, Furtado M, Parrot J. ASMBS allied health nutritional guidelines for the surgical weight loss patient. Surg Obes Relat Dis 2008;4(5): 73–108.

[13] Tabesh MR, Maleklou F, Ejtehadi F, Alizadeh Z. Nutrition, physical activity, and prescription of supplements in pre- and post-bariatric surgery patients: a practical guideline. Obes Surg 2019;29(10):3385–400.

[14] Mechanick JI, Youdim A, Jones DB, Garvey WT, Hurley DL, Mcmahon MM, Heinberg LJ, Kushner R, Adams TD, Shikora S. Clinical practice guidelines for the perioperative nutritional, metabolic, and nonsurgical support of the bariatric surgery patient—2013 update: cosponsored by American Association of Clinical Endocrinologists, The Obesity Society, and American Society for Metabolic & Bariatric Surgery. Surg Obes Relat Dis 2013;9(2):159–91.

[15] Moizé VL, Pi-sunyer X, Mochari H, Vidal J. Nutritional pyramid for post-gastric bypass patients. Obes Surg 2010;20(8):1133–41.

[16] Tsai AG, Wadden TA. The evolution of very-low-calorie diets: an update and meta-analysis. Obesity 2006;14(8):1283–93.

[17] Hwang KO, Childs JH, Goodrick GK, Aboughali WA, Thomas EJ, Johnson CW, Yu SC, Bernstam EV. Explanations for unsuccessful weight loss among bariatric surgery candidates. Obes Surg 2008;19(10):1377–83.

[18] Mohopatra S, Gangadharan K, Pitchumoni C. Malnutrition in obesity before and after bariatric surgery, Disease-a-month. Elsevier; 2019. p. 305–32.

[19] Srtrain GW, Torghabeh MH, Gagner M, Ebel F, Dakin GF, Connolly D, Gildenberg E, Pomp A. Nutrient status 9 years after biliopancreatic diversion with duodenal switch (BPD/DS): an observational study. Obes Surg 2017;27(7):1709−18.

[20] Kanerva N, Larsson I, Peltonen M, Lindroos A, Carlsson LM. Changes in total energy intake and macronutrient composition after bariatric surgery predict long-term weight outcome: findings from the Swedish Obese Subjects (SOS) study. Am J Clin Nutr 2017;106(1):136−45.

[21] Billeter A, Fischer L, Wekerle A, Senft J, Müllerstich B. Malabsorption as a therapeutic approach in bariatric surgery. Viszeralmedizin 2014;30(3):2.

[22] Steenackers N, Van Der Schueren B, Mertens A, et al. Iron deficiency after bariatric surgery: what is the real problem? Proc Nutr Soc 2018;77(4):445−55. https://doi.org/10.1017/S0029665118000149.

[23] Punchai S, Hanipah ZN, Meister KM, Schauer PR, Brethauer SA, Aminian A. Neurologic manifestations of vitamin B deficiency after bariatric surgery. Obes Surg 2017;27(8):2079−82. https://doi.org/10.1007/s11695-017-2607-8.

[24] Dijkhorst PJ, Boerboom AB, Janssen IMC, et al. Failed sleeve gastrectomy: single anastomosis duodenoileal bypass or roux-en-Y gastric bypass? A multicenter cohort study. Obes Surg 2018;28(12):3834−42.

[25] Zaveri H, Surve A, Cottam D, et al. Mid-term 4-year outcomes with single anastomosis duodenal-ileal bypass with sleeve gastrectomy surgery at a single US center. Obes Surg 2018;28(10):3062−72.

[26] Parrott J, Frank L, Rabena R, Craggs-dino L, Isom KA, Greiman L. American Society for Metabolic and Bariatric Surgery integrated health nutritional guidelines for the surgical weight loss patient 2016 Update: micronutrients. Surg Obes Relat Dis 2017;13(5):727−41.

[27] Shoar S, Poliakin L, Rubenstein R, Saber AA. Single anastomosis duodeno-ileal switch (SADIS): a systematic review of efficacy and safety. Obes Surg 2018;28(1):104−13.

[28] Topart P, Becouarn G. The single anastomosis duodenal switch modifications: a review of the current literature on outcomes. Surg Obes Relat Dis 2017;13(8):1306−12.

[29] Ceha CMM, van Wezenbeek MR, Versteegden DPA, Smulders JF, Nienhuijs SW. Matched short-term results of SADI versus GBP after sleeve gastrectomy. Obes Surg 2018;28(12):3809−14.

[30] Homan J, Schijns W, Aarts EO, Janssen IMC, Berends FJ, Boer H. Treatment of vitamin and mineral deficiencies after biliopancreatic diversion with or without duodenal switch: a major challenge. Obes Surg 2017;28(1):234−41.

[31] Quesada-Gomez JM, Bouillon R. Is calcifediol better than cholecalciferol for vitamin D supplementation? Osteoporos Int 2018;29:1697−711.

[32] Busetto L, Dicker D, Azran C, Batterham RL, Farpour-lambert N, Fried M, et al. Practical recommendations of the obesity management task force of the European association for the study of obesity for the post-bariatric surgery medical management. Obes Facts 2017;10(6):597−632.

[33] Rousseau C, Jean S, Gamache P, et al. Change in fracture risk and fracture pattern after bariatric surgery: a nested case-control study. BMJ 2016;354:i3794.

[34] Yu EW, Lee MP, Landon JE, Lindeman KG, Kim SC. Fracture risk after bariatric surgery: roux-en-Y gastric bypass versus adjustable gastric banding. J Bone Miner Res 2017;32:1229−36.

[35] Sukumar D, Ambia-Sobhan H, Zurfluh R, et al. Areal and volumetric bone mineral density and geometry at two levels of protein intake during caloric restriction: a randomized, controlled trial. J Bone Miner Res 2011;26:1339—48.

[36] Zaveri H, Surve A, Cottam D, et al. Does bismuth subgallate affect smell and stool character? A randomized double-blinded placebo-controlled trial of bismuth subgallate on loop duodenal switch patients with complaints of smelly stools and diarrhea. Obes Surg 2018;28(11):3511—7. https://doi.org/10.1007/s11695-018-3369-7.

CHAPTER 13

Postoperative vitamin and mineral supplementation

Ma Jose Castro Alija[1,2], Jose María Jiménez Perez[1,2], Ana García del Rio[3]

[1]*Faculty of Nursing, University of Valladolid, Valladolid, Spain;* [2]*Endocrinology and Clinical Nutrition Research Center (ECNRC), Valladolid, Spain;* [3]*CIC bioGUNE, Bizkaia Technology Park, Derio, Spain*

Chapter outline

Introduction	173
Nutritional deficiencies according to the different surgical techniques in bariatric surgery	174
Restrictive techniques	175
Malabsorptive techniques	175
Mixed procedures	175
Recommendations for vitamin and mineral supplementation after bariatric surgery	177
Thiamine	178
Folate acid	178
Vitamin B12	178
Vitamin D	179
Vitamin A	179
Vitamin K	179
Vitamin E	180
Iron	180
Calcium	181
Zinc	181
Implications and decision making. Supplementation, consensus, and evidence	181
References	184

Introduction

Nutritional alterations, including vitamin and mineral deficiencies, are the most common complications after bariatric surgery, as different surgical techniques can lead to altered intake patterns, decreased tolerance, food consumption and selection, and malabsorption, resulting in an increased risk of frequent short- and long-term nutritional deficiencies [1].

Bariatric surgery, whether by restrictive, malabsorptive, or mixed techniques, can produce a deficit of micronutrients due to surgical complications or to the lack of follow-up of nutritional recommendations by the patient or intensify preoperative nutritional deficiencies, generally due to unbalanced diets, which increase with surgical procedure and rapid weight loss and can even produce severe malnutrition. For this reason, after this type of intervention, monitoring and adequate supplementation is required for life with programmed follow-up by the therapeutic team.

The nutritional recommendations for the bariatric surgery patient may vary slightly according to the type of surgical technique used [2], but it is essential that there are adequate concentrations of vitamins and minerals, for optimal health, especially when losing weight, and during weight maintenance.

The need for supplementation will depend on the type of technique used, the type of feeding performed by the patient, his or her clinical characteristics, age, and the coexistence of pathologies that favor deficiencies. Although the most influential factor is the surgical procedure, which induces anatomical changes in the digestive system, it is also frequent that nutritional deficiencies occur due to the lack of follow-up of the nutritional treatment or due to the lack of knowledge of the dietary pattern to be followed, or due to the need for dietary modifications and the nonattendance of nutritional controls.

It is a fact that all patients will require permanent vitamin and mineral supplements, so after surgery it is important: to provide a complete vitamin-mineral complex that covers at least 100% of the recommended dietary allowance (RDA) [3]; and specifically supplement those vitamins that tend to be more deficient depending on the bariatric technique chosen. Thus, in malabsorptive techniques, attention must be paid to deficiencies of iron, calcium, vitamin B12, and vitamin D [4]. In cases of emesis, thiamine is the most deficient vitamin; and if there is a malabsorptive component, attention must be paid to liposoluble vitamins (A, D, E, K) among other micronutrients.

In most cases, metabolic and nutritional complications are predictable, and therefore can be addressed prophylactically and therapeutically through patient supplementation and follow-up.

Difficulties in maintaining supplementation are conditioned by the fact that when the patient achieves the lost weight they do not continue with the supplement or resume inadequate eating habits, or they do not receive nutritional education, which leads to their not considering nutrition as an integral part of their treatment and the failure of the initial weight loss and after a few years a weight regain occurs. This is why nutritional preparation before surgery is essential to optimize postoperative results [5].

Nutritional education is required before and after surgery to detect preexisting nutritional deficiencies that may become acute after surgery and to correct them, to avoid failure to follow nutritional treatment or because dietary modifications are required, and to avoid nonattendance at nutritional checks.

Nutritional deficiencies according to the different surgical techniques in bariatric surgery

The main techniques approved by the international federation for surgery of obesity and metabolic disorders (IFSO), we can distinguish the following restrictive techniques: adjustable gastric banding (AGB), sleeve gastrectomy (SG). biliopancreatic biversion (BPD) as malabsortive technique and Roux-en-Y gastric bypass (RYGB) and one-anastomosis gastric bypass (OAGB) as mixed techniques.

Restrictive techniques [4]

In restrictive procedures, there is no malabsorption, but the passage of the bolus through the digestive tract is restricted [6], reducing the speed and capacity of ingestion, producing before the sensation of satiety, and reducing the capacity of food consumed. For that reason, a dietetic adjustment is required so that the nutritional contribution is sufficient because otherwise it can be produced deficit mainly of thiamine, iron, folate, and calcium [7].

Although deficiencies in iron, vitamin B12, and calcium are not common in this type of technique, the decrease in gastric acid can reduce the absorption of calcium and, in some cases, lactose intolerance can result in lower oral calcium intake.

In sleeve gastrectomy, by excluding the gastric body: there is a possibility of vitamin B12 malabsorption due to the absence of intrinsic factor.

In these restrictive procedures, monitoring of nutritional status is recommended and routine supplementation is required, through a multivitamin complex and the rest according to individual evolution when intake is not sufficient or nutritional deficiencies are observed.

Malabsorptive techniques [4]

These techniques alter the anatomy of the digestive tract and the stomach is reduced, producing a sensation of satiety more quickly. In addition, a large part of the small intestine becomes inactive and the sections of absorption are reduced, both at the proximal level (duodenum, jejunum) and distal level (jejunum and terminal ileum) restricting the amount of calories and nutrients absorbed by the body. So, it is very important to control the supply of minerals such as iron and calcium, zinc and vitamins such as vitamin B12, thiamine and also, since the daily absorption of fat is diminished, we must pay attention to fat-soluble vitamins (A, D, E, K).

Mixed procedures

This type of bariatric surgery shares the recommendations of the restrictive techniques and, in addition, most of the gastric cavity, duodenum, and first jejunum handles are excluded from the food passage, limiting significantly the absorption mainly of iron, calcium, and some vitamins (folate, thiamine). It is, therefore, necessary to cover the requirements, paying special attention to possible deficiencies of iron, calcium, and some vitamins such as folic acid, thiamine, and vitamin B12.

With these techniques, there is a late contact of the food with the biliopancreatic secretions, which leads to the malabsorption of fats and limits the absorption of fat-soluble vitamins [8].

In these techniques, the effect of malabsorption on phosphocalcic metabolism must be highlighted. Calcium is mainly absorbed in the duodenum and the proximal jejunum so its bypass causes a malabsorption of this micronutrient. Therefore, the administration of calcium and vitamin D is recommended to prevent a negative calcium balance and the risk of osteopenia and secondary hyperparathyroidism.

Calcium is absorbed in the proximal duodenum and jejunum, which is usually excluded in gastric bypass, which in turn is dependent on vitamin D concentrations. This anatomical situation after surgery together with the low intake of dairy products to cover daily requirements can lead to a deficiency in calcium absorption with repercussions on phosphocalcic metabolism (Fig. 13.1).

In a gastric bypass, vitamin B12 deficiency is very common (30%) [9], due to a decrease in the secretion of pepsin required to obtain cobalamin from the meats that contain it and also due to a lack of intrinsic factor, since the stomach is excluded. The deficiency of this vitamin usually appears as soon as the body's reserves are reduced, which is usually after a year of surgery.

Iron deficiency is also quite common after bariatric surgery (50%–70%), due to the anatomical conditions of a gastric bypass [9], as well as other factors such as decreased consumption of red meat, intolerance to this food, and a low intake of iron-rich foods, to which is added a decrease in gastric acidity that hinders the absorption of iron, which in women of childbearing age is even more evident.

In general, nutritional deficiencies are more common in patients undergoing mixed techniques (RYGB, OAGB) or malabsorptive techniques (BPD) than in those undergoing restrictive techniques (SG, AGB).

A review by Shankar et al. [10] identifies micronutrient deficiencies that occur after bariatric surgery. The authors conclude that bariatric surgery patients, especially after mixed and malabsorptive techniques, are at risk for deficiencies of the following nutrients: vitamin B12, vitamin B1, vitamin C, folic acid, vitamin A, vitamin D, and vitamin K, as well as the following minerals: iron, zinc, selenium, and copper. It is recommended that all patients undergoing bariatric surgery receive vitamin and mineral supplements, although the level of evidence from studies is not stated.

Taking into account *Via clinica de cirugía Bariatrica 2017* [11], with the collaboration of the AEC (Spanish association of surgeons), SECO (Spanish society for the surgery of obesity), FUNSECO (foundation of the Spanish society for the surgery of obesity), indicates that the routine control of thiamine, pyridoxine, fat-soluble

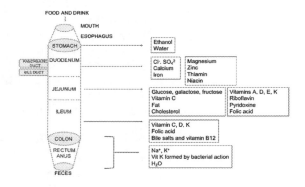

FIGURE 13.1

Location of absorption of each nutrient.

vitamins (A, E, K), zinc (Zn), selenium (Se), copper (Cu) is not required, except in cases of inadequate intake, persistent vomiting or data indicating intestinal malabsorption.

In contrast, deficiencies of vitamin E and vitamin K have been described after BPD, as well as zinc and copper deficiency frequent after mixed procedures (RYGB, OAGB).

Recommendations for vitamin and mineral supplementation after bariatric surgery

Nutritional deficiencies that may occur after bariatric surgery can have serious consequences. Therefore, a prompt identification and adequate treatment through nutritional supplements are recommended, as well as a regular preventive use of such supplements in patients who are candidates for bariatric surgery.

There is little evidence of recommendations for micronutrient supplementation after bariatric surgery. There is no unanimity, and most recommendations are based on judgment and consensus among experts from different scientific societies. However, most assume the need for micronutrient supplementation throughout life after bariatric surgery, although there are no controlled studies on the type and doses that should be used [12] and the form of administration of the supplements, so prospective studies are required to specify these data.

In general, there is an agreement that a continuous nutritional evaluation, adapted to the circumstances of each patient and the type of technique used, should be carried out. This evaluation should be more exhaustive in procedures with a malabsorptive component because the nutritional risk is greater, and therefore the use of supplements is indicated on a routine basis. It is essential to use polyvitamin and multimineral supplements systematically as prophylaxis and to control patient adherence through prolonged follow-up. In some situations where the polyvitamin supplement is insufficient, specific supplementation is also required.

The vitamin and mineral supplements used must contain iron, folic acid and thiamine, calcium, vitamin D, and vitamin B12 among other micronutrients.

The guide developed by the American Association of Clinical Endocrinologists, the Obesity Society and the American Society for Metabolic and Bariatric Surgery [13] update the data from previous guidance conducted in 2008 recommends a nutritional study before bariatric surgery, which should be more extensive for malabsorptive or mixed procedures compared to purely restrictive procedures (Grade A). The recommendations include a weight reduction and preoperative nutritional supplementation in situations where this is required. This guide recognizes that the general recommendations on micronutrient deficiencies and their treatment were designated as Grade A based on expert consensus, but that there are no relevant studies with evidence level 1 for all vitamins and minerals.

The Spanish Society of Bariatric Surgery (SECO) and the Spanish Society for the Study of Obesity (SEEDO) [14] recommend preventive supplementation of all micronutrients through the administration of multivitamin and multimineral preparations in all patients undergoing bariatric surgery.

There are risk factors that favor the appearance of nutritional deficiencies after bariatric surgery; in general, the techniques that generate restriction or malabsorption will be a determining factor, but also the lack of adherence to the dietary treatment of patients, the appearance or reappearance of eating disorders, as well as the presence of surgical complications.

Recommendations for water-soluble and fat-soluble vitamins include the following:

Thiamine

The RDA [3] of thiamine is 1.2 mg/day for the adult male, 1.1 mg/day for the female (approximately 0.5 mg/1000 kcal), and 1.4 mg/day during pregnancy and lactation. Thiamine supplementation is recommended on a routine basis, with at least 1.5 mg/day, present in currently available multivitamins [15].

The reserve of thiamine in the body of an adult is approximately 30 mg with a half-life of 9—18 days so that the lack is evident in the first months after surgery, related to the existence of other risk factors such as inadequate intake, emesis, and enolism.

Folate acid

The recommended RDA for adults is 400 mcg/day, which is the amount present in polyvitamin and multimineral supplements. The total content of folates in the body is between 5 and 10 mg.

The prevalence of folic acid deficiency after bariatric surgery is variable [16], although it is not very frequent. The causes may be a decrease in intake, malabsorption, and, above all, poor adherence to recommended supplementation, especially in patients who have undergone surgery using restrictive techniques.

Vitamin B12

The RDA is 2.4 mcg/day for adults. Vitamin B12 deficiency is common after bariatric surgery, especially after RYGB.

The main causes of the deficit are due to the process of malabsorption and poor digestion mainly due to a deficient acid secretion, an accelerated intestinal transit by the bypass, and a low bioavailability of the intrinsic factor. Another conditioning factor is the decreased intake of foods rich in this vitamin.

As there is a high prevalence of subclinical deficit, prophylactic vitamin B12 supplementation has been proposed universally in patients undergoing bariatric surgery.

The occurrence of deficiencies does not usually occur before the year of intervention as the body's reserves are much higher than the daily needs.

Polyvitamins are not enough, for this reason specific supplementation is required. It could be oral at high doses 1000 mcg/day, subcutaneous or intramuscular

1000 mcg/month. Intramuscular administration of vitamin B12 is the most recommended guideline compared to oral supplementation due to the decreased availability of intrinsic factor after bariatric surgery [5].

Vitamin B12 concentrations should be monitored in surgeries where the lower stomach is partially or totally excluded as in SG and RYGB.

Vitamin D

The current RDA for 25-OH vitamin D is 5—15 μg/day or 400 international units (IU). Vitamin D deficiency must be distinguished: if the serum levels are less than 20 ng/mL it is diagnosed deficiency and with levels between 21 and 29 ng/mL it is diagnosed insufficiency.

In the liposoluble vitamins, vitamin D deficiency is the most frequent, mainly in techniques with a malabsorptive component. In BPD, a minimum of 2000—3000 IU/day is recommended, and higher doses of up to 50,000 IU per week can be reached. Vitamin D deficiency is also evident with restrictive techniques such as SG and AGB, which is why 800—1200 IU/day of vitamin D is recommended [17].

Low levels of vitamin D are associated with a decrease in serum calcium, which causes an increase in parathormone (PTH) and consequently secondary hyperparathyroidism that can lead to osteomalacia.

Many obese patients present a preoperative deficit of 25-OH-cholecalciferol and a secondary hyperparathyroidism that may be due to several factors: deficit in the intake, poor sun exposure, or alterations in the synthesis by hepatic steatosis. The doses of vitamin D (calcifediol or cholecalciferol) to be administered in patients with vitamin D levels < 30 ng/dL should be higher than 2000—3000 IU/day to ensure adequate supplementation and that secondary hyperparathyroidism does not occur.

Vitamin A

The RDA is at 700—900 μg/day or 5000 UI/day. Vitamin A deficiency is more common after malabsorptive procedures. Vitamin A deficiencies have also been described in patients with RYGB or BPD [15]. A contribution from 25,000 IU to high doses of 50,000 IU is recommended. The use of retinol is recommended in patients with low levels of retinol, although excess supply must be controlled because it carries risks due to accumulation, monitoring plasma concentrations to control possible hepatotoxicity. In malabsorptive techniques, some authors recommend a preventive supplementation with 50,000 IU/day [18].

The decrease is related to the deficit of proteins, and it is necessary to adjust the contribution according to levels of prealbumin and to take into account if there is a deficit of iron or copper since they can make it difficult to solve the deficit of vitamin A.

Vitamin K

The RDA is 90—120 μg/day. Although the deficiency is infrequent, a lower bioavailability may occur when accompanied by a decrease in prothrombin time that usually occurs after RYGB [19].

It may also occur after BPD in relation to fat malabsorption and limitation of common channel length. Recommendations for postsurgical supplementation are unclear, although 25% of the RDA has been suggested for restrictive techniques and RYGB, and 100% of the RDA after BPD [18].

Vitamin E

The RDA is 15—20 mg/day. The deficit is rare.

There may be a decrease in vitamin E after bariatric surgery in relation to a decrease in total lipids, and this should be adjusted according to cholesterol levels.

Some authors recommend supplementing with the RDA (15—20 mg/day) after pure restrictive techniques and RYGB, and with 150—200 mg/day in BPD [20].

With regard to the recommendations for mineral supplementation, the main emphasis is on the following:

Iron

The adult RDA for iron is 8 mg/day for men and women over 50 years of age, and 18 mg per day for women under 50 years of age.

Anemia in obese patients is not uncommon before bariatric surgery.

Iron deficiency and postsurgical iron-deficiency anemia depend on the type of technique used, the follow-up time, and the type of polyvitamin supplements used.

In pure restrictive techniques such as AGB [21] or SG it is usual, while in BG or DBP, anemia is diagnosed quite frequently not only because of the anatomical conditions of a gastric bypass but also because of other factors that contribute to further aggravation of iron deficiency [22].

The factors that favor iron deficiency are as follows:

- Reduced intake of red meat mainly due to intolerance or due to iron-rich mollusks
- The decrease of gastric acidity by resection of the proximal stomach that prevents the passage of the ferric to ferrous form necessary to favor its absorption
- The decrease in iron absorption by the exclusion of the duodenum.

The risk of ferropenia is even more important in women of childbearing age. In women of childbearing age, the dose should be increased to 390 mg/day.

The iron contained in multivitamins is not sufficient if there are significant deficiencies, so a specific supplement is required in addition to the iron contained in the multivitamin supplement. Iron supplementation [23] should be carried out with ferrous compounds, such as fumarate, sulfate, or gluconate, at a dose of 150—300 mg/day of elemental iron, divided into two or three intakes accompanied by vitamin C simultaneously, to improve absorption and on an empty stomach, avoiding foods that interfere with absorption (foods with fiber and foods rich in calcium). If there is intolerance by the oral route, it will be necessary to resort to intravenous administration in a single dose of up to 1000 mg/week.

Calcium

The RDA of calcium for adults is 1000–1300 mg/day. Absorption may be impaired by the presence of foods rich in phytates and oxalates, vitamin D deficiency, and certain drugs [23].

Although a standard dose of calcium is not established, it is recommended to provide supplements in doses of 1000–2000 mg/day, depending on dietary intake. The use of calcium citrate is preferable to calcium carbonate because it is better absorbed in situations of hypochlorhydria. After RYGB and BPD, the use of supplements including oral calcium and vitamin D is generally and prophylactically recommended to prevent secondary hyperparathyroidism and loss of bone mass [24].

Zinc

The RDA is 8 mg/day. Zinc deficiency after gastric by-pass is due to the fact that its absorption occurs in the duodenum and proximal jejunum, and also due to a low intake, as its food sources are generally poorly tolerated.

After bariatric surgery, it is recommended to ingest four times the RDA of zinc, depending on the type of procedure.

In malabsorptive techniques, a multivitamin containing 200% of the RDA (16–22 mg/day) is recommended when using mixed procedures such as RYGB. The multivitamin should contain 100%–200% of the RDA (8–22 mg/day). In restrictive techniques SG or AGB, a multivitamin with minerals containing 100% of the RDA (8–11 mg/day) is reeommended [25,26].

Routine vitamin and mineral supplementation after bariatric surgery is effective in controlling possible nutritional deficiencies. Commercial preparations offer different alternatives in the supply of RDAs depending on the surgical technique, although as shown there is no unanimous recommendation, proposing the supplementation shown in Table 13.1.

Implications and decision making. Supplementation, consensus, and evidence

The use of nutritional supplements in patients undergoing bariatric surgery is a recommendation supported by the different clinical guidelines for bariatric surgery highlighting both the guides developed by the American Association of Clinical Endocrinologists, the Obesity Society and the American Society for Metabolic and Bariatric Surgery [13] as the guides developed by the European Chapter of the International Federation for the Surgery of Obesity (IFSO-EC), the European Association for the Study of Obesity (EASO), and the EASO Obesity Management Task Force (EASO OMTF) [27]. among others, which highlight the need for early identification of possible nutritional deficiencies and appropriate therapy through the use of nutritional supplements in patients in which bariatric surgery is indicated.

Table 13.1 Recommended dietary allowance (RDA): postoperative vitamin and mineral supplementation.

Vitamins	Restrictive techniques Doses	%RDA	Malabsorptive techniques Doses	%RDA	Mixed techniques Doses	%RDA
Vitamin A (Retinyl palmitate)	800 µg	100%	2,4 mg	300%	600 µg –1.2 mg	75% –150%
Vitamin B1 (Thiamine)	2,75 mg	250%	3,0 mg	273%	2.75 –3 mg	250% –273%
Vitamin B2 (Riboflavin)	2 mg	143%	3,5 mg	250%	3.5 mg	250%
Vitamin B3 (Nicotinamide)	25 mg	156%	32 mg	200%	32 mg	200%
Vitamin B5 (Calcium pantothenate)	9 mg	150%	18 mg	300%	18 mg	300%
Vitamin B6 (Piridoxal 5'phosphate)	2 mg	143%	1,4 mg	100%	0.98 –1.12 mg	70%–80%
Vitamin B8 (biotine)	150 µg	300%	100 µg	200%	100 µg	200%
Vitamin B9 (Folate acid)	500 µg	250%	600 µg	300%	600 –800 µg	300% –400%
Vitamin B12 (Cyanocobalamin)	100 µg	4000%	500 µg	20,000%	350 –500 µg	14,000% –20000%
Vitamin C (Ascorbic acid)	100 mg	125%	120 mg	150%	120 –140 mg	150% –175%
Vitamin D3 (Cholecalciferol)	75 µg	1500%	75 µg	1500%	75 µg	1500%
Vitamin E (Tocopherol succinate)	15 mg	100%	150 mg	1000%	24–36 mg	100% –200%
Vitamin K	–		300 µg	400%	75 µg	100%
Minerals	**Doses**	**%RDA**	**Doses**	**%RDA**	**Doses**	**%RDA**
Chromium	40 µg	100%	160 µg	400%	160 µg	400%
Iron	28 mg	200%	91 mg	650%	70–85 mg	500% –607%
Iodine	150 µg	100%	225 µg	150%	225 µg	150%
Copper	1,9 mg	190%	3 mg	300%	3 mg	300%
Magnesium	–		–		–	
Manganese	3 mg	150%	3 mg	150%	3 mg	150%
Molybdenum	50 µg	100%	112.4 µg	225%	112.4 µg	225%
Selenium	55 µg	100%	105 µg	191%	105 µg	191%
Potassium	–		–		–	
Phosphorus	–		–		–	
Zinc	8 –15 mg	100%	22.5 mg	225%	22.5 –30 mg	225% –300%

These guidelines recommend an extensive nutritional evaluation before surgery to correct existing deficiencies that can be corrected before the operation and monitoring after surgery, and also establish recommendations for the minimum daily amounts to be provided by supplements according to the various techniques used both those with a malabsorptive component and for cases subjected to purely restrictive techniques.

The SECO and the SEEDO recommend preventive supplementation of all micronutrients through the administration of multivitamin and multimineral preparations in all patients undergoing bariatric surgery [28].

Follow-up after surgery is essential to reinforce eating patterns, control comorbidities, and detect and treat vitamin and mineral deficiencies.

The follow-up schedule depends on each institution. However, it is recommended that a set of tests be performed before surgery and then periodically at 3, 6, 9, and 12 months during the first year; in the second and third year, it is recommended twice a year and then once a year [29].

To achieve these objectives, it is necessary to remember the importance of nutritional education and lifestyle modifications, as well as the need for support from the multidisciplinary team [30].

In general, there is an agreement that a continuous nutritional evaluation, adapted to the circumstances of each patient and the type of technique used, should be carried out. This evaluation should be more exhaustive in procedures with a malabsorptive component, as the nutritional risk is greater, and therefore the use of supplements is indicated on a routine basis. The use of polyvitamin and multimineral supplements is essential as systematic prophylaxis and to control patient adherence through prolonged follow-up. In some situations where multivitamin supplementation is insufficient, specific supplementation is also required.

Almost all guidelines agree to recommend in patients undergoing mixed and malabsorptive procedures two adult multivitamin and mineral supplements (containing iron, folic acid, and thiamine); 1200–1500 mg/day of elemental calcium (in diet and as a citrate supplement in divided doses); at least 3000 (IU) of vitamin D; and vitamin B12 needed to maintain B12 levels in the normal range [31].

Bariatric surgery in general is safe and effective, but it can present new clinical problems associated with possible nutritional deficiencies resulting from the surgical intervention, so after the intervention there should be a multidisciplinary follow-up program [32].

Bariatric surgery entails a modification of the anatomy of the gastrointestinal tract and a modification of the dietary guidelines that must be adapted to the new physiological conditions, both in relation to the volume of the intakes and to the needs of the macronutrients and micronutrients that the patient requires. Furthermore, this adaptation may be accompanied by certain problems, most of which can be alleviated and/or solved, so the supplementation must be individualized and each patient will have a personalized supplementation depending on the diet he or she consumes.

References

[1] Fujioka K, DiBaise J, Martindale RG. Nutrition and metabolic complications after bariatric surgery and their treatment. JPEN (J Parenter Enteral Nutr) 2011;35:S52–9.

[2] Rubio MA, Moreno C. Implicaciones nutricionales de la cirugía bariatrica sobre el tracto gastrointestinal. Nutr Hosp 2007;22(Suppl. 2):124–34.

[3] IOM (Institute of Medicine). Dietary reference intakes: applications in dietary assessment. Washington DC: National Academy Press; 2000b.

[4] Ballesteros MD, González de Francisco T, Cano I. Prevención y manejo de las deficiencias nutricionales tras la cirugía bariátrica. In: Rubio MA, editor. Manual de obesidad mórbida. Madrid: Editorial Médica Panamericana; 2006. p. 309–21.

[5] Majumder SDM, Soriano J, Cruz AL, Dasanu CA. Vitamin B 12 deficiency in patients undergoing bariatric surgery: Preventive strategies and key recommendations. Surg Obes Relat Dis 2013;9:1013–9.

[6] Mason EE. Development and future of gastroplasties for morbid obesity. Arch Surg 2003;138:361–6.

[7] Buchwald H, Williams SE. Bariatric surgery worldwide 2003. Obes Surg 2004;14: 1157–64.

[8] RIED M, Yumuk V, Oppert JM, Scopinaro N, Torres A, Weiner R, et al. Interdisciplinary European guidelines on metabolic and bariatric surgery. Obes Surg 2014; 24(1):42–55. Springer US.

[9] Brolin RE, Gorman JH, Gorman RC, Petschenik AJ, Bradley LJ, Kenler HA, et al. Are vitamin B12 and folate deficiency clinically important after Roux-en-gastric bypass? J Gastrointest Surg 1998;2(5):436–42. No longer published by Elsevier.

[10] Shankar B, Sriram K. Micronutrient deficiencies after bariatric surgery. Nutrition 2010; 26(11–12):1031–7.

[11] Martín García-Almenta E, Ruiz-Tovar Polo J, Sánchez Santos R. Vía Clínica de Cirugía Bariátrica 2017. 2017. SECO [online]. Available from: https://www.seco.org/guiasconsensos_es_27.html.

[12] Fried M, Hainer V, Basdevant A, Buchwald H, Deitel M, Finer N, et al. Interdisciplinary European guidelines on surgery of severe obesity. Int J Obes 2007;31:569–77.

[13] Mechanick JI, Youdim A, Jones DB, et al. Clinical practice guidelines for the perioperative nutritional, metabolic, and nonsurgical support of the bariatric surgery patient — 2013 update : cosponsored by American Association of Clinical Endocrinologists. Obes Soc Am Soc 2013;21:1–27.

[14] Obesity Surgery A Spanish Society joint SECO and SEEDO approach to the postoperative management of the patients undergoing surgery for obesity https://doi.org/10.1007/s11695-019-04043-8.

[15] Isom KA, Andromalos L, Ariagno M, et al. Nutrition and metabolic support recommendations for the bariatric patient. Nutr Clin Pract 2014;29:718–39.

[16] Weng TC, Chang CH, Dong YH, et al. Anaemia and related nutrient deficiencies after Roux-en-Y gastric bypass surgery: a systematic review and meta-analysis. BMJ Open 2015;5:e006964.

[17] Chakhtoura MT, Nakhoul N, Akl EA, et al. Guidelines on vitamin D replacement in bariatric surgery: identification and systematic appraisal. Metabolism 2016;65:586–97.

[18] Aasheim ET, Björkman S, Sovik TT, Engström M, Manvold SE, Mala T, et al. Vitamin status after bariatric surgery: a randomized study of gastric bypass and duodenal switch. Am J Clin Nutr 2009;90:15–22.

[19] Coupaye M, Puchaux K, Bogard C, Msika S, Jouet P, Clerici C. Nutritional consequences of adjustable gastric banding and gastric bypass: a 1-year prospective study. Obes Surg 2009;19:56—65.
[20] Madan, et al. Vitamin and trace mineral levels after laparoscopic gastric bypass. Obes Surg 2006;16:603—6.
[21] Von Dygralsky A, Andris DA. Anemia alter bariatric surgery: more than just iron deficiency. Nutr Clin Pract 2009;24:217—26.
[22] Amaya García MJ, Vilchez López FJ, Campos Martín C, Sánchez Vera P, Pereira Cunill JL. Revisión Micronutrientes en cirugía bariátrica. Nutr Hosp 2012;27(2): 349—61.
[23] Malone M. Recommended nutritional supplements for bariatric surgery patients. Ann Pharmacother 2008;42:1851—8.
[24] Mechanick JI, Kushner RF, Sugerman HJ, Gonzalez-Campoy JM, Collazo-Clavell ML, Guven S, et al. AACE/TOS/ASMBS Bariatric surgery guidelines. Endocr Pract 2008; 14(Suppl. 1):1—83.
[25] Rubio C, González Weller D, Martín-Izquierdo RE, Revert C, Rodríguez I, Hardisson A. El zinc: oligoelemento esencial. Nutr Hosp 2007;22:101—7.
[26] Balsa JA, Botella-Carretero JI, Gómez-Martín JM, Peromingo R, Arrieta F, Santiuste C, et al. Copper and zinc serum levels after derivative bariatric surgery: differences between Rouxen-Y Gastric bypass and biliopancreatic diversion. Obes Surg 2011;21: 744—50.
[27] Fried M, Yumuk V, Oppert JM, et al. Interdisciplinary European guidelines on metabolic and bariatric surgery. Obes Surg 2014;24(1):42-55. https://doi.org/10.1007/s11695-013-1079-8.
[28] Vilallonga R, Pereira-Cunill J, Morales-Conde S, et al. A Spanish Society joint SECO and SEEDO approach to the Post-operative management of the patients undergoing surgery for obesity. Obes Surg 2019;29:3842—53. https://doi.org/10.1007/s11695-019-04043-8.
[29] Malinowski S. Nutritional and metabolic complications of bariatric surgery. Am J Med Sci 2006;331:219—25.
[30] Guisado JA, Vaz FJ, Alarcón J, López-Ibor JJ, Rubio MA, Gaite L. Psycopathological status and interpersonal function following weight loss in morbidly obese patients undergoing bariatric surgery. Obes Surg 2002;12:835—40.
[31] American Society for Metabolic and Bariatric Surgery Integrated Health Nutritional Guidelines for the Surgical Weight Loss Patient 2016 Update: Micronutrients. Surgery for Obesity and Related Diseases 13. 2017. p. 727—41. https://doi.org/10.1016/J.SOARD.2016.12.018.
[32] Busetto L, Dicker D, Azran C, et al. Obesity Management Task Force of the European Association for the study of obesity released "practical recommendations for the post-bariatric surgery medical management". Obes Surg 2018;28:2117—21. https://doi.org/10.1007/s11695-018-3283-z.

CHAPTER 14

Special nutritional requirements in children and adolescents undergoing bariatric surgery

Pablo Priego[1,2]

[1]*Division of Esophagogastric and Bariatric Surgery, Ramón y Cajal University Hospital, Madrid, Spain;* [2]*Surgery, University Alcalá de Henares, Madrid, Spain*

Chapter outline

Introduction	187
Nutritional assessment	188
Nutrition education	189
Nutritional needs	190
Nutritional monitoring	194
Hunger assessment	194
Academic environment	194
Reproductive health	196
Special cases	196
Conclusion	196
References	197

Introduction

The prevalence of obesity in children and adolescents has quadrupled over the past 30 years [1]. Approximately 18.5% of youth in the United States meet the criteria of obesity (i.e., body mass index [BMI] percentile ≥95th for age and sex) [2,3]. In addition, most adolescents have a 50%–77% risk of becoming obese adults with an increase to approximately 80% given one obese parent [4].

In view of this, the American Society for Metabolic and Bariatric Surgery (ASMBS) has considered that bariatric surgery (BS) is a safe and effective treatment for obesity in adolescents and should be considered standard of care [1].

Children and adolescents present exclusive factors specific to their age-related that must be addressed before BS and that are different from standardized approach for adults.

Based on best practice guidelines, a multidisciplinary team (MDT) approach is mandatory to optimize the care of these adolescent obese patients [5]. MDT composition varies from program to program; however, the ASMBS suggested that a team should include an experienced bariatric surgeon, pediatric specialist (pediatric endocrinologist, gastroenterologist, or adolescent specialist), registered dietician (RD), mental health specialist, coordinator, and an exercise physiologist.

Nowadays, there is a lack of standardization of nutrition management for bariatric adolescent patients, and the existing nutrition recommendations are based on best-practice guidelines [6,7].

The current manuscript presents a consensus of recommendations based on the description by the literature and provides interesting information regarding on how to assess, educate, nourish, and monitor the adolescent patients undergoing BS.

Nutritional recommendations for the treatment of the adolescent undergoing BS can be classified into four areas: nutritional assessment, nutrition education, nutritional needs, and monitoring of nutritional status.

Nutritional assessment

Nutritional assessment for adolescents should undergo the following items:

- Assess their ability to understand the risks/benefits of an invasive, nonreversible, elective surgical procedure. These patients have subjected themselves to many physical and psychological changes in this part of their life.
- Assess nutritional deficiencies: Obesity is a known risk factor for micronutrient deficiencies, and BS can worsen or add to these deficiencies [8]. Deficiencies can be attributed to nutrient-poor food choices, lack of dairy and low fruit and vegetable, and/or whole-grain intake.

  Given that, all obese adolescents' candidates for BS should go through an appropriate nutritional evaluation to diagnose nutritional deficiencies and educational needs, especially when a malabsorptive procedure is planned.

  The recommended laboratory parameters to be considered as part of the nutritional evaluation include complete blood cell count with iron, transferrin, and ferritin, red blood cell folate (homocysteine level recommended in some centers for folate monitoring), vitamins B1, B6, B12, calcium, and 25-hydroxy vitamin D level.

  If preexisting nutritional deficiencies are identified in the initial laboratory test, the RD has to advise the patient and to correct these deficiencies. Anyway, and for all children and adolescents patients, a preoperative multivitamin regimen should be recommended to correct these possible preexisting deficiencies.

- Assess diet and current intake using a food frequency/eating behavior questionnaire (eating out, portions, beverages, timing of meals, fluid intake, eating habits, attitudes, and patterns). In addition, the RD has to encourage patients to eat in

small plates and to use small utensils. A recent meta-analysis indicated that approximately one in four children and adolescents with overweight or obesity report binge eating or loss of control eating (LOC) [9]. Correlates of preoperative binge eating disorder and/or LOC include greater comorbid psychopathology and poorer weight-related quality of life [10], suggesting disordered eating may be a signal for another psychosocial burden. Patients who screen positively for eating disordered behavior should receive appropriate intervention. However, given that it is treatable, LOC eating should not be considered a contraindication to BS [1].
- Evaluate family, family support, and home environment, locations where significant time is spent, locations, where food/meals are eaten, financial restraints in procuring healthy food, culture/traditional foods, and parenting style.

The family and home environment play an important role in the adolescent's life. However, it is important to define "family," because this may not be at the permanent address. Moreover, all caregivers within the "family" network should be invited to attend any nutrition education sessions.

Indeed, it is not surprising that the majority of obese adolescents have a primary caregiver who has obesity, if not severe obesity [11]. Interestingly, approximately one in four adolescents have a primary caregiver who has undergone BS themselves. Rates of problematic family functioning are notable (i.e., one in every two to three families) with adolescents and caregivers reporting unhealthy communication, less interest/involvement with one another, and challenges in working together [11]. In those cases, a psychology consult should be considered. Finally, and another important condition, it is to identify the parenting style because this plays an important role in how families approach nutritional counseling around BS. Baumrind [12] developed four models of parenting: authoritarian, authoritative, permissive, and disengaged. *Authoritarian* style is demonstrated via strict rule setting and abidance and adolescents may be best motivated. The *authoritative* style leads to parents being warm and involved, yet consistent and firm in the limit setting. *Permissive* parents are those who are accepting and impose a few rules and restrictions, so these adolescents may have difficulty around rule setting and may test the guidelines established by the clinician. *Disengaged* parents often present as disinterested and may not provide the support to help the adolescent with adherence.

- Assess physical activity levels (i.e., structured, activities of daily living, hours on TV/computer/phone, physical limitations).
- Review prior weight loss attempts.

Nutrition education

It is important to have a standardized program so that all adolescents receive the same information. However, it has to be noticed that each patient has a different learning style, so information may need to be presented in a range of different teaching models. It is also advisable to educate patients regarding the basics postoperative nutrition principles of BS. Although there is no standardization between the programs on particular outcome goals that should be achieved, both clinician and patient should agree to eliminate sugared beverages consuming three or six meals per day (depending on the procedure), and taking vitamins directly both preoperative and postoperative.

The format can be in a group setting or individual sessions. It takes time to develop affinity and build confidence with adolescents. Ideally, the teenager should have at least one MDT member that he or she regularly sees at each clinical visit.

The RD should teach patients regarding "healthy eating," including appropriate serving sizes and food quality according to the dietary guidelines. Moreover, it is recommended that adolescents be encouraged to maintain some methods of self-monitoring such as food records, recording healthy foods that they are eating because it has been reported to help in weight maintenance [13].

It is recommended that educational information be provided in verbal and written fashion. Due to differing learning styles and family support, the number of visits may require some flexibility. A minimum of six preoperative nutrition visits is recommended to complete the nutritional assessment and educational components in preparation for BS. Anyway, most of the adolescent bariatric centers require at least 6 months of preoperative visits, and the preoperative phase lasts an average of 10 months.

The diet progression regimens for Roux-en-Y gastric bypass (RYGB), vertical gastrectomy (VG), and laparoscopic adjustable gastric banding (LAGB) will vary by the number of meals per day, the consistency, and progression of the amount of food consumed at a meal (Tables 14.1 and 14.2).

The postoperative diet focuses on a high protein diet (1.0–1.5 g protein/kg ideal body weight), low in simple carbohydrates, free of added simple sugars, and with modest fat intake.

Nutritional needs

Nonadherence with medical regimens is frequent between adolescents. BS creates a potential for both macro and micronutrient deficiency [1]. Vitamin and mineral deficiencies are usual in Western diets. The two most common deficiencies noted are

Table 14.1 Postoperative diet food.

Stage	Diet	Duration
Stage one	Full liquid diet	5 days (day 0–5)
Stage two	Pureed diet	1 week
Stage three	Soft foods	2–3 weeks
Stage four	Regularly healthy diet	Continuous

Table 14.2 Dietary tips for adolescents undergoing weight loss surgery.

Dietary tips for adolescents undergoing weight loss surgery

- Avoid high-sugar foods and/or fat content to prevent "dumping syndrome." Symptoms may include cramping, clammy feeling, sweating, tachycardia, vomiting, and/or diarrhea. Late dumping may occur up to 2 h after eating foods high in sugar or fat.
- Meals should be eaten in approximately 20 min.
- Adolescents should be encouraged to stop drinking 30 min before a meal and not to drink until 30 min after a meal. Eating and drinking at the same time may decrease satiety and/or increase the incidence of vomiting.
- Encourage the patient to eat slowly, taking small bites. Make sure food is cut into small pieces. Chew food well until it has a pureed consistency.
- Do not eat or drink past the first feeling of fullness. When feeling full, stop eating and put food away or discard what is left.
- To prevent dehydration, it is important to encourage the patient to continually sip fluids throughout the day, preferably water. Consider limiting caffeinated products.
- Do not lie down within 1 h after meals.

From Fullmer et al. Nutritional strategy for adolescents undergoing bariatric surgery: report of a Working Group of the Nutrition Committee of NASPGHAN/NACHRI. JPGN. 2012;54:125–135.

Table 14.3 Daily recommended intake.

	Daily recommended intake	
	Girls 14–18 y	Boys 14–18 y
Hydration	2.3 L/d	3.3 L/d
Protein	46 gr/d	52 gr/d
Vitamin B1 (thiamin)	1 mg/d	1.2 mg/d
Vitamin B6 (pyridoxine)	1.2 mg/d	1.3 mg/d
Vitamin B9 (folic acid)	400 µg/d	400 µg/d
Vitamin B12 (cobalamin)	2.4 µg/d	2.4 µg/d
Vitamin A	700 µg/d	900 µg/d
Vitamin D	400 IU/d	400 IU/d
Calcium	1300 mg/d	1300 mg/d
Iron	15 mg/d	11 mg/d
Zinc	9 mg/d	11 mg/d
Magnesium	420 mg/d	420 mg/d
Copper	890 µg/d	890 µg/d

d, day; gr, gram; IU, International Units; mg, milligram; µ, micro; L, liters; y, years.

iron and vitamin D. As I have mentioned before, supplementation with a complete multivitamin should occur in all candidates undergoing BS. For those adolescents noted to have a specific micronutrient deficiency, correction of the deficient state should occur before the bariatric procedure. Daily recommended intake for girls and boys ages 14–18 years is presented in Table 14.3.

- Hydration:

    After BS, patients are at risk for dehydration usually because of inadequate intake, vomiting, or diarrhea. Given the nature of restrictive forms of BS, several patients are not able to take in large volumes of water at one point in time and must consume their water in small volumes frequently throughout the day. Adolescents should be advised to consume liquids slowly, ideally 30 min before and after meals to reduce vomiting.

    Diarrhea associated with dumping syndrome may contribute to dehydration in patients undergoing RYGB. These adolescents should be instructed to avoid table sugar, candy, honey, jelly, and other concentrated forms of sugar, which may increase the osmolarity of contents entering the small intestine with subsequent diarrhea.

- Protein:

    Protein intake should be assessed periodically by the clinicians to assure an acceptable education and implementation of the diet. Parenteral supplementation should be considered in patients with severe protein malnutrition that is not responsive to oral protein supplements [14]. Given the current practices in the children population, 60–90 g of protein per day is recommended in adolescents undergoing RYGB, LAGB, and VG procedures.

- Vitamin B1 (Thiamin)

    Moderate-to-severe thiamin deficiency has been previously found in 10%–20% of obese women [15]. High-carbohydrate diets have been associated with thiamin deficiency [16]. After BS, vitamin B1 deficiency occurs in patients with persisting vomiting and/or excessive weight loss [17]. In adolescents, thiamin deficiency has been reported in girls 4–6 months after RYGB with Wernicke's encephalitis, increasing lower extremity weakness and pain, nystagmus, and hearing loss [18]. After surgery, adolescents should receive a minimum of 50 mg of thiamin per day.

- Vitamin B6 (Pyridoxine)

    It is recommended that adolescents undergoing BS take a multivitamin that includes vitamin B6.

- Vitamin B9 (Folic Acid)

    Folic acid is found in breakfast cereals, green vegetables, liver, and kidney. After BS, due to decreased folic acid, increased homocysteine levels were between 32% and 66% of patients. Recommended supplementation after RYGB or biliopancreatic diversion on adults is between 400 μg and 1 mg daily. Because folic acid is absorbed throughout the small intestine, a multivitamin containing folic acid should be enough for restrictive procedures such as LAGB.

- Vitamin B12 (Cobalamin)

    Cobalamin is found in fish, milk, eggs, meat, and poultry serves. It is suggested a supplementation of 500 μg sublingual form or monthly injections. In case of deficiency in an adult after BS, it is recommended as oral (350 μg daily), 1000 μg in q-2 to q-3 months, or 500 μg/week nasal spray.

- Vitamin A

Supplementation with vitamin A is recommended for adolescents post BS as described in Table 14.3. For individuals undergoing more extensive malabsorptive procedures such as duodenal switch or long-limb RYGB, additional supplementation may be required.

- Vitamin D/Calcium

Vitamin D is essential for the normal absorption of calcium in the gastrointestinal tract (normally at duodenum and jejunum). Deficiency in vitamin D leads to hypocalcemia, hypophosphatemia with resultant nutritional rickets in children, and osteomalacia, cardiovascular disease, insulin resistance, and hypertension in adults. Given that, these patients are at risk for developing bone mineral density and metabolism issues after these procedures. Most bariatric programs prescribed calcium with vitamin D in the form of calcium citrate or calcium carbonate with vitamin D. The minimum recommended dose of calcium is 1300 mg/day; the minimum vitamin D intake should be 600 IU [19]. Some pediatric programs prescribe up to 2000 IU/day. If vitamin D deficiency is detected, supplementation of 1000–5000 IU may want to be considered for the correction of deficiency [20].

- Iron

Iron deficiency has been reported in up to 50% after malabsorptive procedures, but this rarely occurred after restrictive surgery. The risk of iron deficiency is higher in obese girls rather than their nonobese counterparts [21]. To prevent it, it is advocated a treatment with ferrous sulfate 300 mg daily with vitamin C (remember that vitamin C may increase iron absorption by 50%) [22]. On the other hand, if adolescents underwent a restrictive surgery and have a good tolerance of liver, beef, grain bread, cereals, eggs, and dried fruit, supplementation may not be required.

- Zinc and Magnesium

Similar to iron deficiencies, zinc and magnesium deficiencies are rarely to happen after restrictive surgery. Minimal reports of zinc deficiency after RYGB associated with alopecia have been described. For this reason, zinc and magnesium supplementation are only recommended as needed based on the clinical suspect and serum levels.

- Copper

Copper deficiency after RYGB is associated with myelopathy, anemia, and neutropenia. Clinician has to offer the adolescent a multivitamin treatment that contains copper, especially if iron deficiency is not easily corrected because it may be cause by copper deficiency.

- Omega-3 fatty acids

Adequate intake of omega-3 fatty acids is vital in adults with cardiovascular disease. The restricted nature of bariatric procedures may reduce the consumption of fatty fish in our adolescent patients. For this reason, the clinician should take in count the intake of adolescents to determine the adequacy of omega-3 in the diet or supplement it to advocate nutritional competence.

Nutritional monitoring

After BS, the RD and the clinician are responsible for assessing nutrition-related laboratory values and recommending adjustments in supplementation as needed. However, it should be considered a transitional program to an adult bariatric care center to provide for long-term monitoring for nutritional deficiencies. Postoperative laboratory analysis should include a complete blood cell count, iron, ferritin, serum folate, thiamin, vitamin B12, methylmalonic acid, 25-hydroxy vitamin D, calcium, parathyroid hormone, alkaline phosphatase, hemoglobin A1c, albumin, magnesium, phosphorus, vitamin A, zinc, copper, and selenium 2 months postsurgery and posterior semiannually and annually.

If concerns for osteomalacia exist, consideration of pre- and postprocedure dual-energy X-ray absorptiometry scan may be beneficial (Table 14.4).

As I have mentioned before, and although there are limited data on the effects of family support in weight loss, it is true that families and caregivers play an important role for providing meals, ensuring that prescriptions are filled, providing vitamin supplements, transporting the adolescent to and from appointments, and providing them a safe living arrangement [23]. Given this, the family should continue to be involved during the monitoring phase.

In addition to individual clinician visits, attendance at support group sessions has been related to a higher adherence to visits postoperatively and a positive influence in long-term outcomes [24]. Given this, support groups should be an integral part of the surgical weight management program.

Hunger assessment

Teaching hunger satiety clue before and after BS may help in recognition of the teenager for the need for less volume of food intake, which may affect postoperative weight loss. This method consists of asking adolescents to record hunger/satiety on a scale of 1—10 before and in the middle of a meal (1 means extreme hunger and 10 means extreme fullness). If they record a number >7 in the middle of the meal, then they should be advised to consider finishing the meal [6].

Academic environment

Adolescent obese patients present topics regarding the academic environment that does not have concurrence in adult patients. Some advice for adolescents may be to carry a water bottle to sip on fluids throughout the day, desire lunch between 11 a.m. and 13 p.m., the possibility to intake a snack or protein supplement during class time, and desirable to take a packed lunch with healthy food. Given this, it should be essential to write a letter to the school administrator to communicate the special requirements of these patients.

The same recommendations should take in count for adolescents attending college on campus. Normally, eating plans at these colleges offer a variety of nutritious

Table 14.4 Age-appropriate laboratory parameters to be monitored post adolescent obesity surgery. This table is a guide. Many laboratories have variability in the parameters that are checked as well as normal values. It is recommended that the clinician become familiar with the laboratory that typically serves their patients. If a deficiency is diagnosed, then it is recommended to repeat the nutrient as per traditional nutrient repletion guidelines (34, 63, 64). 25-OHD, 25-hydroxy vitamin D; PLP, pyridoxal-5-phosphate; RBC, red blood cell.

Nutritional factor	Laboratory parameter	Normal value	Effects of deficiency
Thiamin (B1)	Red blood cell transketolase stimulation	<15%	Beriberi, neuritis, edema, cardiac failure, anorexia, hoarseness, restlessness, aphonia
Pyridoxine (B6)	Plasma PLP	<20 nmol/L	Neuropathy, photosensitivity
Folic acid (B9)	Serum folate, RBC folate, homocysteine	>6 ng/mL, >160 ng/mL	Megaloblastic anemia, irritability, paranoid behavior
Cobalamin (B12)	Urine/serum B12[a]	<3.60 mmol/mol creatinine or 200–900 pg/mL	Pernicious anemia, neurological deterioration
Vitamin A	Plasma retinol	20–72 mg/dL	Night blindness, xerophthalmia, dermatomalacia, impaired resistance to infection, follicular Hyperkeratosis, poor bone growth
Calcium	Ionized calcium	4.48–4.92 mg/dL	Numbness and tingling in the fingers, muscle cramps, convulsions, lethargy, poor appetite, and abnormal Heart rhythms
Vitamin D	Serum 25-OHD	<50 nmol/L	Rickets, osteomalacia
Vitamin C	Plasma vitamin C	0.2–2 mg/dL	Bleeding gums, diarrhea, perifollicular hemorrhage, scurvy
Vitamin E	Plasma a-tocopherol	0.7–10 mg/dL	Hyporeflexia spinocerebellar and retinal degeneration
Zinc	Serum zinc	0.75–1.2 mg/L	Anorexia, hypogeusia, delayed growth or sexual maturation, impaired wound healing
Magnesium	Serum magnesium	1.5–2.0 mg/dL	Convulsions, neuropsychiatric disorders, hypomagnesemia
Copper	Serum copper	1.10–1.45 mg/L	Microcytic, hypochromic anemia, delayed growth osteoporosis, neutropenia

[a] If borderline low level, confirm deficiency with serum methylmalonic acid may be check.

From Fullmer et al. Nutritional strategy for adolescents undergoing bariatric surgery: report of a Working Group of the Nutrition Committee of NASPGHAN/NACHRI. JPGN. 2012;54:125–135.

options, with lean protein sources readily available. Moreover, our patients should have in their rooms a stocked with protein-rich foods, whole-grain snacks, water, and sugar-free drinks that will allow them to make healthy, appropriate choices and minimize unplanned snacking on high-sugar, high-fat foods that provide much energy but few nutrients [6].

Reproductive health

The American College of Obstetrics and Gynecology encourages delaying pregnancy for a period of 12—18 months after BS [25]. The patient should understand that weight loss will improve fertility, and those who were not consistently using contraception before BS without consequences will now need to be more vigilant for pregnancy prevention. Little is known about the safety of a developing fetus in the setting of rapid weight loss and energy and nutrition restriction that occurs after BS [6,7]. Deficiencies of folic acid and vitamin B_{12} increase the risk of an open neural tube defect (spina bifida). Given this, special attention should be focused on girls after malabsorptive procedures. Dietary counseling before, during, and after pregnancy is essential for assessment and prevention of vitamin deficiencies (folic acid, vitamin B12, iron).

Special cases

Success after BS requires significant behavioral changes that are dependent on the patient's ability to implement lifestyle changes [26]. For this reason, many bariatric centers exclude patients with significant cognitive impairment [1].

As recently as 10 years ago, a critical analysis of BS in adolescents with Prader—Willi Syndrome (PWS) suggested that outcomes were not as good as in children without syndromic obesity [27]. Alqahtani published a case-matched study of 24 children with PWS and those without, which confirmed outcomes of more weight regain after VG in patients with PWS; however; the VG was safe and effective showing a 5-year sustained BMI drop of 10 points [28].

The role of BS in adolescents who have hypothalamic obesity (HyOb) as a result of craniopharyngioma (CP) was reviewed in a meta-analysis by Bretault et al. [29]. The authors demonstrated the safety and efficacy of bariatric procedures in patients with HyOb from CP for whom there is no other effective treatment available. Although outcomes were quite variable, the RYGB appeared to be more effective at maintaining long-term weight loss than the VG or LAGB.

Given the lack of other options in children with PWS, other syndromic obesity, or HyOb, BS should be considered, especially when comorbidities exist [1].

Conclusion

Careful considerations should be made when assessing, educating, and monitoring the adolescent for a BS. An MDT should stabilize and treat preexisting eating disorders, assure stable social support, assess and assist with nutrition and activity knowledge, and consider the addition of supplements when appropriate. It should be considered to develop a transitional program to an adult bariatric care center to provide for long-term monitoring for nutritional deficiencies. Further long-term studies in this population will allow for the standardization of nutrition guidelines for the adolescent bariatric patient.

References

[1] Pratt JSA, Browne A, Browne NT, Bruzoni M, Cohen M, Desai A, et al. ASMBS pediatric metabolic and bariatric surgery guidelines, 2018. Surg Obes Relat Dis 2018;14(7):882−901.

[2] Skinner AC, Ravanbakht SN, Skelton JA, Perrin EM, Armstrong SC. Prevalence of obesity and severe obesity in US children, 1999−2016. Pediatrics 2018;141(3): e20173459.

[3] Ogden C, Carroll MD, Fryar CD, Flegal KM. Prevalence of obesity among adults and youth: United States, 2011−2014. NCHS Data Brief 2015;(219):1−8.

[4] Whitaker RC, Wright JA, Pepe MS, et al. Predicting obesity in young adulthood from childhood and parental obesity. N Engl J Med 1997;337:869−73.

[5] Messiah SE, Lopez-Mitnik G, Winegar D, et al. Changes in weight and co-morbidities among adolescents undergoing bariatric surgery: 1-year results from the bariatric outcomes longitudinal database. Surg Obes Relat Dis 2013;9:503−13.

[6] Fullmer MA, Abrams SH, Hrovat K, Mooney L, Scheimann AO, Hillman JB, Suskind DL. Nutritional strategy for adolescents undergoing bariatric surgery: report of a Working Group of the Nutrition Committee of NASPGHAN/NACHRI. JPGN 2012;54:125−35.

[7] Nogueira I, Hrovat K. Adolescent bariatric surgery: review on nutrition considerations. Nutr Clin Pract 2014;29(6):740−6.

[8] McGintya S, Richmond TK, Desai NK. Managing adolescent obesity and the role of bariatric surgery. Curr Opin Pediatr 2015;27(4):434−41.

[9] He J, Cai Z, Fan X. Prevalence of binge and loss of control eating among children and adolescents with overweight and obesity: an exploratory meta-analysis. Int J Eat Disord 2017;50(2):91−103.

[10] Utzinger LM, Gowey MA, Zeller M, et al. Loss of control eating and eating disorders in adolescents before bariatric surgery. Int J Eat Disord 2016;49(10):947−52.

[11] Zeller MH, Hunsaker S, Mikhail C, et al. Family factors that characterize adolescents with severe obesity and their role in weight loss surgery outcomes. Obesity 2016; 24(12):2562−9.

[12] Baumrind D. Patterns of parental authority and adolescent autonomy. N Dir Child Adolesc Dev 2005;108:61−9.

[13] Wing RR, Phelan S. Long-term weight loss maintenance. Am J Clin Nutr 2005;82. 222S−5S.

[14] Mechanick JI, Kushner RF, Sugerman HJ, et al. American Association of Clinical Endocrinologists, The Obesity Society, and American Society for Metabolic & Bariatric Surgery medical guidelines for clinical practice for the perioperative nutritional, metabolic, and nonsurgical support of the bariatric surgery patient. Obesity 2009;17(Suppl. 1):S1−70.

[15] Patrini C, Griziotti A, Ricciardi L. Obese individuals as thiamin stores. Int J Obes Relat Metab Disord 2004;28:920—4.
[16] Ben Ghorbel I, Veit V, Schleinitz N, et al. Acute neuromyocarditis secondary to diet-induced beriberi. Rev Med Intern 2000;21:989—92.
[17] Malone M. Recommended nutritional supplements for bariatric surgery patients. Ann Pharmacother 2008;42:1851—8.
[18] Towbin A, Inge TH, Garcia VF, et al. Beriberi after gastric bypass surgery in adolescence. J Pediatr 2004;145:263—7.
[19] Institute of Medicine. Dietary reference intakes for calcium and vitamin D dietary reference intakes for calcium and vitamin D. Washington, DC: Institute of Medicine; 2010.
[20] Misra M, Pacaud D, Petryk A, et al. Vitamin D deficiency in children and its management: review of current knowledge and recommendations. Pediatrics 2008;122: 398—417.
[21] Tussing-Humphreys LM, Liang H, Nemeth E, et al. Excess adiposity, inflammation, and iron-deficiency in female adolescents. J Am Diet Assoc 2009;109:297—302.
[22] Rhode BM, Shustik C, Christou NV, et al. Iron absorption and therapy after gastric bypass. Obes Surg 1999;9:17—21.
[23] McLean N, Griffin S, Toney K, Hardeman W. Family involvement in weight control, weight maintenance and weight-loss interventions: a systematic review of randomized trials. Int J Obes Relat Metab Disord 2003;27:987—1005.
[24] Sawhney P, Modi AC, Jenkins TM, et al. Predictors and outcomes of adolescent bariatric support group attendance. Surg Obes Relat Dis 2013;95:773—9.
[25] ACOG Committee opinion number 315, September 2005. Obesity in pregnancy. Obstet Gynecol 2005;106:671—5.
[26] Powers PS, Rosemurgy A, Boyd F, et al. Outcome of gastric restriction procedures: weight, psychiatric diagnoses, and satisfaction. Obes Surg 1997;7:471—7.
[27] Scheimann AO, Butler MG, Gourash L, Cuffari C, Klish W. Critical analysis of bariatric procedures in Prader-Willi syndrome. J Pediatr Gastroenterol Nutr 2008;46(1):80—3.
[28] Alqahtani AR, Elahmedi MO, Al Qahtani AR, Lee J, Butler MG. Laparoscopic sleeve gastrectomy in children and adolescents with Prader-Willi syndrome: a matched-control study. Surg Obes Relat Dis 2016;12(1):100—10.
[29] Bretault M, Boillot A, Muzard L, et al. Clinical review: bariatric surgery following treatment for craniopharyngioma: a systematic review and individual-level data meta-analysis. J Clin Enocrinol Metab 2013;98(6):2239—46.

CHAPTER 15

Special nutritional requirements in the elderly patient undergoing bariatric surgery

Andrei Sarmiento[1], Ramiro Carbajal[2], Rosa Lisson[2]

[1]*Surgery at Universidad Privada San Juan Bautista, Lima, Perú;* [2]*Hospital Nacional Edgardo Rebagliati Martins, Lima, Perú*

Chapter outline

Introduction	199
Preoperative clinical evaluation	200
Nutritional profile	200
Aging-related changes in gastric function (could predispose to nutritional issues)	201
Aging-related changes in small intestinal function (could predispose to nutritional issues)	201
Vitamin D	201
Calcium	202
Vitamin B12	202
Iron	202
Protein	202
Laparoscopic sleeve gastrectomy	203
Roux-en-Y gastric bypass	203
One anastomosis/mini gastric bypass	204
Follow-up and supplementation in elderly patients	204
Conclusion	204
References	205

Introduction

The prevalence of obesity in patients aged 60 years old or older has been increasing, and over recent years the number of bariatric and metabolic surgeries within this group experienced an upward trend worldwide [1]. Even though bariatric surgery for patients older than 60 years has formulated some questions, these patients are being regarded for bariatric surgery greater often. Gebhart et al. reported that

10% of bariatric procedures performed in the United States in 2013 were in patients 60 years old or older versus 2.7% in 2006 [2].

In 1991, as is well known, National Institutes of Health consensus panel developed a paper that described the indications in the field of metabolic and bariatric surgery [3]. These indications have remained unchanged over the years; however, more recently, several studies have emerged that offer to expand the limits regarding not only body mass index but also the age of the patients [4–6].

The goal of this chapter is to provide a review of the several factors that may affect the essential nutritional requirements as well as examine the outcomes after different options of bariatric surgery in the elderly population.

Preoperative clinical evaluation

Elderly patients deserve a special approach because of their more complex characteristics with more comorbidities, usually more severe by what they usually take more daily prescription drugs [7]. Along these lines, Dunckle-Blatter et al. evaluated the data of 1065 patients who underwent Roux-en-Y gastric bypass (RYGB) and found that the mean number of comorbidities was 10 in the older group (>60 years) compared with 4.7 in the younger group (<60 years). At the same time, the mean number of preoperative medications was 10 in the older group compared with 6.0 in the younger group [8].

Nowadays, there is broad consensus among surgeons that a multidisciplinary approach is essential for the comprehensive management of obesity, this includes a cautious preoperative evaluation to determinate the profile of candidates to increase its safety, and this point would be essential in terms of safety, especially when treating aged patients [9,10]. Along these lines, it is important to take into mind that the changes relate to normal aging, such as age-related bone changes, skeletal muscle mass, and strength, disability, and frailty. The preoperative evaluation should be carried out in a strict multidisciplinary approach involving medical history, nutritional, psychological, and procedural evaluations [11], within which it should include body composition and bone mass by dual-energy radiographic absorptiometry of hip and spine [12]. All elderly candidates for bariatric procedures should undergo a preoperative evaluation for obesity-related comorbidities and patient condition should be optimized before surgery.

Nutritional profile

With reference to the nutritional profile of patients with obesity before surgery, previous studies have reported that they have at least one vitamin or mineral deficiency [13]. However, thus far there is no specific data in the obese elderly population. Additionally, aged organs and weakened homeostatic controls that could lead to increase morbidity (including nutritional risk) and mortality; nonetheless, according to some systematic review have stimulated the utilization of bariatric surgery in the elderly patients, demonstrating comparable outcomes with the younger population [5,14].

Patients undergone bariatric surgery should take routine mineral and vitamin supplementation; however, despite this fact, some patients will have any deficiency depending upon several factors such as type of surgery, adherence to follow-up and supplementation, food intolerance, physical activity/inactivity, and behavioral modifications [15,16]. Each type of surgery has their own advantages and drawbacks, also is well known that, to a greater or lesser degree, these procedures change the anatomy of the gastrointestinal tract and consequently its physiology, apart from changes in neural and gut hormonal signals, making patients more susceptible to developing nutritional complications in both macronutrients and micronutrients, for example, iron deficiency, vitamin B12 deficiency, calcium deficiency, and other nutritional complications such as hypoalbuminemia [17,18]. Aging affects, to variable degrees, all functions of the gastrointestinal system: motility, enzyme and hormone secretion, digestion, and absorption [19].

Nutritional deficiencies may be more noticeable in elderly patients if we look at the changes in their gastrointestinal tract with normal aging, especially gastric and small intestine.

Aging-related changes in gastric function (could predispose to nutritional issues)

Decreased acid secretion, cytoprotective factors (prostacyclins), pepsin, sodium, fluid secretion, and increased contact time with NSAIDs/other noxious agents. Moreover, decreased gastric motility [19].

Aging-related changes in small intestinal function (could predispose to nutritional issues)

Decreased uptake of vitamin D, folic acid, vitamin B12, calcium, copper, zinc, fatty acids, and cholesterol.

Motility of the small bowel is not significantly different but may vary with medications, polypharmacy, concomitant diseases as is the case with neuropathy from long-standing diabetes [20].

Vitamin D

Hypovitaminosis D may result from fat malabsorption, as the primary absorption sites of liposoluble vitamins in the small intestine are bypassed. Additionally, lower sun exposure affected skin synthesis of previtamin D, and also decreased hydroxylation in the kidney with aging lead to vitamin D deficiency in the elderly population. The serum 25-hydroxy vitamin D (25OHD) levels should be verified after a minimum of 3 months. Treatment guidelines propose that for maintaining appropriate levels of vitamin D after RYGB, at least 5000 IU/d is necessary, though higher doses (up to 50,000 IU) are required after biliopancreatic diversion. Recent studies have indicated that the level of vitamin D should remain above 25—30 ng/mL for the successful prevention of osteoporosis and bone fracture [21,22].

Calcium

Calcium uptake from the gastrointestinal tract decreases significantly after age 60 in both sexes. Individuals older than 70 years old absorb approximately one-third less calcium. Absorption of calcium is dependent on vitamin D; hence, bioavailability depends on the intake and status of vitamin D. The absorption efficiency is related to calcium physiological requirements and is dose-dependent. Bariatric surgery impact on bone metabolism and induce significant changes, above all, caused by bypass the duodenum and proximal jejunum, which are the main sites of absorption of calcium/vitamin D. Regular calcium supplement (preferably as calcium citrate) is recommended from 1200 to 2000 mg daily [22,23]. Oral calcium can also be known to interfere with the absorption of other essential minerals such as iron, zinc, and copper.

Vitamin B12

Vitamin B12 deficiency may be caused by inadequate secretion of the intrinsic factor, limited gastric acidity and, and above all else, bypassing the duodenum, the main site of absorption of vitamin B12.

Iron

Reduced absorption of iron by hypochloridria, bypass duodenum, and proximal.
Jejunum (the principal iron absorption sites). Postoperative changes in food intake, food preferences, for instance, meat intolerance and milk products, are important contributing factors.

Protein

According to one small study, protein absorption occurs slowly and may suppress or delay protein synthesis in the senescent muscle of elderly people [24]. This is one of the known challenges in the elderly not only for the correct supplementation but also for avoiding sarcopenia. In the classical definition, this refers to loss of muscle mass, strength, and performance; according to the literature, these effects could be explained by disuse, changing endocrine function, chronic diseases, inflammation, insulin resistance, and nutritional deficiencies, by which it is important to understand the impact of sarcopenia on physical impairment, injury, fall, and mortality [25].

In this sense, PROT-AGE Study Group claims that elderly people need more dietary protein than younger adults to support good health, promote recovery from illness, and maintain functionality. Several factors could explain this observation: firstly, a declining anabolic response to protein intake; secondly, more protein is also needed to counteract inflammatory and catabolic conditions associated with chronic and acute diseases that occur commonly with aging. PROT-AGE Study Group recommend that older people should consume an average daily intake at least in the range of 1.0—1.2 g/kg BW/d, and most older adults who have an acute or chronic disease need even more dietary protein (i.e., 1.2e1.5 g/kg BW/d). Combined with increased protein intake, exercise is recommended at individualized levels that are safe and tolerated [26]. Not long-ago bariatric surgery was restricted to patients under 60 years old based on the concerns of age-related increased surgical risks; nevertheless, data from more recent studies suggest acceptable risk/benefit ratio. Until now, there is no consensus about the best surgical option for elderly patients; however, the following bariatric surgeries are being undertaken. In contrast, the malabsorptive surgical procedure must be used with utmost care on nutritional status, especially in this population.

Laparoscopic sleeve gastrectomy

Recent studies have shown that sleeve gastrectomy is a safe and effective surgical approach in patients aged above 60 years [27,28]. Laparoscopic sleeve gastrectomy (LSG) is widely known for its shorter operating time, rapid recovery, and low complications rate. However, there are no data about short- and long-term nutritional effects.

Roux-en-Y gastric bypass

RYGB is an effective weight loss procedure for elderly patients and may offer better weight loss compared to LSG; however, it seems to have higher complication rate than LSG [29]. To determine the risk and benefits, Uri Kaplan et al. (2018) carried out a retrospective cohort study for patients older than 60 years in Canadian population at 1-year follow-up, who underwent laparoscopic gastric bypass (LRYGB) or LSG, who found that both procedures were at no greater risk for intraoperative and postoperative complications and also showed a greater reduction in medication use postsurgery when were divided into older (>60) and younger (>60) [30]. Additionally, according to recent reports, RYGB is associated with a substantial increase in the quality of life in the elderly [31].

One anastomosis/mini gastric bypass

Recently, IFSO (International Federation for Surgery of Obesity and Metabolic Disorders) consensus conference statement on one-anastomosis gastric bypass (OAGB-MGB) claims that this procedure is appropriate for the elderly (over 60 years old) [32], in accordance with the first consensus statement on OAGB/mini gastric bypass (OAGB/MGB) in 2017, which indicated that this procedure is an acceptable surgical option for suitable elderly patients even > 70.0 years old, although in both consensus highlight the importance of closer follow-up [33]. Peraglie (2016) showed that OAGB-MGB is safe and efficient as a metabolic and even revisional procedure in patients age 60 and older [34]. With regard to this procedure, variations in the length of the afferent limb have been described (from 180 to 300 cm) depending on some factors such as age, eating habits, and comorbid conditions of the patient, to get better outcomes on nutritional status [35]. Notwithstanding, evidence on nutritional status in elderly patients is limited, so further studies are necessary.

Follow-up and supplementation in elderly patients

Preoperative screening of nutritional deficiency is a critical part of preparing for bariatric surgery. After surgery, a lifelong follow-up of the nutritional profile, appropriate supplementation, monitoring, and early recognition of vitamins and minerals deficiencies is extremely important (this is discussed in detail in another chapter). Appropriate doses of daily multivitamin and mineral tablets in elderly patients are yet unknown, this is particularly so given that there are limited data about the absorption and bioavailability of drugs and nutrients following bariatric surgery. Nevertheless, there are some considerations (apart from changes in gastrointestinal anatomy) that we need to take into account, such as greater vulnerability toward loss of muscle mass, decrease in bone mineral density, vitamin and mineral deficiencies along with impaired absorption, and altered metabolism due to aging of the organs. Considering the aforesaid, short- and long-term data on the nutritional outcome based on the technique performed will help to standardize nutritional supplementation and follow-up for elderly patients. There are some special nutritional requirements in this subpopulation: overall calcium, vitamin D, B12, and proteins.

Conclusion

Bariatric surgery offers a range of benefits for obese elderly patients; however, it should be individualized to the risk profile of particular patients, to improve their quality of life. Additionally, lifelong follow-up (including biochemical follow-up) is needed to obtain better outcomes in terms of weight loss and avoid nutritional deficiencies. Further research should be undertaken to provide answers on the doses of mineral and vitamins in obese elderly after bariatric surgery.

References

[1] Flegal KM, Carroll MD, Kit BK, Ogden CL. Prevalence of obesity and trends in distribution of BMI among US adults, 1999−2010. J Am Med Assoc 2012;307(5):491−7.

[2] Gebhart A, YoungMT, Nguyen NT. Bariatric surgery in the elderly: 2009−2013. Surg Obes Relat Dis 2015;11(2):393−8.

[3] NIH conference. Gastrointestinal surgery for severe obesity. Consensus development conference panel. Ann Intern Med 1991;115(12):956−61.

[4] Ritz P, Topart P, Benchetrit S, Tuyeras G, Lepage B, Mouiel J, et al. Benefits and risks of bariatric surgery in patients aged more than 60 years. Surg Obes Relat Dis 2014. https://doi.org/10.1016/j.soard.2013.12.012.

[5] Giordano S, Victorzon M. Bariatric surgery in elderly patients: a systematic review. Clin Interv Aging 2015;10:1627−35.

[6] Nor Hanipah Z, Punchai S, Karas LA, et al. The outcome of bariatric surgery in patients aged 75 years and older. Obes Surg 2018;28:1498−503. https://doi.org/10.1007/s11695-017-3020-z.

[7] Locher JL, Roth DL, Ritchie CS, et al. Body mass index, weight loss, and mortality in community-dwelling older adults. J Gerontol A Biol Sci Med Sci 2007;62:1389.

[8] Dunkle-Blatter SE, St Jean MR, Whitehead C, et al. Outcomes among elderly bariatric patients at a high-volume center. Surg Obes Relat Dis 2007;3(2):163−9.

[9] De Luca M, Angrisani L, Himpens J, et al. Indications for surgery for obesity and weight-related diseases: position statements from the International Federation for the Surgery of Obesity and Metabolic Disorders (IFSO). Obes Surg 2016;26:1659−96. https://doi.org/10.1007/s11695-016-2271-4.

[10] Kuruba R, Koche LS, Murr MM. Preoperative assessment and perioperative care of patients undergoing bariatric surgery. Med Clin N Am 2007;91(3). 339−351, ix.

[11] Fried M, Yumuk V, Oppert JM, et al. Interdisciplinary European guidelines on metabolic and bariatric surgery. Obes Surg 2014;24:42−55.

[12] Cosman F, de Beur SJ, LeBoff MS, et al. Clinician's guide to prevention and treatment of osteoporosis. Osteoporos Int 2014;25:2359.

[13] Gehrer S, Kern B, Peters T, et al. Fewer nutrient deficiencies after laparoscopic sleeve gastrectomy (LSG) than after laparoscopic roux-Y-gastric bypass (LRYGB)—a prospective study. Obes Surg 2010;20:447−53. https://doi.org/10.1007/s11695-009-0068-4.

[14] Lynch J, Belgaumkar A. Bariatric surgery is effective and safe in patients over 55: a systematic review and meta-analysis. Obes Surg 2012;22:1507−16. https://doi.org/10.1007/s11695-012-0693-1.

[15] Nett P, Borbély Y, Kröll D. Micronutrient supplementation after biliopancreatic diversion with duodenal switch in the long term. Obes Surg 2016;26:2469−74. https://doi.org/10.1007/s11695-016-2132-1.

[16] Mahawar KK, Clare K, O'Kane M, et al. Patient perspectives on adherence with micronutrient supplementation after bariatric surgery. Obes Surg 2019;29:1551−6. https://doi.org/10.1007/s11695-019-03711-z.

[17] Poitou Bernert C, Ciangura C, Coupaye M, et al. Nutritional deficiency after gastric bypass: diagnosis, prevention and treatment. Diabetes Metab 2007;33:13.

[18] Ledoux S, Flamant M, Calabrese D, et al. What are the micronutrient deficiencies responsible for the most common nutritional symptoms after bariatric surgery? Obes Surg 2020;30:1891−7. https://doi.org/10.1007/s11695-020-04412-8.
[19] Dumic I, Nordin T, Jecmenica M, Lalosevic MS, Milosavljevic T, Milovanovic T. Gastrointestinal tract disorders in older age. Chin J Gastroenterol Hepatol 2019;2019: 6757524. https://doi.org/10.1155/2019/6757524.
[20] Rémond D, Shahar DR, Gille D, et al. Understanding the gastrointestinal tract of the elderly to develop dietary solutions that prevent malnutrition. Oncotarget 2015;6(16): 13858−98.
[21] Hollis BW. Circulating 25-hydroxyvitamin D levels indicative of vitamin D sufficiency: implications for establishing a new effective dietary intake recommendation for vitamin D. J Nutr 2005;135:317.
[22] Mechanick JI, Youdim A, Jones DB, Garvey WT, Hurley DL, McMahon MM, Heinberg LJ, Kushner R, Adams TD, Shikora S, Dixon JB, Brethauer S, American Association of Clinical Endocrinologists; Obesity Society; American Society for Metabolic & Bariatric Surgery. Clinical practice guidelines for the perioperative nutritional, metabolic, and nonsurgical support of the bariatric surgery patient−2013 update: cosponsored by American Association of Clinical Endocrinologists, The Obesity Society, and American Society for Metabolic & Bariatric Surgery. Obesity 2013;21(Suppl. 1):S1−27. https://doi.org/10.1002/oby.20461. PMID: 23529939.
[23] Lupoli R, Lembo E, Saldalamacchia G, Avola CK, Angrisani L, Capaldo B. Bariatric surgery and long-term nutritional issues. World J Diabetes 2017;8:464. https://doi.org/10.4239/wjd.v8.i11.464.
[24] Milan AM, D'Souza RF, Pundir S, Pileggi CA, Thorstensen EB, Barnett MPG, Markeworth JF, Canmeron-Smith D, Mitchell CJ. Older adults have delayed amino acid absorption after a high protein mixed breakfast meal. J Nutr Health Aging 2015; 19:839−45. https://doi.org/10.1007/s12603-015-0500-5.
[25] Pasco JA, Mohebbi M, Holloway KL, et al. Musculoskeletal decline and mortality: prospective data from the Geelong Osteoporosis Study. J Cachexia Sarcopenia Muscle 2016;8(3):482−9.
[26] Bauer J, Biolo G, Cederholm T, et al. Evidence-based recommendations for optimal dietary protein intake in older people: a position paper from the PROT-AGE study group. J Am Med Dir Assoc 2013;14:542−59.
[27] Bartosiak K, Różańska-Walędziak A, Walędziak M, et al. The safety and benefits of laparoscopic sleeve gastrectomy in elderly patients: a case-control study. Obes Surg 2019;29:2233−7. https://doi.org/10.1007/s11695-019-03830-7.
[28] Dvir Froylich MD, Omer Sadeh MD, Hagar Mizrahi MD, Naama Kafri RD, Guy Pascal MD, Christopher R, Daigle MD, Nisim Geron MD, David Hazzan MD. Midterm outcomes of sleeve gastrectomy in the elderly, surgery for obesity and related diseases. Surg Obes Relat Dis 2018. https://doi.org/10.1016/j.soard.2018.07.020.
[29] Abbas M, Cumella L, Zhang Y, et al. Outcomes of laparoscopic sleeve gastrectomy and roux-en-Y gastric bypass in patients older than 60. Obes Surg 2015;25(12):2251−6.
[30] Kaplan U, Penner S, Farrokhyar F, et al. Bariatric surgery in the elderly is associated with similar surgical risks and significant long-term health benefits. Obes Surg 2018; 28:2165−70. https://doi.org/10.1007/s11695-018-3160-9.
[31] Almerie MQ, Rao VSR, Peter MB, et al. The impact of laparoscopic gastric bypass on comorbidities and quality of life in the older obese patients (age >60): our UK experience. Obes Surg 2018;28:3890−4. https://doi.org/10.1007/s11695-018-3414-6.

[32] Ramos AC, Chevallier J, Mahawar K, et al. IFSO (International Federation for Surgery of Obesity and Metabolic Disorders) consensus conference statement on one-anastomosis gastric bypass (OAGB-MGB): results of a modified Delphi study. Obes Surg 2020;30:1625−34. https://doi.org/10.1007/s11695-020-04519-y.

[33] Mahawar KK, Himpens J, Shikora SA, et al. The first consensus statement on one anastomosis/mini gastric bypass (OAGB/MGB) using a modified delphi approach. Obes Surg 2018;28:303−12. https://doi.org/10.1007/s11695-017-3070-2.

[34] Peraglie C. Laparoscopic mini-gastric bypass in patients age 60 and older. Surg Endosc 2016;30:38−43.

[35] Ahuja A, Tantia O, Goyal G, et al. MGB-OAGB: effect of biliopancreatic limb length on nutritional deficiency, weight loss and comorbidity resolution. Obes Surg 2018;28(11): 3439−45.

CHAPTER 16

Special nutritional requirements in specific situations in women: pregnancy, lactancy, and postmenopausal status

Irene Bretón Lesmes, Cynthia González Antigüedad, Clara Serrano Moreno

Department of Endocrinology and Nutrition, Hospital General Universitario Gregorio Marañón, Madrid, Spain

Chapter outline

Introduction	209
Obesity and reproductive function in women	210
Bariatric surgery and pregnancy	211
Dietary recommendations	213
Nutritional supplements	213
Gestational diabetes	215
Specific complications of pregnancy after bariatric surgery	216
Neonatal care	216
Lactation	217
Bariatric surgery and menopause	217
Pregnancy, lactation, and menopause in women with previous bariatric surgery: summary of recommendations	218
References	219

Introduction

Bariatric surgery (BS) is increasingly used in the treatment of morbid obesity, especially in women. When compared to medical treatment, BS can induce a significant and maintained weight loss and a remission or improvement of most comorbidities, such as diabetes mellitus, hypertension, sleep apnea, and osteoarthritis.

Pregnancy and lactation can be a matter of concern in childbearing women with morbid obesity when bariatric surgery is proposed. It is well known that obesity decreases fertility and increases the risk of maternal–fetal complications in pregnancy, such as gestational diabetes, hypertension and preeclampsia, problems in childbirth, and macrosomia. Bariatric surgery can decrease the risk of these obesity-related complications. However, and mainly because of its effect on nutrient intake and absorption, it may also induce adverse consequences on both maternal and fetal health. Close clinical monitoring is recommended in these situations and should be performed by a multidisciplinary team.

Menopause should also be taken into account in bariatric patients, as there is a higher risk of metabolic bone disease and sarcopenia in these populations, especially when malabsorptive techniques are used.

This chapter describes the main recommendations on pregnancy, lactation, and menopause in relation to bariatric surgery.

Obesity and reproductive function in women

Obesity directly affects reproductive function in both men and women through complex and not entirely known mechanisms. In women, obesity is related to a greater risk of infertility and is a factor in poor prognosis when assisted reproduction techniques are used [1]. Obesity is independently associated with increased time to pregnancy, even in women with normal menstruation. The relationship between obesity, metabolic disorders, and infertility is especially evident in polycystic ovary syndrome (PCOS). Women with PCOS are at increased risk of pregnancy complications such as gestational diabetes, pregnancy-related hypertension, macrosomia, intrauterine growth retardation, and prematurity [2].

Recommended weight gain during pregnancy is shown in Table 16.1. Both obesity and excess weight gain during pregnancy increase the risk of maternal and fetal complications (Table 16.2). Up to 25% of the total risk of adverse outcomes during pregnancy and delivery can be attributed to maternal overweight. The maternal complications that are most often associated with obesity are gestational diabetes, pregnancy-related hypertension, including preeclampsia, thromboembolic disease, and weight retain after pregnancy [3]. Excess maternal weight increases the risk of prolonged pregnancy, prematurity, and the need for a C-section [4]. There is greater difficulty in breastfeeding. Women with severe obesity have the highest risk of complications [5].

Table 16.1 Recommendations for weight gain during pregnancy. IOM, 2009.

Pregestational BMI	Maternal weight gain
<18.5 kg/m^2	12.5–18 kg
18.5–25 kg/m^2	11.5–16 kg
25–30 kg/m^2	6.8–11.3 kg
>30 kg/m^2	5.0–9.1 kg

Table 16.2 Clinical consequences of maternal overweight and excess weight gain in pregnancy.

Maternal	
Preconception	Higher risk of diabetes, high blood pressure, and infertility
Pregnancy	Previous metabolic diseases, gestational diabetes, hypertension, deep vein thrombosis, pulmonary thromboembolism, depression
Delivery	Higher risk of complications, instrumental delivery, ccaesarean, higher anesthetic risk
Postpartum	Infection, depression, failure in breastfeeding, weight retain after delivery, obesity

Newborn and infant
Macrosomia, large for gestational age newborn, prematurity, shoulder dystocia, birth defects, neonatal hypoglycemia

Long term
Higher risk of obesity, metabolic complications. Higher vascular risk for both the mother and offspring

Bariatric surgery and pregnancy

The effect of bariatric surgery on future pregnancies is an issue that concerns both morbidly obese women seeking treatment with bariatric surgery and physicians. Pregnancy after bariatric surgery generally presents a lower risk of obesity-related complications, such as gestational diabetes, gestation-related hypertension, and macrosomia [6–8]. These benefits of BS are most evident when maternal–fetal outcomes are compared with those of severely obese women. On the contrary, there is a higher risk of small-for-gestational-age newborn and prematurity. The effect of the previous BS on the risk of cesarean is not consistent in different studies, as it depends mainly on the clinical setting. An increased risk of iron deficiency anemia and other complications such as gastrointestinal bleeding, band migration, and intestinal obstruction have been described (Table 16.3). Some studies have shown that malabsorptive bariatric surgery is associated with a greater decrease in the risk of macrosomia and a higher risk of low-weight newborns, in comparison to restrictive techniques [9,10].

Table 16.3 Complications of pregnancy after bariatric surgery.

Pregnancy after bariatric surgery: risk of complications

• Nutritional deficiency
  • Low weight gain, malnutrition
  • micronutrient deficiency
• Dumping's syndrome, hypoglycemia
• Gastroesophageal reflux, esophagitis, GI bleeding
• Internal hernia
• Band complications

Pregnancy in women with a history of bariatric surgery requires a protocolized follow-up, and some clinical decisions should be taken in advance. It is important to ensure an appropriate selection of the bariatric surgical technique in women of child-bearing age with morbid obesity, according to clinical characteristics, associated comorbidity, and the team's experience. There are no scientific data to recommend a particular surgical technique for women of childbearing age requiring bariatric surgery. In young women with a desire for pregnancy, nonmalabsorptive techniques, such as sleeve gastrectomy, will generally be preferred. In case of extreme obesity, with BMI >50 kg/m^2, mixed or malabsorptive bariatric techniques can be considered to favor greater weight loss and decrease the risk of complications associated with obesity in future pregnancies. In these patients, it must be taken into account that the risk of nutritional complications will be higher. Women should be informed of the risks of surgical complications, such as internal hernia, after procedures involving the small intestine, the possibility of band problems after adjustable gastric banding, and the higher frequency of nutritional deficiencies after malabsorptive bariatric procedures [11,12].

It is mandatory to perform an adequate follow-up after bariatric surgery that includes dietary advice and micronutrient supplementation, to prevent and treat possible nutritional deficiencies. If pregnancy is desired, an antenatal consultation is mandatory. Follow-up during pregnancy should be carried out by a multidisciplinary team, which includes gynecology and obstetrics specialists, endocrinologists, surgeons, dietitians, and specialized nurses and midwives.

Contraception should start before bariatric surgery. Is should be noted that all contraceptive methods are efficacious in obese patients. Long-acting reversible contraceptives, such as intrauterine devices or etonogestrel implants, appear to be the best options before and after BS. If these methods are not used, it should be noted that there can be a higher risk of contraception failure if nausea, vomiting, or diarrhea is present. There is also a high risk of thrombotic complications with oral contraceptives that should be discontinued from 6 weeks before BS to 4–6 weeks after surgery [11,13].

Most clinical guidelines advise to delay pregnancy to 12–18 months after bariatric surgery, a period when most weight loss after surgery occurs, tolerance to oral diet is lower and may increase the risk of nutritional deficiencies. It will be taken into account, in any case, that this higher risk in early pregnancies has not been clearly shown, so pregnancy occurring before 12–18 does not necessarily imply an increased risk of complications. A shorter interval between bariatric surgery and gestation may be considered in older women, with closer monitoring during pregnancy and provided there is adequate clinical stability [11–13].

Clinical and nutritional evaluation, at least every 3 months during pregnancy, with a careful assessment of dietary intake and biochemical evaluation to identify possible nutritional deficiencies. Closer monitoring is needed in case of oral diet intolerance, nausea, or vomiting.

Maternal nutritional factors are of great importance in fetal development. Energy and nutrient requirements are increased during gestation, to allow for adequate embryonic and fetal development and the necessary changes in the mother for pregnancy and lactation. A balanced diet, providing a sufficient amount of energy, contains a sufficient amount of essential nutrients. However, during pregnancy, requirements are often not met by oral diet and specific supplementation is required to prevent deficiencies. This fact is especially relevant in pregnancy after bariatric surgery. Pregnant women after BS should follow the same weight gain recommendations of the general population [11].

Dietary recommendations

There are very few studies that have evaluated the adequacy of dietary intake during pregnancy in women with previous BS [14]. Dietary advice should be provided, and adapted to the surgical technique and to the clinical condition and GI symptoms. Constipation can be observed in restrictive techniques, such as gastric banding or sleeve gastrectomy; diarrhea can occur in malabsorptive procedures. Close monitoring of maternal weight gain and intrauterine growth is mandatory. Oral nutritional supplements and/or treatment with pancreatic enzymes should be considered in case of low maternal weight gain or fetal growth, in malabsorptive bariatric surgery or in case of twin pregnancy.

Small and frequent meals are recommended in case of postprandial nausea, gastroesophageal reflux, or early satiety, especially in late pregnancy. Adequate fluid intake must be ensured, as well as an appropriate consumption of high protein meals, vegetables, and fruits. The intake of rapidly absorbed carbohydrates, such as soft drinks, juices, sweets, and pastries, should be restricted. Legumes and whole grains are recommended, as well as high protein foods: dairy products, eggs, fish, meat, or chicken. Protein requirements in pregnant women after BS depend on body weight and increase in malabsorptive bariatric procedures. Dietary recommended intake of protein during pregnancy is 1.1 g/kg of prepregnancy body weight per *day*. Although some clinical guidelines recommend a protein intake of 60 g per *day* [15], a dose of 1.1–1.5 g/kg/day can be more appropriate in pregnancy after BS. Smoking and alcoholic beverages should be strictly prohibited.

Nutritional supplements

Micronutrients are essential in fetal development, especially in women at risk of deficiency, as is the case with post-BS gestation. Micronutrients deficiency can have deleterious effects in both mother and fetus (Table 16.4). Preventive supplementation with minerals and micronutrients is needed, in an appropriate dose, according to previous nutritional deficiency and to the technique of bariatric surgery. In general, micronutrient supplementation should be started before pregnancy, with adjustment of the dose of iron, calcium, zinc, and vitamin D and other nutrients, if necessary, to maintain adequate plasma levels [11,12,15]. It should be taken into

Table 16.4 Clinical consequences of micronutrient deficiency during pregnancy.

Micronutrient	Clinical consequences of deficiency on maternal/fetus health
Folate	Neural tube defects, miscarriage, abruptio placentae, prematurity
Iron	Increases maternal and fetal morbidity and mortality, and decreases weight and fetal development
Vitamin B12	Abortion, prematurity, growth retardation, neural tube defects, cognitive impairment
Vitamin D	Gestational diabetes, preeclampsia, low birth weight, long-term complications
Zinc	Delayed fetal growth and maturation, prematurity
Copper	Abortion, prematurity, low weight
Selenium	Preclampsia
Thiamine	Risk of thiamine deficiency in hyperemesis gravidarum
Vitamin A	Fetal malformations, pulmonary dysplasia, anemia
Vitamin E	Preeclampsia, neural tube defects, cognitive impairment, hemolytic disease of the newborn
Vitamin K	Periventricular and intraventricular hemorrhage

account that the normal values of serum levels of minerals and micronutrients are different during pregnancy, as a result of hemodilution and other factors.

Anemia in pregnancy, defined as hemoglobin below 11 g/dl in the first and third quarters and below 10 g/dl in the second quarter, increases maternal morbidity and mortality, impairs fetal growth and maturation, and is associated with an increased risk of low birth weight and impaired neurocognitive development. In the long term, it favors obesity and metabolic problems in the offspring, including increased cardiovascular risk. Bariatric surgery increases the risk of iron deficiency anemia during pregnancy and that this increase is greater as time goes by after the surgery. The prevalence of this complication can be as high as 70% in some series [16]. There is no agreement on the most appropriate iron supplementation regimen in pregnancy after BS. The recommended dose ranges from 40 to 600 mg/day; serum ferritin should be above 30 μg/l [11,12,15]. It should be noted that treatment with intravenous iron during the first trimester of pregnancy is not indicated.

Folic acid is a very relevant nutrient during pregnancy and its deficiency is associated with neural tube defects, anencephaly and encephalocele, spina bifida, abortion, abruptio placentae, and prematurity. Data on the prevalence of folate deficiency in pregnancy after BS are very scarce and just a few cases of neural tube defects have been described. A dose of 400–800 mg/day has been proposed. Vitamin B12 deficiency should be prevented in every patient after bariatric surgery; a dose of 1000 μg/1–3 months i.m. is recommended.

Vitamin D deficiency is common in the general population, especially in obese patients and after BS and can have adverse consequences on maternal and fetal

Table 16.5 Micronutrient supplementation in pregnancy after bariatric surgery.

Micronutrient	Proposed dose	Comments
Folate	400–800 mcg	Consider a higher dose in obese women
Iron	100–200 mg	Gradual increase of dose, between meals, consider vit. C to enhance absorption. Ferritin >30 mg/l
Iodine	200–250 μg	Iodine deficiency is not increased after BS
Vitamin B12	1000–2000 μg/1–3 m	Can be administered orally (>350–500 μg/day)
Calcium	1000–1500 mg	Increase dietary intake. Supplements should be taken distant to Fe dose
Vitamin D	2000–4000 UI	Vitamin D > 30 ng/ml
Zinc	12–30 mg	Can decrease copper absorption
Copper	1–2 μg	Separated from the zinc supplements
Selenium	50–60 mg	
Thiamine	12 mg	Increase to 100 mg/d if nausea/vomiting
Vitamin A	800–1500 μg	A dose below 3000 μg (10,000 IU) per day is safe in pregnancy
Vitamin E	15 mg	
Vitamin K	50–120 μg	Higher risk of deficiency in premature newborn

health. Vitamin D deficiency has been described in up to 70% of pregnancies after BS. A dose or 2000–4000 IU/day is recommended, to maintain vitamin D serum levels above 30 ng/ml [17].

Other micronutrients, such as zinc, copper, vitamin A and E, are especially relevant in malabsorptive bariatric surgery. Thiamine dose should be increased to 50–100 mg/day.

Table 16.5 includes recommended micronutrient supplementation in pregnancy after BS. It should be borne in mind that some of the standard multivitamins or those designed for pregnancy do not provide all the nutrients or the dose necessary for pregnancy after bariatric surgery. A daily vitamin A dose of less than 10,000 IU/day is safe during pregnancy.

Gestational diabetes

Several studies have observed that bariatric surgery can prevent the development of gestational diabetes (GD), especially when compared to morbidly obese women or the same women before BS. The screening of GD in women who have had previous bariatric surgery is not well established; usual criteria may overestimate the diagnosis of GD. Plasma glucose responds to oral glucose stimulation in a different way in gastrectomized patients, especially in the absence of pylorus and if there is a gastrojejunal anastomosis. There is a rapid increase in plasma glucose after oral overload, frequently followed by reactive hypoglycemia. On the other hand, due to the physiopathological characteristics of bariatric surgery, especially gastric by-pass, oral glucose overload in pregnant women may trigger side effects, such as nausea, diarrhea, hypotension, dizziness, or severe hypoglycemia.

Plasma glucose cut-off points for the diagnosis of a GD after bariatric surgery are not well defined and the clinical impact of hyperglycemia after an oral glucose overload (75–100 g), according to the current criteria, is not known. Data on the diagnosis of GD after sleeve gastrectomy, that is being used with increasing frequency in women of childbearing age, are limited. In this technique, pyloric functionality is maintained and may result in less fluctuation of blood glucose.

Taking into account the risk of side effects and the fact that diagnostic criteria for GD in women with previous BS have not been established following the usual criteria, some authors recommend avoiding oral glucose overload with 75 and 100 g, especially in the case of gastric bypass. As an alternative, capillary glucose testing can be performed before and after meals for 7 days, between 24 and 28 weeks of gestation, or in the first trimester in patients at risk. A diagnosis of gestational diabetes will be considered if fasting blood glucose is > 95 mg/dl and/or postprandial blood glucose is > 140 mg/dl (1 h after meals) or >120 mg/dl (2 h after meals) [18,19].

Specific complications of pregnancy after bariatric surgery

Pregnancy may promote internal hernia, as a result of increased intraabdominal pressure. This is a rare complication that should be suspected in women with abdominal pain and/or vomiting. Early diagnosis is essential and should not be delayed due to pregnancy. A magnetic resonance imaging scan is recommended as a first option, and, if not available, a CT scan should be performed. A systematic review of the literature published in 2016 [20] reports 52 cases; nine of them required bowel resection; it includes two cases of maternal death and three of perinatal death, in which surgical treatment was performed with a delay of more than 48 h after the onset of symptoms. Gastroesophageal reflux can occur, especially in late pregnancy and in patients with previous sleeve gastrectomy. Band migration is also a matter of concern in pregnant patients. Postprandial hypoglycemia is a complication that can affect up to 15% of patients after BS, especially in derivative techniques (gastric by-pass, biliopancreatic diverssion), and has been also described during pregnancy [21]. Postprandial hypoglycemia can also complicate the treatment of gestational diabetes. In these situations, continuous monitoring of interstitial glucose may facilitate clinical management.

Neonatal care

Pregnancy after BS is associated with a lower risk of macrosomia, in comparison to that of morbidly obese patients. However, an increase of low birth weight and, in some studies, prematurity has been observed [11,12,15].

The effect of bariatric surgery on the risk of fetal malformations has been evaluated in various studies, with inconclusive results, as obesity itself increases the risk of birth defects. Bariatric surgery-induced weight loss may decrease this risk, but it may also increase the risk of nutritional deficiencies, that can impair fetal growth and development. Fetal malformations have been described in pregnancy after BS, in relation to malnutrition and micronutrient deficiency. A study carried out in Sweden, based on data from a national registry, evaluated 270,0805 pregnancies, 341 of them with previous BS, and did not observe an increased risk of birth defects [22]. A systematic review has recently been published, including 15 studies; the results do not indicate that there is a greater or lesser risk of malformations after bariatric surgery [23].

Newborns of women with previous bariatric surgery should follow local protocols of postnatal care, and routine screening of malformations or nutritional deficiencies is not recommended, except in case of complications. Anyway, pediatricians should be informed about maternal previous bariatric surgery and eventual secondary complications during pregnancy. Data on the long-term effect of maternal bariatric surgery on offspring health are scarce.

Lactation

Breastfeeding is recommended in women with previous bariatric surgery, as in the general population, due to its well-recognized benefits to both mother and newborn health.

It has been observed that milk macronutrient composition and vitamin A content is similar in women with or without previous BS. It should be noted that nutrient requirements in lactating women are higher than those in pregnancy, so there is a risk of malnutrition and micronutrient deficiency, especially after malabsorptive bariatric surgery. Several reports on micronutrient deficiency in infants have been described, especially regarding vitamin B12 [24].

Dietary advice is mandatory.

Bariatric surgery and menopause

In the climacteric period, there is a progressive decrease in estrogen levels due to age-related ovarian failure, which causes an increase in gonadotropin levels (FSH and LH), and a series of metabolic changes that predispose to weight gain. Changes in the regions of the hypothalamus that regulate intake and basal metabolism cause changes in body composition, with an increase in visceral and abdominal fat [25,26]. This leads to increased insulin resistance and changes in the lipid profile and blood pressure, resulting in increased cardiovascular risk. All these changes cause the basal metabolic rate to drop, and weight loss in postmenopausal women is more difficult than in premenopausal women. Menopause also influences bone health, as the decrease in estrogen causes a decrease in bone mineral density and a higher risk of osteoporosis in most women.

All these effects can also be seen in patients who have undergone bariatric surgery. Women operated in the postmenopausal period, lose less weight than premenopausal women, both with restrictive and mixed techniques [27]. In addition, bone health may be affected to a greater extent, especially in malabsorptive techniques, due to calcium and vitamin D malabsorption, and secondary hyperparathyroidism. Women operated on in the postmenopausal period experience greater loss of bone mass than young women, and this is visible in the early stages after surgery [28]. However, this loss of bone mass has not been shown to be different from nonoperated women of the same age [29].

Bariatric surgery in postmenopause does have benefits in terms of weight improvement and other cardiovascular risk factors, and may improve some menopause-related symptoms [30], so it remains an effective treatment in these patients.

Physical exercise is mandatory in menopausal women after bariatric surgery, to prevent sarcopenia and osteopenia/osteoporosis. An adequate protein consumption, 1.2—1.5 g/kg/day, is also recommended, as well as an appropriate intake of calcium and vitamin D, both from diet and from nutritional supplements.

Pregnancy, lactation, and menopause in women with previous bariatric surgery: summary of recommendations

- Follow-up during pregnancy and lactation should be carried out by a multidisciplinary team, which includes gynecology and obstetrics specialists, endocrinologists, surgeons, dietitians, and nursing.
- An appropriate selection of the bariatric surgical technique should be performed, according to BMI, associated comorbidity, team's experience, and patient's preferences. Women should be informed about the risk and benefits of BS in relation to pregnancy.
- An adequate contraception should be ensured before bariatric surgery.
- It is advisable to delay pregnancy to 12—18 months after bariatric surgery.
- An adequate follow-up after bariatric surgery is mandatory, which includes dietary advice and micronutrient supplementation. Antenatal consultation is also recommended. Close clinical monitoring of both maternal and fetal health is needed.
- Preventive supplementation with minerals and micronutrients is recommended, in an appropriate dose, according to previous nutritional deficiency and to the technique of bariatric surgery. In the case of oral diet intolerance, nausea, or vomiting, thiamine dose should be increased.
- Screening of pregnancy complications, following specific protocols, should be performed. It is recommended to avoid the use of oral glucose tolerance tests, especially in women the previous gastric bypass and biliopancreatic diversion.
- Surveillance of the appearance of surgical complications, such as internal hernia, is required.

- Breastfeeding should be advised. A clinical and nutritional monitoring during lactation is also recommended.
- In menopausal women, the possible deleterious effect of BS on bone mass and the higher risk of osteoporosis and sarcopenia should be considered, especially when malabsorptive techniques are used.

References

[1] Broughton DE, Moley KH. Obesity and female infertility: potential mediators of obesity's impact. Fertil Steril 2017;107(4):840−7. https://doi.org/10.1016/j.fertnstert.2017.01.017.

[2] Palomba S, de Wilde MA, Falbo A, Koster MP, La Sala GB, Fauser BC. Pregnancy complications in women with polycystic ovary syndrome. Hum Reprod Update 2015;21(5):575−92. https://doi.org/10.1093/humupd/dmv029.

[3] LifeCycle Project-Maternal Obesity and Childhood Outcomes Study Group, Voerman E, Santos S, et al. Association of gestational weight gain with adverse maternal and infant outcomes. J Am Med Assoc 2019;321(17):1702−15. https://doi.org/10.1001/jama.2019.3820.

[4] Yang Z, Phung H, Freebairn L, Sexton R, Raulli A, Kelly P. Contribution of maternal overweight and obesity to the occurrence of adverse pregnancy outcomes. Aust N Z J Obstet Gynaecol 2019;59(3):367−74. https://doi.org/10.1111/ajo.12866.

[5] Crane JM, Murphy P, Burrage L, Hutchens D. Maternal and perinatal outcomes of extreme obesity in pregnancy. J Obstet Gynaecol Can 2013;35(7):606−11. https://doi.org/10.1016/S1701-2163(15)30879-3.

[6] Akhter Z, Rankin J, Ceulemans D, et al. Pregnancy after bariatric surgery and adverse perinatal outcomes: a systematic review and meta-analysis. PLoS Med 2019;16(8):e1002866. https://doi.org/10.1371/journal.pmed.1002866. Published 2019 Aug 6.

[7] Galazis N, Docheva N, Simillis C, Nicolaides KH. Maternal and neonatal outcomes in women undergoing bariatric surgery: a systematic review and meta-analysis. Eur J Obstet Gynecol Reprod Biol 2014;181:45−53. https://doi.org/10.1016/j.ejogrb.2014.07.015.

[8] Kwong W, Tomlinson G, Feig DS. Maternal and neonatal outcomes after bariatric surgery; a systematic review and meta-analysis: do the benefits outweigh the risks? Am J Obstet Gynecol 2018;218(6):573−80. https://doi.org/10.1016/j.ajog.2018.02.003.

[9] Sheiner E, Balaban E, Dreiher J, Levi I, Levy A. Pregnancy outcome in patients following different types of bariatric surgeries. Obes Surg 2009;19(9):1286−92. https://doi.org/10.1007/s11695-009-9920-9.

[10] González I, Rubio MA, Cordido F, et al. Maternal and perinatal outcomes after bariatric surgery: a Spanish multicenter study. Obes Surg 2015;25(3):436−42. https://doi.org/10.1007/s11695-014-1387-7.

[11] Ciangura C, Coupaye M, Deruelle P, et al. Clinical practice guidelines for childbearing female candidates for bariatric surgery, pregnancy, and post-partum management after bariatric surgery. Obes Surg 2019;29(11):3722−34. https://doi.org/10.1007/s11695-019-04093-y [published correction appears in obes surg. 2020 Jun 5;:].

[12] Falcone V, Stopp T, Feichtinger M, et al. Pregnancy after bariatric surgery: a narrative literature review and discussion of impact on pregnancy management and outcome. BMC Pregnancy Childbirth 2018;18(1):507. https://doi.org/10.1186/s12884-018-2124-3. Published 2018 Dec 27.

[13] Mengesha B, Griffin L, Nagle A, Kiley J. Assessment of contraceptive needs in women undergoing bariatric surgery. Contraception 2016;94(1):74–7. https://doi.org/10.1016/j.contraception.2016.02.027.

[14] Maslin K, James A, Brown A, Bogaerts A, Shawe J. What is known about the nutritional intake of women during pregnancy following bariatric surgery? A scoping review. Nutrients 2019;11(9):2116. https://doi.org/10.3390/nu11092116. Published 2019 Sep. 5.

[15] Shawe J, Ceulemans D, Akhter Z, et al. Pregnancy after bariatric surgery: consensus recommendations for periconception, antenatal and postnatal care. Obes Rev 2019; 20(11):1507–22. https://doi.org/10.1111/obr.12927.

[16] Rottenstreich A, Elazary R, Goldenshluger A, Pikarsky AJ, Elchalal U, Ben-Porat T. Maternal nutritional status and related pregnancy outcomes following bariatric surgery: a systematic review. Surg Obes Relat Dis 2019;15(2):324–32. https://doi.org/10.1016/j.soard.2018.11.018.

[17] Chakhtoura MT, Nakhoul N, Akl EA, Mantzoros CS, El Hajj Fuleihan GA. Guidelines on vitamin D replacement in bariatric surgery: identification and systematic appraisal. Metabolism 2016;65(4):586–97. https://doi.org/10.1016/j.metabol.2015.12.013.

[18] Freitas C, Araújo C, Caldas R, Lopes DS, Nora M, Monteiro MP. Effect of new criteria on the diagnosis of gestational diabetes in women submitted to gastric bypass. Surg Obes Relat Dis 2014;10(6):1041–6. https://doi.org/10.1016/j.soard.2014.03.013.

[19] Benhalima K, Minschart C, Ceulemans D, et al. Screening and management of gestational diabetes mellitus after bariatric surgery. Nutrients 2018;10(10):1479. https://doi.org/10.3390/nu10101479. Published 2018 Oct 11.

[20] Vannevel V, Jans G, Bialecka M, Lannoo M, Devlieger R, Van Mieghem T. Internal herniation in pregnancy after gastric bypass: a systematic review. Obstet Gynecol 2016; 127(6):1013–20. https://doi.org/10.1097/AOG.0000000000001429.

[21] Nor Hanipah Z, Punchai S, Birriel TJ, et al. Clinical features of symptomatic hypoglycemia observed after bariatric surgery. Surg Obes Relat Dis 2018;14(9):1335–9. https://doi.org/10.1016/j.soard.2018.02.022.

[22] Josefsson A, Bladh M, Wiréhn AB, Sydsjö G. Risk for congenital malformations in offspring of women who have undergone bariatric surgery. A national cohort. BJOG 2013;120(12):1477–82. https://doi.org/10.1111/1471-0528.12365.

[23] Benjamin RH, Littlejohn S, Mitchell LE. Bariatric surgery and birth defects: a systematic literature review. Paediatr Perinat Epidemiol 2018;32(6):533–44. https://doi.org/10.1111/ppe.12517.

[24] Wardinsky TD, Montes RG, Friederich RL, Broadhurst RB, Sinnhuber V, Bartholomew D. Vitamin B12 deficiency associated with low breast-milk vitamin B12 concentration in an infant following maternal gastric bypass surgery. Arch Pediatr Adolesc Med 1995;149(11):1281–4. https://doi.org/10.1001/archpedi.1995.02170240099020.

[25] Mastorakos G, Valsamakis G, Paltoglou G, Creatsas G. Management of obesity in menopause: diet, exercise, pharmacotherapy and bariatric surgery. Maturitas 2010; 65(3):219–24.

[26] Ambikairajah A, Walsh E, Tabatabaei-Jafari H, Cherbuin N. Fat mass changes during menopause: a metaanalysis. Am J Obstet Gynecol 2019;221(5):393–409. e50.

[27] Ochner CN, Teixeira J, Geary N, Asarian L. Greater short-term weight loss in women 20-45 versus 55-65 years of age following bariatric surgery. Obes Surg. octubre de 2013;23(10):1650–4.
[28] Schafer AL, Kazakia GJ, Vittinghoff E, Stewart L, Rogers SJ, Kim TY, et al. Effects of gastric bypass surgery on bone mass and microarchitecture occur early and particularly impact postmenopausal women. J Bone Miner Res 2018;33(6):975–86.
[29] Valderas JP, Velasco S, Solari S, Liberona Y, Viviani P, Maiz A, et al. Increase of bone resorption and the parathyroid hormone in postmenopausal women in the long-term after Roux-en-Y gastric bypass. Obes Surg 2009;19(8):1132–8.
[30] Goughnour SL, Thurston RC, Althouse AD, Freese KE, Edwards RP, Hamad GG, et al. Assessment of hot flushes and vaginal dryness among obese women undergoing bariatric surgery. Climacteric J Int Menopause Soc 2016;19(1):71–6.

CHAPTER 17

Follow-up and screening of postoperative nutritional deficiencies

Natalia Pérez-Ferre, Clara Marcuello-Foncillas, Miguel Ángel Rubio-Herrera
Endocrinology and Nutrition Department, Hospital Clinico San Carlos, Madrid, Spain

Chapter outline

Introduction	223
Pathophysiology of nutritional deficiencies after weight loss surgery	224
Micronutrient deficiencies after weight loss surgery	226
Iron	227
Vitamin D and calcium	228
Vitamin B12 (cobalamine)	230
Folic acid	230
Vitamin B1 (thiamin)	231
Fat-soluble vitamins: A, E, K	232
Trace elements	233
Copper	233
Zinc	234
Selenium	236
Suggested protocol for the follow-up and screening of nutritional deficiencies after weight loss surgery	236
Further reading	236

Introduction

An adequate nutritional status is essential for a successful result of the weight loss process after surgery. Nutritional supplementation is a necessary therapy, contributing to weight loss in a healthy manner. Candidates to weight loss surgery (WLS) must be informed and agree to be adherent to nutritional recommendations, take the supplements for life, attend to medical appointments, and take blood tests periodically. If the patient fails to any of these commitments, important complications can arise in the medium term and long term, even malnutrition syndromes or irreversible consequences of a severe nutritional deficiency.

For the prevention of nutritional deficiencies, the keys are an adequate diet in the postoperative period and the prescription of appropriate doses of supplements of vitamins and minerals from the first month after surgery. We must emphasize the importance of compliance with multivitamin supplements in the long term. Patients usually stop taking supplements after 1–2 years after surgery for different reasons, sometimes economical issues, or just because they do not see any direct benefit on their own health. That is why we must ask in every visit about the compliance with the prescribed treatment and explain to the patient the possible consequences of a nutritional deficiency.

In other cases, despite the daily use of supplements, the level of some nutrients may decrease, and we will have to adapt the doses individually.

Early detection of subclinical deficiencies must be performed with laboratory testing with the appropriate frequency according to the technique and clinical evolution. We must take into account the potential interactions among micronutrients: a deficiency in one specific micronutrient may cause the deficiency of another one, and the replacement of one micronutrient level may cause disorders in another micronutrient. That is why the evaluation of deficiencies must be *complete* and the interpretation must be *global*.

Follow-up with laboratory testing must be performed for life in most of the cases. For that purpose, the collaboration of the Endocrinology and Nutrition Unit with Primary Care physician will be very useful.

The treatment of deficiencies must be performed on time to avoid overt syndromes that can be severe or cause irreversible consequences.

There are no absolutely strong recommendations to prevent or treat most nutritional deficiencies after weight loss surgery. In some cases, we must consider micronutrient mega-doses because of the lower bioavailability resulting from physiological changes provided by the surgical technique.

In this chapter, we will discuss the pathophysiology of nutritional deficiencies after weight loss surgery and the basis for the follow-up of the most frequent micronutrient deficiencies, with recommendations and tips for the clinical practice.

Pathophysiology of nutritional deficiencies after weight loss surgery

Anatomical and physiological changes after weight loss surgery may lead to nutritional deficiencies. The prevalence and severity of the different nutritional deficiencies depend on the characteristics of the specific technique: the extent of the gastric and intestinal resection, the duodenum exclusion, the malabsorptive grade of the procedure, and the biliopancreatic diversion.

There are specific locations in the gut for preferred absorption of micronutrients, that we must remember to understand the pathophysiology of nutritional deficiencies (Fig. 17.1).

Other important factors that may influence the prevalence of nutritional deficiencies in the postoperative period depend on the patient: preexisting deficiencies before surgery that must be screened and treated (vitamin D, vitamin B12, folic acid), tolerance and adherence to an adequate diet, and, of course, the compliance

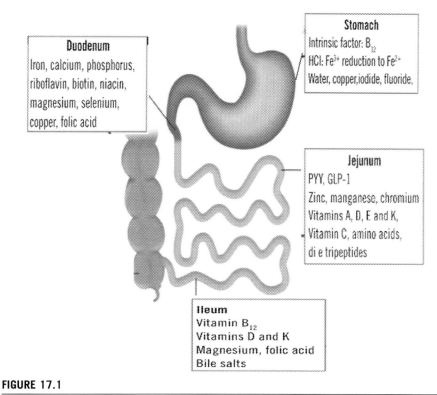

FIGURE 17.1

Locations of preferred absorption of nutrients in the gut.

to the intake of supplements of vitamins and minerals. In addition, we must take into account the intestinal adaptation after surgery. Patients over 60 years old undergoing a WLS will have less and slower adaptation of their intestinal absorption than a younger patient, being a special risk group for nutritional deficiencies.

Restrictive techniques (sleeve gastrectomy) may lead to nutritional deficiencies due to a reduction in the intake because of the smaller gastric reservoir or due to a not optimal tolerance to the prescribed diet because of early satiety, nausea or vomiting, or dietary aversions after surgery.

Nutritional deficiencies after a **gastric bypass** may occur through two different mechanisms: restrictive and malabsorptive component. The reduction in the gastric reservoir compromises the intake. The exclusion in the contact of nutrients with the duodenum and proximal jejunum leads to malabsorption of several micronutrients. The length of the alimentary limb (between 100 and 120 cm) will determine the absorptive capacity for all the nutrients. The length of the common limb (from 150 to 300 cm) will determine the time of contact of the nutrients with bile and pancreatic secretions, and therefore will determine fat absorption.

Table 17.1 Prevalence of nutritional deficiencies depending on the surgical technique. Data are shown as percentages, resulting from the summary of the literature.

	LAGB	LSG	RYGB	BPDDS	SADI-S
Iron	0–32	15–45	20–55	30–40	30–40
Vitamin B12	10	10–20	30–70	5–20	5–20
Folic acid	10	10–20	9–35	1.3–22	5–20
Vitamin B1	0	0	12–49	10–15	–
Vitamin D	30	30–70	30–50	40–100	40–100
Vitamin A	10	10–20	10–50	60–70	60–70
Vitamin E	0	0–5	10	10–70	10–70
Vitamin K	0	0	0	60–70	–
Zinc	–	7–15	20–37	10–50	10–50
Copper	–	10	10	70–90	10–50
Selenium			14–42	–	–

BPDDS, *biliopancreatic diversion with duodenal switch*; LAGB, *laparoscopic-assisted gastric banding*; LSG, *laparoscopic sleeve gastrectomy*; RYGB, *Roux Y gastric bypass*; SADI-S, *single anastomosis duodeno-ileal with sleeve gastrectomy*

Biliopancreatic diversion with duodenal switch has a main malabsorptive component with a length of the common limb between 50 and 100 cm. The resulting fat malabsorption compromises the absorption of fat-soluble vitamins and trace elements.

Single anastomosis duodeno-ileal with sleeve gastrectomy (SADI-S) procedure combines a restrictive component (sleeve gastrectomy) with a malabsorptive component (single anastomosis duodeno-ileal) that can vary according to the length of the common limb (from 200 to 300 cm). For instance, a common limb of 250 cm will be more malabsorptive than a common limb of 300 cm, so the first one will have more probably deficiencies in fat-soluble vitamins and trace elements.

The prevalence of the different nutritional deficiencies has a wide variability according to the series. These differences in outcomes underscore the methodological limitations of existing studies, such as small sample sizes and heterogeneity of study design and outcomes, with most of these studies relying upon self-report to assess multivitamin intake. Most data are based on retrospective studies. In addition, the level of a specific micronutrient to consider deficiency or normal range is different among studies (Table 17.1).

Micronutrient deficiencies after weight loss surgery

Following the guidelines from the American Society for Metabolic and Bariatric Surgery updated in 2017, we summarize the recommendations for the most prevalent deficiencies in micronutrients after weight loss surgery. Macronutrient deficiency will be exposed in another chapter.

Table 17.2 Grading scheme for recommendations, per the AACE protocol for production of clinical practice guidelines. step III: grading of recommendations.

Best evidence level	Subjective factor impact	Consensus	Recommendation grade
Strong			
1	None	Yes	A
2	Positive	Yes	A
Intermediate			
2	None	Yes	B
1	Negative	Yes	B
3	Positive	Yes	B
Weak			
3	None	Yes	C
2	Negative	Yes	C
4	Positive	Yes	C
No evidence			
4	None	Yes	D
3	Negative	Yes	D
1,2,3,4	N/A	No	D

For the recommendations on screening and doses of micronutrients, we used the grading strategy published by AACE to provide consistent and systematic grades, with strongest to weakest levels noted as A through D and best evidence level (BEL) from strongest to weakest noted as 1—4 for each recommendation (Table 17.2).

Iron

Iron absorption occurs mainly in the duodenum and proximal jejunum.

The main causes of iron deficiency after bariatric surgery are as follows: the bypassing of absorption sites in the gastrointestinal tract (duodenum and proximal jejunum); decreased intake of iron-rich foods due to intolerance or preference (red meat); inadequate supplement adherence; and/or altered absorption due to interaction of iron with calcium supplements or certain food components. In addition, gastric hypochlorhydria makes difficult iron release from food. There is a decreased reduction of ferric iron to ferrous iron, being this last one more soluble for its absorption in duodenum.

The most affected groups are as follows: women of childbearing age are (due to prolonged menses and/or hypermenorrhea), individuals with iron deficiency before bariatric surgery and duodenal exclusion techniques (gastric bypass and Scopinaro biliopancreatic diversion). It can also reflect imperceptible, but persistent losses, due to esophagitis, gastroesophageal reflux, or through the intestine (diverticula, polyps, hemorrhoids, and even colon cancer), therefore, in certain cases, endoscopic examinations are recommended.

We must assess the iron status in all patients postbariatric surgery, using both physiological signs and symptoms and laboratory results.

The following are the recommendations from the guidelines of the American Society for Metabolic and Bariatric Surgery[a]:

Recommendations for postoperative screening of iron deficiency
- Routine post-WLS screening of iron status is recommended for all patients within 3 months after surgery, and then every 3—6 months until the 12-month visit, and annually thereafter (Grade B, BEL 2).
- Iron status in post-WLS patients should be monitored at regular intervals using an iron panel, complete blood count, total iron-binding capacity, ferritin, and soluble transferrin receptor if available, along with clinical signs or symptoms (Grade C, BEL 3).
- Additional iron screening in post-WLS patients who should be conducted as warranted by clinical signs or symptoms and or laboratory findings, or in other instances in which a deficiency is suspected (Grade B, BEL 2).

Recommendations for supplementation of iron for preventing deficiency
- Patients at low risk of postoperative iron deficiency should receive at least 18 mg of iron from their multivitamin (Grade C, BEL 3).
- Menstruating females who have had RYGB, SG, or BPD/DS should take 45—60 mg of elemental iron daily (cumulative from all vitamin and mineral supplements) (Grade C, BEL 3).
- Oral supplementation should be taken in divided doses separately from calcium supplements, acid-reducing medications, and foods high in phytates or polyphenols (Grade D, BEL 3).

Vitamin D and calcium

Calcium absorption occurs mainly in the duodenum and proximal jejunum, and it is mediated by vitamin D in an acid environment. Vitamin D is absorbed in jejunum and ileum. Calcium absorption is decreased in RYGB and SG because of a less production of gastric acid. In addition, there is a decrease in the intake of calcium because of a not optimal tolerance to dairy products and the reduction in the global intake. Vitamin D deficiency is highly prevalent before surgery in obese patients (21%—80%) and may become higher after surgery because of the malabsorptive component in RYGB, BPD, and SADI-S. Deficiency in vitamin D and calcium may cause acute clinical hypocalcemia, and, in the long term, osteoporosis and risk of bone fracture.

The metabolism of vitamin D (cholecalciferol) is altered in obese patients, showing lower values than the general population due to various causes:

---

[a] Adapted from: Parrott J, Frank L, Rabena R, Craggs-Dino L, Isom KA, Greiman L. American society for metabolic and bariatric surgery integrated health nutritional guidelines for the surgical weight loss patient 2016 update: micronutrients. Surg Obes Relat Dis 2017;13(5):727—41.

(A) sequestration in adipose tissue (it is more fat-soluble); (B) worse intestinal absorption after surgery, since it is necessary to follow the fat absorption process through the lymphatic system; (C) the enzyme that converts cholecalciferol to calcifediol (CYP2R1) is less expressed in obesity and is interfered with by the action of various drugs (anticonvulsants, antiretrovirals, antipsychotics, etc.). Therefore, it is preferred to administer Calcifediol after bariatric surgery because it is better absorbed at the intestinal level, reaching the liver via the portal (water-soluble) and does not depend on CYP2R1 enzymatic activity. Dose distributed (daily, weekly), in the form of drops, drinkable vials, or capsules, in an amount> 1000−2000 IU/day, as necessary, to maintain concentrations between 20 and 50 ng/mL. Biliopancreatic shunts may require high doses of calcifediol (up to 150,000−200,000 IU/month) if malabsorption is marked. In some cases, it may be necessary to resort to parenteral administration (im or sc) every 15−30 days.

One of the objectives of the treatment will be to prevent or minimize secondary hyperparathyroidism without inducing hypercalciuria. Monitoring of urine calcium levels is recommended in the follow-up to control if the intake and the intestinal absorption of calcium are optimal.

Hypophosphatemia is usually due to vitamin D deficiency. We can use oral phosphate supplementation for mild to moderate hypophosphatemia (1.5−2.5 mg/dL).

We must take special attention when the patient is taking calcium lowering medication (bisphosphonates) because of the risk of severe acute hypocalcemia with potential clinical titania. Fixed combinations of calcium and vitamin D are very commonly used in clinical practice.

Recommendations for postoperative screening of vitamin D and calcium
- Routine post-WLS screening of vitamin D status is recommended for all patients (Grade B, BEL 2).
- More research is needed before a recommendation can be made regarding the use of vitamin D binding protein assays as an additional tool for determining vitamin D status in post-WLS patients (Grade C, BEL 3).

Recommendations for supplementation of vitamin D and calcium for preventing deficiency
- All post-WLS patients should take calcium supplementation (Grade C, BEL 3).
- The appropriate dose of calcium varies by surgical procedure:
    - BPD/DS: 1800−2400 mg/day
    - LAGB, SG, RYGB: 1200−1500 mg/day
- The recommended preventative dose of vitamin D in post-WLS patients should be based on serum vitamin D levels:
    - Recommended vitamin D3 dose is 3000 IU daily, until blood levels of 25(OH)D are greater than sufficient (30 ng/mL) (Grade D, BEL 4).
    - As compared to recommended vitamin D2 doses, a 70%−90% smaller vitamin D3 bolus dose is needed to achieve the same effects in healthy nonbariatric surgical patients (Grade A, BEL 1).
- To enhance calcium absorption in post-WLS patients, the following dosing considerations apply (Grade C, BEL 3):
    - Calcium should be given in divided doses
    - Calcium carbonate should be taken with meals, and the tolerance is better.
    - Calcium citrate may be taken with or without meals and is more soluble when a reduction in the gastric acid is present.

Vitamin B12 (cobalamine)

Risk for vitamin B12 deficiency after WLS is dependent upon a number of factors: type of surgical procedure (procedures that involve bypass or removal of all or part of the stomach, such as the SG, RYGB, and BPD/DS, put patients at higher risk for deficiency); preoperative B12 deficiency; postsurgical timeframe; adequacy of dietary intake; concomitant use of medications that interfere with B12 bioavailability; and adherence to B12 supplementation.

Disruption of B12 absorption may occur when a WLS procedure leads to a significantly decreased intake of dietary protein and/or impairs hydrolysis of free colbalamine by reducing pepsin and HCl production. In purely restrictive procedures such as the LAGB, B12 deficiency is less likely as there is no effect on gastric acid or IF production. However, due to food intolerances, restriction of dietary protein intake, and chronic use of PPIs seen in some LAGB patients, B12 deficiency can be seen in this population as well.

The delayed manifestation of vitamin B12 deficiency is explained because of the long-term hepatic storage of B12 (approximately 2000 mcg), so low values typically emerge 2–3 years after surgery.

Recommendations for postoperative screening of vitamin B12
- Routine postoperative screening of vitamin B12 is recommended in patients who have undergone RYGB, SG, or BPD/DS (Grade B, BEL 2).
- More frequent screening in the first postoperative year, every 3 months and then at least annually or as clinically indicated is recommended for post-WLS patients who are chronically using medications that exacerbate the risk of B12 deficiency: nitrous oxide, neomycin, metformin, colchicine, PPIs, or seizure medications (Grade B, BEL 2).
- Serum B12 may not be adequate to identify B12 deficiency. It is recommended to include serum MMA with or without homocysteine to identify metabolic deficiency of B12 in symptomatic or asymptomatic patients, and in those patients with a history of B12 deficiency or preexisting neuropathy (Grade B, BEL 2).

Recommendations for supplementation of vitamin B12 for preventing deficiency
- All post-WLS patients should take vitamin B12 supplementation (Grade B, BEL 2).
- The recommended supplement dose for vitamin B12 varies based on the route of administration (Grade B, BEL 2):
    - Orally by disintegrating tablet, sublingual, or liquid: 350–500 mcg daily
    - Nasal spray: as directed by the manufacturer
    - Parenteral (IM or SQ): 1000 mcg monthly.

Folic acid

Folate absorption from dietary sources occurs mainly in the jejunum. Only a small amount of folate is stored. The total amount of body folate is estimated to be approximately 10–30 mg, with the liver containing approximately half of the total folate pool.

The primary symptom of folate deficiency is megaloblastic anemia. This rarely occurs independent of vitamin B12 deficiency because the two vitamins work synergistically in hematopoiesis. Folate deficiency can manifest in clinical signs such as oral mucosal ulcerations, changes in skin and nail pigmentation, and elevated homocysteine serum levels.

The risk for folate deficiency is reported in all currently performed WLS procedures and may be secondary to low intake of folate-rich foods, poor adherence to supplement regimens, taking vitamin regimens that contain less than 400 mcg of folate, chronic use of medications that interfere with the bioavailability of folate, alcoholism, preexisting medical or surgical conditions that interfere with folate absorption, and/or an existing preoperative folate deficiency.

Similar to the case with B12, most post-WLS patients who are folate deficient are asymptomatic or suffer from subclinical symptoms, so these deficient states may not be easily identified.

Folate deficiency can occur even in the context of routine supplementation, especially if multivitamins do not contain the proper dosage of folic acid and the dietary intake of folate is inadequate. Folate supplementation above 1 mg per day is not recommended due to the potential masking of vitamin B12 deficiency.

Recommendations for postoperative screening of folate
- Routine post-WLS screening of folate status is recommended in all patients (Grade B, BEL 2).
- Particular attention should be paid to female patients of childbearing age (Grade B, BEL 2).

Recommendations for supplementation of folate for preventing deficiency
- Post-WLS patients who are not female and childbearing age should take 400—800 mcg oral folate daily from their multivitamin (Grade B, BEL 2).
- Women of childbearing age should take 800—1000 mcg oral folate daily (Grade B, BEL 2).

Vitamin B1 (thiamin)

The prevalence of thiamin deficiency has been estimated between <1% and 49%, with variations based on the type of procedure, the follow-up time, and risk factors. Proton inhibitors, antacids, can inhibit the absorption of thiamin, as well as alcohol, tea, coffee, and raw fish. Chronic diuretic treatment increases renal thiamin losses.

Risk factors associated with neurological complications following surgery include the absolute amount of weight loss, malnutrition, prolonged GI symptoms, poor postoperative nutritional follow-up, and reduced serum albumin and transferrin. A recent systematic review suggests that bariatric beriberi generally occurs 1—3 months after surgery. However, thiamin deficiency can occur at any time if risk factors are present. Symptomatic B1 deficiency occurs in up to 49% of patients postsurgery, varying by the procedure. Several systematic reviews on the risk of Wernicke encephalopathy after all types of WLS have been published. A primary determinant and predictor of this major neurological complication is persistent vomiting.

Monitoring is recommended in patients at high risk of presenting thiamin deficiency such as persistent vomiting, alcohol consumption, malnutrition, and bacterial overgrowth.

> **Recommendations for the postoperative screening of thiamin**
> - Routine postoperative screening of thiamin is recommended for high-risk groups:
>   - Patients with risk factors for TD (Grade B, BEL 2).
>   - Patients with concomitant medical conditions such as cardiac failure (especially those receiving furosemide) (Grade B, BEL 2).
>   - Females (Grade B, BEL 2).
>   - African Americans (Grade B, BEL 2).
>   - Patients not attending a nutritional clinic after surgery (Grade B, BEL 2).
>   - Patients with GI symptoms (intractable nausea and vomiting, jejunal dilation, mega-colon, or constipation) (Grade B, BEL 2).
>   - Patients with small bowel bacterial overgrowth (SBBO) (Grade C, BEL 3).
> - If signs and symptoms or risk factors are present in post-WLS patients, thiamin status should be assessed at least during the first 6 months, then every 3—6 months until symptoms resolve (Grade B, BEL 2).
>
> **Recommendations for supplementation of thiamin for preventing deficiency**
> - Thiamin supplementation above the RDA is suggested to prevent TD:
>   - Post-WLS patients should take at *least* **12 mg thiamin daily** (Grade C, BEL 3) and
>   - *preferably* **a 50 mg dose of thiamin from a B-complex supplement or multivitamin once or twice daily** (Grade D, BEL 4) to maintain blood levels of thiamin and prevent TD.

Fat-soluble vitamins: A, E, K

Lipid digestion is delayed in post-WLS patients, especially in patients who undergo RYGB, and BPD/DS. In these procedures, the fats do not pass through the duodenum impairing the release of bile and pancreatic lipase. Limited production of these enzymes leads to the malabsorption of fat; thus, fat-soluble vitamin deficiency may result. Water-soluble vitamin deficiencies tend to occur early in the postoperative period, but fat-soluble deficiencies develop more slowly, based on the rate of the progression of fat malabsorption.

Vitamin A deficiency is relatively common (**up to 70%**) in LAGB, RYGB, and BPD/DS patients within 4 years after surgery. Vitamin A deficiency may cause night blindness (xeroftalmia). We must adjust for prealbumin levels (carrier protein): ratio retinol/prealbumin. A low prealbumin may result in a nonreal vitamin A low level. Iron and copper deficiency may be difficult to the recovery of vitamin A levels.

There is a small risk of hepatic toxicity with vitamin A, mainly in the case of fatty liver.

Prevalence of vitamin E and K deficiency is rare, so its postsurgical monitoring is not recommended. For vitamin E evaluation, we must use ratio Vit E/Cholesterol. A normal ratio means an adequate antioxidant status. It is unusual and rare to observe complications related to vitamin K deficiency post-WLS; however, any malabsorptive procedure (BPD/DS or RYGB) does confer an elevated risk for vitamin K deficiency.

Low prothrombin time has been used as an indicator of vitamin K deficiency. It is recommended to maintain an INR <1.4. If vitamin K deficiency is suspected (probably together with other vitamins) parenteral vitamin K should be administered until normalization.

> **Recommendations for postoperative screening of vitamins A, E, K deficiency**
> - Post-WLS patients should be screened for vitamin A deficiency within the first year after surgery, particularly those who have had BPD/DS, whether symptoms are present or not (Grade B, BEL 2).
> - Vitamin A should be measured in patients who have had RYGB or BPD/DS, particularly in those patients with evidence of protein-calorie malnutrition (Grade B, BEL 2).
> - Although vitamin E and K deficiencies are uncommon after WLS, patients who are symptomatic should be screened (Grade B, BEL 2).
>
> **Recommendations for supplementation of vitamins A, E, K for preventing deficiency**
> - Post-WLS patients should take vitamins A, E, and K, with the dosage based upon the type of procedure:
>   - LAGB: Vitamin A (5000 IU/d) and vitamin K (90–120 ug/day) (Grade C, BEL 3).
>   - RYGB, and SG: Vitamin A (5000–10,000 IU/d) and vitamin K (90–120 ug/day) (Grade D, BEL 4).
>   - LAGB, SG, RYGB, BPD/DS: Vitamin E (15 mg/d) (Grade D, BEL 4).
>   - DS: Vitamin A (10,000 IU/d) and vitamin K (300 μg/d) (Grade B, BEL 2).
> - Higher maintenance doses of fat-soluble vitamins may be required for post-WLS patients who have a previous history of vitamin A, E, or K deficiency (Grade D, BEL 4).
> - Water-miscible forms of fat-soluble vitamins are also available to improve absorption (Grade D, BEL 4).
> - Special attention should be given to prenatal supplementation of vitamin A and K in pregnant women who have had WLS (Grade D, BEL 4).

Trace elements
Copper

It is estimated that copper deficit after bariatric surgery is between 10% and 20% after gastric bypass and up to 90% in patients undergoing malabsorptive surgery. Systematic monitoring of copper and ceruloplasmin is recommended in all surgeries with malabsorptive component (RYGB, BPD, SADI-S) at least once a year, but with greater emphasis in patients with suggestive symptoms such as neuropathy, myeloneuropathy, anemia not related to iron deficiency, and healing difficulties.

> **Recommendations for postoperative screening of copper deficiency**
> - Routine screening of copper status in post-WLS patients is recommended at least annually after BPD/DS and RYGB, even in the absence of clinical signs or symptoms of deficiency (Grade C, BEL 4).

Continued

> **—cont'd**
> - In post-WLS patients, serum copper and ceruloplasmin are the recommended biomarkers for determining copper status, as they are closely correlated with physical symptoms of copper deficiency (Grade C, BEL 4).
>
> **Recommendations for supplementation of copper for preventing deficiency**
> - All post-WLS patients should take copper as part of routine multivitamin and mineral supplementation, with dosage based upon the type of procedure (Grade C, BEL 3):
>   - BPD/DS or RYGB patients should supplement with 200% of the RDA for copper (2 mg/day)
>   - SG or LAGB patients should supplement with 100% of the RDA for copper (1 mg/day)
> - In post-WLS patients, supplementation with 1 mg copper is recommended for every 8—15 mg of elemental zinc to prevent copper deficiency (Grade C, BEL 3).
> - In post-WLS patients, copper gluconate or sulfate is the recommended source of copper for supplementation (Grade C, BEL 3).

Zinc

The prevalence of Zn deficiency in patients with bariatric surgery varies between 40% and 70%. Zn is absorbed in the duodenum and the first jejunal loops so that subjects with the exclusion of this anatomical area and those with a higher malabsorptive component are at greater risk of deficiency.

The possibility of Zn deficiency should be routinely monitored in malabsorptive techniques (gastric bypass, biliopancreatic diversión, SADI-S) (level of evidence: moderate), but should also be analyzed in any bariatric technique if the subject manifests chronic diarrhea, hair loss, itches, dysgeusia, and among men with unexplained data on hypogonadism or erectile dysfunction (low level of evidence).

> **Recommendations for postoperative screening**
> - Although the evidence does not suggest that all post-WLS patients should be screened for zinc deficiency, patients who have RYGB or BPD/DS should be screened at least annually for zinc deficiency (Grade C, BEL 3).
> - Serum or plasma zinc is the most appropriate biomarkers for zinc screening in post-WLS patients. The same biomarkers should be used in preoperative and postoperative patients (Grade C, BEL 3).
> - Zinc should be evaluated in all post-WLS patients when the screening results for iron deficiency anemia are negative (Grade C, BEL 3).
> - Post-WLS patients who have chronic diarrhea should be evaluated for zinc deficiency (Grade D, BEL 4).
>
> **Recommendations for supplementation of zinc for preventing deficiency**
> - All post-WLS patients should take zinc, with the dosage based upon the type of procedure (Grade C, BEL 3):
>   - BPD/DS: Supplement with 16—22 mg/day of zinc.
>   - RYGB: Supplement with 8—22 mg/day of zinc.
>   - SG/LAGB: Supplement with 8—11 mg/day of zinc.
> - To minimize the risk of copper deficiency in post-WLS patients, it is recommended that the supplementation protocol contain a zinc-to-copper ratio of 8—15 mg of supplemental zinc per 1 mg of copper (Grade C, BEL 3).
> - Formulation and composition of zinc supplements must be taken into account for accurate calculation of elemental zinc levels. (Grade D, BEL 4).

Table 17.3 Suggested follow-up protocol after bariatric surgery.

	3 months post	6 M	12 M	18 M	24 M	Every year
Blood count	✓	✓	✓	✓	✓	✓
Total proteins, albumin, prealbumin	✓	✓	✓	✓	✓	✓
Glucose, A1C, lipidic and hepatic profile	✓	✓	✓	✓	✓	✓
Iron, ferritin	✓	✓	✓	✓	✓	✓
Calcium, P, Mg	✓	✓	✓	✓	✓	✓
Vitamin D, PTH	✓	✓	✓	✓	✓	✓
Vitamin B12, folate	✓	✓	✓	✓	✓	✓
Vitamin A, retinol-binding protein			✓		Recommended in RYGB, BPD, and SADI-S	Recommended in RYGB, BPD, and SADI-S
Vitamin E, ratio vitamin E/Cholesterol			✓		Recommended in BPD and SADI-S	Recommended in BPD and SADI-S and in case of deficiency or suspected deficiency
Selenium, zinc, copper, ceruloplasmin						
Vitamin B1	In case of suspected deficiency					

BPD, biliopancreatic diversion; LAGB, laparoscopic-assisted gastric banding; LSG, laparoscopic sleeve gastrectomy; RYGB, *Roux Y gastric bypass*; SADI-S, single anastomosis duodeno-ileal with sleeve gastrectomy.

Selenium

Selenium deficiency is in most of the cases subclinical, not causing any symptoms. Selenium levels should be checked in patients with unexplained anemia or fatigue, persistent diarrhea, cardiomyopathy, or metabolic bone disease.

Suggested protocol for the follow-up and screening of nutritional deficiencies after weight loss surgery

As a general recommendation, in patients undergoing bariatric surgery, we should perform blood testing at 3, 6, 12, 18, and 24 months after surgery and annually thereafter. The laboratory parameters recommended in every visit are displayed in Table 17.3. However, in malabsorptive techniques (such as duodenal switch, distal gastric bypass, or SADI-S), it is recommended to extend laboratory testing with the evaluation of trace elements (zinc, copper-ceruloplasmin, and selenium).

Along with the follow-up, the frequency of blood tests must be individualized according to the patient and deficiencies detected. Patients with a high risk of nutritional deficiencies must be screened more often, for example, patients over 60 years old (with less capacity of intestinal adaptation), women on childbearing age, and women during pregnancy. As nutritional requirements are increased during gestation, providing adequate doses of supplements is essential for the correct fetus development and growth. In this situation, controls at least every 3 months will be necessary.

Further reading

[1] Parrott J, Frank L, Rabena R, Craggs-Dino L, Isom KA, Greiman L. American society for metabolic and bariatric surgery integrated health nutritional guidelines for the surgical weight loss patient 2016 update: micronutrients. Surg Obes Relat Dis 2017;13(5): 727−41.

[2] Mechanick JI, Apovian C, Brethauer S, Garvey WT, Joffe AM, Kim J, et al. Clinical practice guidelines for the perioperative nutrition, metabolic, and nonsurgical support of patients undergoing bariatric procedures - 2019 update: cosponsored by american association of clinical endocrinologists/american college of endocrinology, the obesity society, american society for metabolic & bariatric surgery, obesity medicine association, and american society of anesthesiologists. Endocr Pract November 4, 2019. https://doi.org/10.4158/GL-2019-0406 [Epub ahead of print].

[3] Busetto L, Dicker D, Azran C, Batterham RL, Farpour-lambert N, Fried M, et al. practical recommendations of the obesity management task force of the european association for the study of obesity for the post-bariatric surgery medical management. Obes Facts 2017;10(6):597−632.

[4] Moizé V, Andreu A, Flores L, Torres F, Ibarzabal A, Delgado S, et al. Long-term dietary intake and nutritional deficiencies following sleeve gastrectomy or roux-en-y gastric bypass in a mediterranean population. J Acad Nutr Diet 2013;113(3):400−10.

[5] Shoar S, Poliakin L, Rubenstein R, Saber AA. Single anastomosis duodeno-ileal switch (SADIS): a systematic review of efficacy and safety. Obes Surg 2018;28(1):104−13. https://doi.org/10.1007/s11695-017-2838-8.

[6] Topart P, Becouarn G. The single anastomosis duodenal switch modifications: a review of the current literature on outcomes. Surg Obes Relat Dis 2017;13(8):1306−12. https://doi.org/10.1016/j.soard.2017.04.027.

[7] Gudzune KA, Huizinga MM, Chang HY, Asamoah V, Gadgil M, Clark JM. Screening and diagnosis of micronutrient deficiencies before and after bariatric surgery. Obes Surg 2013;23(10):1581−9.

[8] Patel JJ, Mundi MS, Hurt RT, Wolfe B, Martindale RG. Micronutrient deficiencies after bariatric surgery: an emphasis on vitamins and trace minerals [formula: see text]. Nutr Clin Pract 2017;32(4):471−80.

[9] Arias PM, Domeniconi EA, García M, Esquivel CM, Martínez Lascano F, Foscarini JM. Micronutrient deficiencies after roux-en-Y gastric bypass: long-term results. Obes Surg 2020;30(1):169−73.

[10] Nett P, Borbély Y, Kröll D. Micronutrient supplementation after biliopancreatic diversion with duodenal switch in the long term. Obes Surg 2016;26(10):2469−74.

[11] Roizen JD, Long C, Casella A, O'Lear L, Caplan I, Lai M, et al. Obesity decreases hepatic 25-hydroxylase activity causing low serum 25-hydroxyvitamin D. J Bone Miner Res 2019;34:1068−73.

[12] Cesareo R, Falchetti A, Attanasio R, Tabacco G, Naciu AM, Palermo A. Hypovitaminosis D: is it time to consider the use of calcifediol? Nutrients May 6, 2019;11(5). pii: E1016.

[13] Lewis CA, de Jersey S, Hopkins G, Hickman I, Osland E. Does bariatric surgery cause vitamin A, B1, C or E deficiency? A systematic review. Obes Surg 2018;28(11):3640−57.

CHAPTER 18

Postoperative management of specific complications: anaemia, protein malnutrition and neurological disorders

Manuel Ferrer-Márquez[1], Mercedes Vázquez-Gutiérrez[2], Pablo Quiroga-Subirana[3]

[1]*Bariatric Surgery Department, Hospital Universitario Torrecárdenas, Almería, Spain;*
[2]*Endocrinology and Clinical Nutrition Department, Hospital Universitario Torrecárdenas, Almería, Spain;* [3]*Neurology Department, Hospital Universitario Torrecárdenas, Almería, Spain*

Chapter outline

Anemia	240
Protein malnutrition	244
Neurological complications	245
Vitamin B1 or thiamine deficiency	247
Vitamin B12 deficiency	248
Copper deficiency	249
Vitamin B6 deficiency (pyridoxine)	250
Folate deficiency	251
Vitamin E deficiency	251
Vitamin D deficiency	252
Recommendations	252
References	253
Further reading	256

Obesity has become a worldwide epidemic of the 21st century. It is associated with a high number of comorbidities, significantly affecting the quality of life of patients suffering from it [1,2]. If trends continue, it is estimated that in 2030, 38% of the population will be overweight and another 20% will be obese. Currently, bariatric surgery (BS) remains the most effective therapeutic alternative for achieving sustained weight loss over time and resolving or improving most of its associated diseases, with good results in the medium and long term [3]. Depending on the techniques performed, type 2 DM can be controlled in 50%–85% of cases, even before significant weight loss has occurred, and biliopancreatic diversions (BPD) are the techniques that achieve the best resolution percentages. In relation to dyslipidemia, it improves in about 70%—90% of cases. Similarly, marked control of arterial hypertension is achieved following bariatric surgery, between 43% and 83% depending on the techniques performed [4,5]. However, the negative effects of BS have been observed as a result of the anatomical modifications made, both restrictive and malabsorptive. BS carries a risk of morbidity and mortality due to technical, nutritional, and even psychiatric complications, and multidisciplinary follow-up in the short and long term is essential. Patient follow-up by an endocrine nutritionist after bariatric surgery is essential to avoid possible complications and to treat those that appear from the beginning and therefore avoid greater repercussions [6,7].

Considering that BS constitutes a nutritional risk situation, it is necessary to make an adequate nutritional diagnosis before surgery, as many patients have deficiencies, such as in iron or vitamin D, which must be corrected before the intervention. Although folate and/or vitamin B12 deficiencies are not uncommon in BS candidates, iron deficiency is the most frequent cause of anemia in these patients and may be present in up to 60% of cases [8,9] associated with a higher rate of post-surgical complications.

As mentioned in previous chapters, possible complications that patients may develop depend, in part, on the technique performed (laparoscopic sleeve gastrectomy (SG), gastric bypass (RYGB), duodenal switch (DS) ...), so we must take them into account in the follow-up in the medium to long term, to either avoid or treat them correctly. Clinical practice guidelines recommend that all patients are administered with chronic micronutrients after surgery, depending on the technique carried out. The most frequent deficiencies are vitamin B12, calcium and vitamin D, and iron [9]. Throughout the next chapter, we will discuss three of the possible complications to be taken into account with these patients, and protocolize their treatment.

Anemia

Although CB is associated with a low risk of bleeding, it increases the risk of the development of anemia and iron deficiency after surgery. The anemia presented by these patients tends to be multifactorial and due to different mechanisms, which will be discussed in the following.

- **Iron deficiency:** The prevalence of iron deficiency and iron deficiency anemia is estimated in various studies to be at 30%—50% and 20%—30%, respectively [10,11], and increases with time elapsed since surgery, as well as in women of reproductive age. Any bariatric procedure can cause iron deficiency through different mechanisms, although it is more frequent in techniques with a malabsorptive component [12,13]. Although iron is absorbed throughout the small intestine, the area of greatest absorption is the duodenum and proximal jejunum. Derivative techniques prevent the passage of food through these sections, thus causing a general decrease in iron absorption. In the case of a malabsorptive technique, the acceleration of intestinal transit decreases the contact time between ingested iron and intestinal lumen, further decreasing its absorption [14]. When comparing the two procedures, different studies find conflicting results regarding iron deficiency. One study found that patients who underwent RYGB were more susceptible to developing postsurgical iron deficiency (15% post-op vs. 2% pre-op; $P < .01$) than those undergoing SG (0% post-op vs. 0.0% pre-op), while two others found no differences in a year of follow-ups [15,16]. On the other hand, iron absorption is carried out in the form of ferrous iron ($Fe2+$), and the conversion of ferric ion ($Fe3+$), ingested in the diet, into ferrous iron is facilitated by a low pH. Any surgical technique that decreases the volume of parietal cells and causes a decrease in gastric acid secretion will also lead to a decrease in absorption. A significant percentage of patients have intolerances to certain foods after derivative techniques. Tolerance to red meat is very poor, but it can even occur with chicken or fish. Other factors that can influence the risk of deficiency are complications such as surgical bleeding or marginal ulcers.

Many studies include an inaccurate diagnosis of anemia. Ferritin is the fundamental parameter to assess total body iron deposits and the reduction in its serum levels is diagnostic of iron deficiency. Ferritin also behaves as an acute phase reactant and can vary with age, inflammatory conditions (such as obesity), and infections. An adequate interpretation of the parameters of iron metabolism is required for a correct differential diagnosis between iron deficiency anemia and anemia associated with chronic inflammation (total iron fixation capacity, serum iron, and complete blood count).

The clinical practice guidelines recommend chronic supplementation of micronutrients for all postoperative patients, adjusted according to the technique used and patient characteristics. In the case of iron, a dose of 45–60 mg is generally recommended, including content in multivitamins [11]. However, as there may not be a good tolerance to oral iron in the first few weeks, it might be advisable to customize the start time of the supplementation schedule and the dose. To do this, we will take into account factors such as previous iron deposits, blood loss in the perioperative period, the characteristics of the surgery (greater requirements in the techniques that exclude the duodenum and the first loops of the jejunum), diet tolerance (with foods containing iron), and the existence of blood loss (for example, menstrual) [17–20]. We recommend determining the hemoglobin level (Hb) 24–48 h after surgery. If Hb values are normal (Hb > 12 g/dL in women or > 13 g/dL in men), supplementation with 40–65 mg of elemental iron may be sufficient, included in or in conjunction with a multivitamin complex. If moderate postoperative anemia is detected (Hb 10–12 g/dL in women or 10–13 g/dL in men), we should consider treatment with an intravenous (IV) iron infusion if it is considered that there has been a significant development of anemia (intra/perioperative loss > 500 mL or decrease in Hb > 3 g/dL). In the remaining cases with Hb > 10 g/dL, the use of oral ferrotherapy is recommended, at a dose of 100–200 mg per day, preferably with a liquid formulation or in sachets [21].

Regarding medium-term follow-up, the Bariatric Surgery European Clinical Practice Guidelines advise carrying out a periodic analytical evaluation that includes blood count and iron tests from the month of intervention [7], and to start treatment with oral iron (100–200 mg/d) in the case of isolated iron deficiency or moderate iron-deficiency anemia (Hb > 10 g/dL), until the reassessment of its efficacy at 8–12 weeks of treatment. In the case of Hb < 10 g/dL, with intolerance or ineffectiveness before oral iron, significant concomitant blood losses (e.g., gynecological), or BS malabsorptive techniques, it is advisable to administer IV iron treatment until the calculated iron deficiency is completed, especially if the anemia is symptomatic. Patients may have very low Hb levels with high clinical tolerance, due to its chronic establishment that allows the development of adaptive mechanisms. In these cases, IV iron treatment is especially recommended to minimize the possibility of requiring a transfusion. It must be taken into account that anemia following BS may be caused by other deficiencies in, for example, B12, folates, copper, selenium, and zinc (as later discussed), which should be evaluated when the diagnostic parameters of iron deficiency are negative. In general, patients who do not have anemia or iron deficiency in the postoperative control (ferritin > 30 ng/mL and IST > 20%), or those who were treated, need to have a follow-up with quarterly analysis and continue with the usual micronutrient supplementation, which includes iron. In certain groups of patients at risk such as women of childbearing age, those with a limited intake due to intolerance to certain food groups or patients subjected to techniques with a malabsorptive component, as well as in those in which oral iron was not effective, periodic treatment may be considered with parenteral iron to maintain stable iron deposits [21,22]. It is important to consider that the iron deficiency itself induces villous atrophy that makes intestinal iron absorption even more difficult. In the case of recurrence of anemia and/or iron deficiency, treatment with oral or IV iron must be restarted, and it is advisable to rule out blood loss or other causes of anemia (such as vitamin B12 or folic acid deficiency [15]). One year following intervention, stable patients without alterations in iron metabolism can have follow-ups semiannually or annually depending on their characteristics.

- **Vitamin B12 or cobalamin deficiency:** The preoperative prevalence of vitamin B12 deficiency is between 0% and 18% and the different techniques used in BS can also cause vitamin B12 deficiency. Vitamin B12 deficiency is one of the most frequently observed after RYGB. Its frequency varies between 26%–70% in RYGB and 5%–14.6% in BPD. Vitamin B12 deficiency in 18% of patients following SG has been recorded by some authors [23]. Cobalamin is absorbed in the terminal ileum attached to the intrinsic factor produced in gastric parietal cells. Its deficiency is due to a decrease in both the release of vitamin B12 from the foods that contain it (meat intolerance in certain patients) and the formation of the intrinsic factor-vitamin B12 complex. The decrease in hydrochloric acid prevents the change from pepsinogen to pepsin, which is necessary for the release of vitamin B12 from protein. Intrinsic factor is produced by parietal stomach cells and, under conditions such as gastric and intestinal resections, deficiency occurs, preventing vitamin B12 absorption. Preoperative vitamin B12 deficiency occurs in less than 5% of patients undergoing CB BS. Vitamin B12 body reserves normally exceed the daily requirements so that there is no deficiency in the early postoperative period. Low levels of B12 can be detected approximately 6 months into the postoperative period, but they are most commonly diagnosed after a year, when liver reserves are depleted. Vitamin B12 deficiency can manifest as megaloblastic anemia, thrombopenia, leukopenia, and glossitis, which are reversible with supplements. It can also cause weakness or fatigue secondary to megaloblastic anemia, polyneuropathy, paresthesia, delusions, and permanent neurological damage. Therefore, it is essential to control its levels, which can be done in different ways; the deficiency is usually diagnosed when levels below 200 pg/mL are present or by means of the serum measurement of methylmalonic acid and homocysteine concentrations (which makes it possible to distinguish between folate deficiency and vitamin B12).

As a consequence of the high prevalence of subclinical deficiency and the severity of symptoms if no treatment is established, prophylactic vitamin B12 supplementation has been considered universally in patients undergoing CB [15]. Most groups recommend it at 6 months after surgery when body reserves begin to deplete, although there are currently no controlled studies on this intervention. The administration of a multivitamin is not sufficient in many cases, requiring the addition of a minimum dose of 350–600 μg/day to correct the deficiency in 81% –95% of patients. When a deficiency appears, it is treatable with 1000 μg weekly for 4–8 weeks until hemoglobin normalization is established, and with 1000 μg/month for maintenance [11,18].

- **Folic acid deficiency**: This is rare because folic acid absorption occurs throughout the entire intestine, but since it is water-soluble and does not provide the body with important deposits, deficiency can be caused by an inadequate intake. It is estimated that folic acid deficiency ranges between 9%–35% in RYGB, and 1.3%–22% in BPD. Some series have reported this vitamin deficiency in up to 22% of patients with SG [15]. These techniques increase the risk of developing folic acid deficiency within a few months, in relation to decreased intake, malabsorption, and mainly due to poor adherence to the recommended vitamin supplementation. Folic acid deficiency is asymptomatic in most patients and, therefore, difficult to diagnose. It can cause macrocytic anemia, leukopenia, thrombocytopenia, or glossitis. Homocysteine increases when there are low levels of folate and also in cases of vitamin B12 deficiency. This amino acid is an independent risk factor for cardiovascular diseases and/or oxidative stress. As folic acid deficiency does not affect the myelin sheath, neurological damage is less frequent than in vitamin B12 deficiency, but it can produce neurological symptoms such as memory loss, irritability, and even paranoid behavior in severe cases. A daily intake of 800 μg/day of folic acid (200 μg included in a multivitamin tablet)[11,18] is recommended for prevention. If a deficiency appears, it should be treated with 1000 μg/day of folic acid, up to 5 mg/day, for 4 months and maintenance with 5 mg/week. All women with a wish to become pregnant should be treated with folic acid supplements because of the risk of neural tube defects caused by a deficiency in this vitamin.

Protein malnutrition

Protein malnutrition is an uncommon but potentially serious metabolic complication that occurs primarily in the late postoperative period, especially in the first year after surgery. Its frequency can reach 13% at 2 years in patients with RYGB with a Roux or alimentary limb greater than 150 cm, and 5% with a limb less than 150 cm (largest common limb). In BPD, a prevalence of protein malnutrition of 7.7% has been observed, even increasing up to 21%, when the gastric pouch is less than 200cc. In most patients, an onset event (ulceration of the gastro-intestinal anastomosis, chronic diarrhea, intestinal obstruction...) [24] can be identified. The risk of protein malabsorption decreases over time owing to the progressive intestinal adaptation that increases the absorptive capacity of the rest of the small intestine and the colon. From a clinical point of view, it can be asymptomatic or cause ascites, arterial hypotension, and increased susceptibility to infections with lymphocytopenia and even cutaneous energy, hair discoloration, muscular atrophy, asthenia, as well as edemas that can cause false weight gain.

There are several factors, some related to the surgical technique, that may lead to its occurrence [24—28]:

- Poor compliance with the prescribed diet with decreased protein intake
- Vomiting or eating disorders
- Bacterial overgrowth
- Malabsorption due to the surgical technique: maldigestion and malabsorption cause a loss of protein from the diet and a loss of endogenous protein from the biliopancreatic secretions themselves
- Very small gastric reservoir
- Depressive symptoms
- Concomitance of major surgery, infections or malignancies

Different surgeons have argued that the length of the common intestinal limb determines the degree of intestinal malabsorption. Based on these considerations, it has been noted that due to the high risk of nutritional deficiencies in the long-term postoperative period, patients undergoing RYGB need more frequent nutritional care than patients undergoing gastric restrictive surgery, such as vertical laparoscopic gastrectomy surgery. Although the guidelines on the length of the Roux-en-Y limb are relevant, it is essential to keep in mind that the different anatomical segments of absorption of the gastrointestinal tract have specific characteristics. As the initial portion of the small intestine is an important site of amino acid absorption, the exclusion of the duodenum and the proximal part of the jejunum is sufficient to expose the individual to the risk of protein deficiency.

The prevention of protein malabsorption includes adequate follow-up, monitoring, and supervision of clinical and laboratory parameters, to be able to act before complications appear. The necessary protein requirement estimated to maintain lean mass during the active phase of weight loss is 1.2 g/kg of weight [24]. Due to the malabsorption that the BPD/DS entails, it is recommended to increase the daily contribution to 1.5—2.0 g of protein/kg of weight, which means an average requirement of 90 g per day [25]. In the first months after surgery, it is difficult to achieve the protein objectives through diet and it is essential to monitor protein intake at each visit. Food intake based on a diet rich in eggs and dairy products (added to purees, creams, salads, fruit smoothies, etc.) should be recommended. As these food groups are often poorly tolerated, protein powder supplements can be prescribed to enrich the diet, or hyperprotein nutritional supplements in the case of the recommendations not being reached in the diet, or confirmed hypoproteinemia. From an analytical point of view, monitoring of serum albumin and prealbumin may be useful for assessing visceral protein levels; however, they may be decreased in seriously ill patients with systemic inflammation after BS. The test to detect protein malabsorption is fecal clearance of alpha-1-antitrypsin. The stool may have compatible organoleptic characteristics, namely, creatorrhea.

Treatment will depend on the severity and the cause needs to be investigated to correct the determining factors as much as possible. In most cases, protein deficiency is reduced to mild hypoalbuminemia (3—3.5 mg/dL), which is usually resolved with dietary advice, pancreatic enzymes, and protein supplements. In more severe cases, support with enteral nutrition, alone or with parenteral treatment, may be necessary. In case of a lack of response, conversion surgery would be advised, differing depending on the aforementioned techniques. In the case of RYGB, its conversion is possible and thus described [29]. In the case of malabsorptive techniques, Dr. Baltasar outlines three possible ways to treat it:

- Reversion of the small intestine to a normal state, reinstating its normal form and function. The disadvantage of this may be weight gain if the restrictive component is not enough.
- Perform a lateral-lateral anastomosis between the food loop and biliopancreatic loop at 60—70 cm aboral and the Y-de-Roux to increase the absorptive area, which is called "anastomosis in kiss-in X".
- Lengthen the common limb by moving the food limb > 100 cm aboral in the biliopancreatic limb above the Y-de-Roux.

Severe hypoalbuminemia after CB should be considered as a serious condition that requires timely attention by professionals with nutritional experience. Regular monitoring of serum albumin is strongly recommended to prevent the development of severe protein malnutrition after the most serious malabsorptive procedures, such as SADIs, distal RYGB, and BPD. In our experience, hyperprotein supplements combined with pancreatic enzymes may be useful for treating mild hypoalbuminemia, but they are ineffective for the treatment of severe hypoalbuminemia. In these cases, enteral nutritional support, home parenteral nutrition, or even reversal may be necessary.

Neurological complications

Owing to the improvement of BS and the emergence of specialized centers to develop these types of interventions, the different surgical and medical complications have decreased in recent years [1,2,30,31]. Nevertheless, neurological complications can be present between 5% and 16%, affecting both the central and peripheral nervous systems [30].

Neurological complications can be divided into early and late, the latter being the most common. We can also divide the neurological complications in relation to time after BS [30,31]:

1. Neurological complications in the immediate perioperative period
   - Compression neuropathy.
   - Stretch injuries of the brachial plexus.
   - Rhabdomyolysis.
2. Neurological complications that occur weeks or months after bariatric surgery:
   - Vitamin B1 or thiamine deficiency that can produce:
     (a) Wernicke's encephalopathy.
     (b) Peripheral neuropathy.
   - Guillain Barré syndrome.
   - Episodic encephalopathy.
3. Neurological complications that occur months or years after BS, related to a deficiency in the following nutrients: Vitamin A, B3, B6, B12, vitamin D, E, folate, and copper.

We can compare the different neurological manifestations after BS with the different nutrient deficiencies [30,31]:

- Encephalopathy: Thiamine (Vitamin B1), Vitamin B12 and, less frequently, folate and niacin (Vitamin B3).
- Myelopathy: Vitamin B12, copper and, less frequently, folate and vitamin E.
- Optic neuropathy: Vitamin B12, thiamine, copper and, less frequently, folate.
- Polyradiculopathy or variant of Guillain Barré: Thiamine.
- Neuropathy: Vitamin B12, thiamine, copper and, more rarely, folate, pyridoxine, niacin, and vitamin E, D.

The mechanisms related to neurological complications are diverse [30–37]:

- Postsurgical complications such as compression neuropathies or brachial plexus stretching injuries.
- Rapid and high weight loss percentage.
- Prolonged gastrointestinal symptoms: nausea, vomiting, diarrhea, dumping syndrome.
- Technique or type of surgical procedure used.
- Subclinical presurgical deficiency of vitamins and other nutrients.
- Postsurgical deficiency of vitamins and other nutrients.
- Inadequate nutritional monitoring without adherence to the recommended replacement treatment.
- Immune-mediated and/or inflammatory mechanism.

In some patients with neurological complications after BS, greater synthesis of immunoglobulin G has been found in the cerebrospinal fluid, which may explain the suggested immune-mediated and/or inflammatory mechanism [31,33].

The rapidity and percentage of weight loss is another mechanism related to compression mononeuropathies, such as peroneal nerve entrapment at the fibular head at the knee level [31,38].

The nutrient deficiencies most common in patients who have undergone CB, and who have neurological complications, are related to deficiencies in vitamin B12, vitamin B1, and copper and will be described in more depth in this review. The neurological relevance in relation to other vitamin deficiencies such as vitamin B6 or pyridoxine, folate, vitamin B3 or niacin, vitamin B2 or riboflavin, vitamin E, and vitamin D is unclear. Likewise, few studies have been carried out on the minerals calcium, phosphorus, magnesium, and trace elements such as zinc, iodine, and selenium in patients undergoing BS [31,33,34].

Vitamin B1 or thiamine deficiency

Thiamine is an important coenzyme in the metabolism of carbohydrates, lipids, and amino acids. It has a role in the synthesis of adenosine triphosphate, the maintenance of the myelin sheath, and the production of neurotransmitters [31,39].

Body reserves of thiamine after BS can be depleted in 4—6 weeks and neurological manifestations related to its deficiency can be observed in 4—12 weeks [31,40,41]. Thiamine deficiency may be due to a decrease in intake, decreased absorption, defective transport as well as increased losses, and maybe aggravated by intractable vomiting, rapid weight loss, inadequate vitamin supplements, glucose administration without previous thiamine administration, parenteral feeding, or bacterial overgrowth [31,39].

Thiamine deficiency affects the CNS, the peripheral nervous system, and the cardiovascular system [31,39,42,43]. Peripheral neuropathy associated with thiamine deficiency is called beriberi and is characterized by a sensitive motor distal axonal polyneuropathy, often associated with calf cramps, muscle pain, neuropathic pain, and dysautonomic abnormalities. A rapid progression of polyneuropathy that simulates Guillain—Barré syndrome has also been described. The symptoms of subclinical thiamine deficiency may go unnoticed as they are often nonspecific and include fatigue, lethargy, irritability, restlessness, and headaches [31,39,44].

Wernicke's encephalopathy and Korsakoff syndrome are the best characterized neurological disorders caused by thiamine deficiency. The term Wernicke—Korsakoff syndrome is commonly used. Wernicke's encephalopathy is a consequence of severe short-term thiamine deficiency, while peripheral neuropathy is usually the result of prolonged (mild to moderate) thiamine deficiency. It is characterized by subacute onset of the classic triad of ocular abnormalities, gait ataxia, and changes in mental state. The onset can be gradual and the classic triad is not always evident. Ocular abnormalities include nystagmus, ophthalmoparesis, and conjugate gaze paralysis. Gait and truncal ataxia are consequences of cerebellar and vestibular dysfunction. If left untreated, it can progress to coma (which, rarely, may be the only manifestation of Wernicke's encephalopathy) and death. In addition, Wernicke's encephalopathy after BS has been associated with atypical features that include optic neuropathy, papilledema, deafness, paresis, seizures, myoclonus, and asterixis [31,39,42,43,45].

About 80% of patients who survive Wernicke's encephalopathy develop Korsakoff syndrome (most probable when encephalopathy is secondary to alcohol abuse). In this syndrome, memory is more affected in relation to other aspects of cognitive function such as attention and alertness [31,45,46].

The diagnosis is largely clinical. Complementary tests should include an analysis and brain MRI. The analysis must include blood count and thiamine levels. A normal serum thiamine level does not exclude Wernicke's encephalopathy and thiamine levels in whole blood are more sensitive than in plasma. As laboratory abnormalities normalize rapidly, it is advisable to take a blood sample before starting treatment [31,39,42,43]. The MRI is of great importance for the diagnosis, although sometimes abnormalities may not be found. Typical findings of magnetic resonance include increased T2 signal, FLAIR in the periventricular regions [31,39,46].

In relation to treatment, patients with a history of BS who present gastrointestinal complications or difficulties should receive thiamine in a preventive manner. Patients at risk should receive parenteral thiamine before administration of glucose or parenteral nutrition. Patients suspected of having beriberi or Wernicke's encephalopathy should immediately receive parenteral thiamine [31,37].

One way to perform thiamine treatment is to administer 100 mg through IV every 8 h. Higher doses may be required, and it has been suggested that patients with signs of Wernicke's encephalopathy receive up to 500 mg of infused thiamine hydrochloride for 30 min three times a day for 3 days. Thereafter the dose may be reduced to 250 mg/day of thiamine, IV or IM, for 5 days. Finally, for long-term oral maintenance, 50—100 mg of thiamine per day is administered, with regular checks. The response in Wernicke's encephalopathy is variable; ocular symptoms improve in a few hours, although fine horizontal nystagmus may persist, and improvement in gait ataxia and memory may take longer. Immediate treatment of Wernicke's encephalopathy prevents the development of Korsakoff syndrome. Korsakoff syndrome often does not respond to thiamine therapy. The recovery of consciousness can be seen even in patients in a deep coma. In wet beriberi, cardiac symptoms may disappear within a few days, although improvement in motor and sensory symptoms may take months [31,37,39,41,47].

Vitamin B12 deficiency

The clinical manifestations related to vitamin B12 deficiency are observed months or years after the CB, due to body reserves. Neurological disorders may be the first and only signs of vitamin B12 deficiency and can be observed in the following neurological manifestations: myelopathy with the involvement of the dorsal spine and corticospinal tract, myeloneuropathy, peripheral neuropathy such as mononeuropathy, multiple mononeuropathy, or symmetric polyneuropathies of the lower and upper limbs, and optic neuropathy. In addition, it can be associated with observed neuropsychiatric clinical manifestations, including memory problems, personality changes, psychosis, emotional lability, and occasionally even coma [31,42,43,48−51].

The diagnosis is clinical, requiring the assistance of the previously mentioned complementary laboratory tests, neurophysiological tests, and MRI [31,42]. The neurophysiological study includes electroneurography, electromyography, and somaesthetic evoked potentials (SEPs), which can show sensory and motor axonal polyneuropathy data and abnormalities in the conduction of SEPs at the level of the posterior cords.

The brain and pan-medullary column MRI indicates signal changes in the posterior and lateral columns of the spinal cord and, less frequently, the subcortical white matter.

The goal of treatment is to reverse the signs and symptoms produced by the deficiency, replenish body reserves, and gain control of prolonged treatment [31,51]. The response of neurological manifestations is variable, may be incomplete, and often begins in the first week. In the absence of controlled studies, the most commonly recommended initial routine is with vitamin B12 supplements after BS. In addition, as a consequence of the high prevalence of subclinical deficiency and the severity of symptoms, if no treatment is established, prophylactic vitamin B12 supplementation has been considered universally in postoperative patients [15].

Copper deficiency

The most frequent cause of acquired copper deficiency is BS 32. Copper plays an important role in the function of multiple enzymes that have a critical role in the structure and function of the nervous system [42,52].

Copper is absorbed in the stomach and proximal intestine. Alteration of gastric acidity is related to copper deficiency, as it facilitates its solubilization [31,53]. Other causes of copper deficiency can coexist, such as excessive zinc supplementation, gastrointestinal diseases that cause malabsorption, prolonged parenteral nutrition, and bacterial overgrowth [31,42].

The coexistence of multiple causes of copper deficiency, associated with other nutrient deficiencies (vitamin B12, E, D …) increases the chances of clinical neurological abnormalities with a worse prognosis. For example, it is important to consider copper deficiency (or other nutrients) in situations of persistent neurological deterioration such as myelopathy related to vitamin B12 deficiency. Furthermore, neurological alterations continue to be observed despite B12 levels normalizing [31,52−57].

The time of onset of neurological clinical manifestations related to copper deficiency in BS is variable, ranging from approximately 1 year to more than 2 decades. The most characteristic neurological manifestations are myelopathy, myeloneuropathy resembling subacute combined degeneration observed with vitamin B12 deficiency, peripheral neuropathy, and optic neuropathy [31,53,55−57].

In relation to laboratory tests, the decrease in serum copper or ceruloplasmin and the decrease in urinary excretion of copper in 24 h should be taken into consideration. Copper in urine decreases when copper in the diet is low. Changes in blood copper levels are generally parallel to the concentration of ceruloplasmin. However, we must bear in mind that ceruloplasmin is an acute phase reagent and its increase is probably responsible for the increase in blood copper observed in conditions such as pregnancy, use of oral contraceptives, and various inflammatory, infectious, and systemic diseases. These conditions could, therefore, mask a deficiency. In addition, it is recommended to monitor serum zinc levels and zinc excretion in urine for 24 h, and if these are increased, the search for an external source of zinc should be instigated [31,54,55,58].

The neurophysiological study includes electroneurography, electromyography, and somaesthetic evoked potentials, which may show data of sensory and motor axonal polyneuropathy and abnormalities in the conduction of somatosensory evoked potentials at the level of the posterior cords [31,54,55].

The MRI of the spine may show increased T2 signal affecting the posterior cords, with the cervical cord being most commonly involved [31,54,55,59].

There are no studies on the most effective dose, time, and administration route for the replacement of copper in CB 32. Due to the need for long-term replacement therapy, oral treatment is preferred. One of the recommendations would be an oral regime: 8 mg/day of elemental copper orally for 1 week, 6 mg/day during the second week, 4 mg/day during the third week, and 2 mg/day thereafter. A commonly used initial parenteral treatment plan is 2 mg of elemental copper administered intravenously (for 2 h) daily for 5 days. Periodic monitoring of copper status in high-risk patients after CB should be considered. The response to the replacement treatment of hematological parameters (including bone marrow findings) is rapid and complete. The recovery of neurological signs and symptoms is variable. It has been observed that the normalization of serum copper leads to clinical improvement in neurological symptoms, improvement in the controls of neurophysiological and imaging studies, and the halting of progression [31,42,54,55].

Vitamin B6 deficiency (pyridoxine)

Vitamin B6 deficiency has been found in patients undergoing BS [31], although there are other additional causes of deficiencies that include gastrointestinal diseases associated with malabsorption and alcoholism.

The most evident chronic shortage of vitamin B6 is in a clinical manifestation of related peripheral neuropathy (sensory motor sensory dominance). Other clinical manifestations include microcytic hypochromic anemia, secondary hyperoxaluria and nephrolithiasis, glossitis, stomatitis, cheilosis, and dermatitis [31].

In the laboratory, we can assess levels of vitamin B6 in the blood or urine. The most commonly used measure is plasma pyridoxal phosphate [31]. The neurophysiological study includes electroneurography and electromyography, which can show data on sensory and motor axonal polyneuropathy (sensory predominance) [31].

There are no studies on dose and time of treatment or the most effective administration route for the replacement treatment of B6 in CB. However, it is advised that vitamin B6 can be prescribed orally in doses of 50—100 mg daily to prevent the development of neuropathy. The administration of higher doses has been associated with sensory polyneuropathies [31].

Folate deficiency

Folate deficiency can cause the same changes as those observed for vitamin B12 deficiency, due to its importance in the production of methionine, S-adenosyl-L-methionine, and tetrahydrofolate. However, it has been observed that the deficiency of pure folic acid does not affect the myelin sheath, therefore neurological alterations are less frequent than in vitamin B12 deficiency [31,42,60,61].

The diagnosis is clinical to a large extent. Folate deficiency can coexist with other nutrient deficiencies, so the neurological manifestations attributed to folate deficiency require the exclusion of other potential causes. In the laboratory, it may be found that plasma homocysteine levels are elevated. Serum folate fluctuates daily and does not correlate with tissue stores, so red blood cell folate is more reliable than plasma folate [31,42,60,61].

The coexistence of vitamin B12 deficiency before folate treatment should be ruled out. It is recommended that due to acute neurological abnormalities caused by documented folate deficiency, parenteral administration of 1—5 mg daily, or 1—5 mg orally on a daily basis, should be considered. For maintenance treatment, between 400 µg/day and 1 mg/day orally can be prescribed. The best tool for monitoring the response to treatment is homocysteine, which decreases within a few days of administering folate treatment [31,42,60,61].

Vitamin E deficiency

Vitamin E deficiency has been observed after CB (BPD). Its reserves run out after many years. In addition, vitamin E deficiency can be observed in the presence of chronic cholestasis, pancreatic insufficiency, intestinal diseases associated with malabsorption, and inadequate replacement therapy in patients with total parenteral nutrition [31].

In neurological manifestations caused by vitamin E deficiency, we can find a myeloneuropathy or a spinocerebellar syndrome with variable involvement of peripheral polyneuropathy, with a phenotype similar to that of Friedreich's ataxia [31,42].

The diagnosis is clinical to a large extent. With laboratory assistance, we can observe undetectable levels of vitamin E in patients with neurological manifestations. In addition, we can observe increased stool fat and decreased serum carotene levels as additional markers of intestinal malabsorption in patients with vitamin E deficiency. Spine MRIs in patients with myeloneuropathy may reveal increased signal in the dorsal cervical spine region [31,42].

The recommended treatment in asymptomatic postsurgical patients is a standard multivitamin-mineral formulation containing vitamin E. Treatment with higher doses may be necessary for the presence of severe deficiencies [31].

Vitamin D deficiency

Vitamin D deficiency has been observed after CB with RYGB. Obesity alone is associated with plasma 25-hydroxyvitamin D deficiency (25 [OH] D)[31].

Vitamin D deficiency causes hypocalcemia with secondary hyperparathyroidism that further deteriorates bone mineralization, which can cause osteomalacia as a delayed side effect in some CB techniques. In addition, vitamin D deficiency can cause proximal myopathy associated with osteomalacia, pathological fractures, and bone pain. The pelvic and thigh muscles are more engaged than the arms, which can lead to a swinging gait. The neck muscles may be involved without compromising bulbar and eye muscles. In addition, severe hypocalcemia can cause tetany and may be associated with hypomagnesemia [31,42].

The diagnosis is largely clinical. In the laboratory, vitamin D deficiency may be accompanied by a decrease in serum calcium and an increase in PTH levels. Vitamin D status is best assessed with 25 (OH) D levels. Other laboratory abnormalities may include increased alkaline phosphatase of bone origin, hypocalcemia, hypophosphatemia, elevated PTH, urinary excretion reduced calcium, and elevated urinary hydroxyproline [31,42].

Vitamin D can be administered orally as vitamin D2 or vitamin D3. In patients with minimal sun exposure, 400 IU/day of vitamin D is sufficient to prevent deficiency. If there is a clinical vitamin D deficiency, 50,000 IU of vitamin D2 or vitamin D3 may be required weekly for 6–8 weeks. The maintenance treatment can be carried out with 800 IU a day up to 1000 IU a day. A higher dose may be necessary orally (or even parenteral administration) in the presence of intestinal malabsorption [31].

An understanding of the neurological disorders related to CB is of great importance. Rare but serious, and potentially reversible, neurological complications require immediate treatment, particularly rhabdomyolysis (a rapidly progressive neurological emergency), Wernicke's encephalopathy, and polyneuropathy that simulates Guillain Barré Syndrome [30,31].

Recommendations

- Patient follow-up by a multidisciplinary team after bariatric surgery is essential to avoid possible complications and to treat those that appear from the beginning and therefore avoid greater repercussions.
- Considering that BS constitutes a nutritional risk situation, it is necessary to make an adequate nutritional diagnosis before surgery, as many patients have deficiencies, such as in iron or vitamin D, which must be corrected before the intervention

- The clinical practice guidelines recommend chronic supplementation of micronutrients for all postoperative patients, adjusted according to the technique used and patient characteristics.
- Iron status should be monitored in all patients undergoing bariatric surgery. Intravenous iron infusion (preferably with ferric gluconate or sucrose) may be needed for patients with severe intolerance to oral iron or refractory deficiency due to severe iron malabsorption.
- Baseline and postoperative evaluation for vitamin B12 deficiency is recommended in all bariatric surgery and annually in those with procedures that exclude the lower part of the stomach. The administration of vitamin B12 and folic acid supplements in these patients should be considered.
- Nutritional anemias resulting from malabsorptive bariatric surgical procedures might also involve deficiencies in vitamin B12, folate, protein, copper, selenium, and zinc and should be evaluated when routine screening for iron deficiency anemia is negative.
- The prevention of protein malabsorption includes adequate follow-up, monitoring, and supervision of clinical and laboratory parameters, to be able to act before complications appear. Treatment will depend on the severity and the cause needs to be investigated to correct the determining factors as much as possible. In most cases, protein deficiency is reduced to mild hypoalbuminemia, which is usually resolved with dietary advice, pancreatic enzymes, and protein supplements.
- An understanding of the neurological disorders related to CB is of great importance. Rare but serious, and potentially reversible, neurological complications require immediate treatment, particularly rhabdomyolysis (a rapidly progressive neurological emergency), Wernicke's encephalopathy, and polyneuropathy that simulates Guillain Barré Syndrome.

References

[1] Hruby A, Hu FB. The epidemiology of obesity: a big picture. Pharmacoeconomics 2015;33(7):673—89.
[2] Kelly T, Yang W, Chen C-S, Reynolds K, He J. Global burden of obesity in 2005 and projections to 2030. Int J Obes 2008;32(9):1431—7.
[3] Colquitt JL, Pickett K, Loveman E, Frampton GK. Surgery for weight loss in adults. Cochrane Database Syst Rev 2014;(8):CD003641.
[4] Evolución de las comorbilidades tras la cirugía. García-Orian Serrano MJ, Muros Bayo J. Cirugía de la obesidad mórbida. Ruíz de Adana JC, Sánchez.
[5] Burguera B, Ruiz de Adana JC. Long term effects of bariatric surgery. Cir Esp 2012; 90(5):275—6.
[6] Aarts MA, Sivapalan N, Nikzad SE, Serodio K, Sockalingam S, Conn LG. Optimizing bariatric surgery multidisciplinary follow-up: a focus on patient-centered care. Obes Surg 2017;27(3):730—6.

[7] Fried M, Yumuk V, Oppert JM, Scopinaro N, Torres A, Weiner R, et al. International federation for surgery of obesity and metabolic disorders-European chapter (IFSO-EC); European association for the study of obesity (EASO); European association for the study of obesity management task force (EASO OMTF). Interdisciplinary European guidelines on metabolic and bariatric surgery. Obes Surg 2014;24(1):42−55.

[8] Moizé V, Deulofeu R, Torres F, de Osaba JM, Vidal J. Nutritional intake and prevalence of nutritional deficiencies prior to surgery in a Spanish morbidly obese population. Obes Surg 2011;21:1382−8.

[9] Careaga M, Moizé V, Flores L, Deulofeu R, Andreu A, Vidal J. Inflammation and iron status in bariatric surgery candidates. Surg Obes Relat Dis 2015;11(4):906−11.

[10] Muñoz M, Botella-Romero F, Gómez-Ramírez S, Campos A, García-Erce JA. Iron deficiency and anaemia in bariatric surgical patients: causes, diagnosis and proper management. Nutr Hosp 2009;24:640−54.

[11] Mechanick JI, Youdim A, Jones DB, Garvey WT, Hurley DL, McMahon MM, et al. Clinical practice guidelines for the perioperative nutritional, metabolic, and nonsurgical support of the bariatric surgery patient−2013 update: cosponsored by American Association of Clinical Endocrinologists, the Obesity Society, and American Society for Metabolic & Bariatric Surgery. Endocr Pract 2013;19:337−72.

[12] Salgado Jr W, Modotti C, Nonino CB, Ceneviva R. Anemia and iron deficiency before and after bariatric surgery. Surg Obes Relat Dis 2014;10:49−54.

[13] Obinwanne KM, Fredrickson KA, Mathiason MA, Kallies KJ, Farnen JP, Kothari SN. Incidence, treatment, and outcomes of iron deficiency after laparoscopic Roux-en-Y gastric bypass: a 10- year analysis. J Am Coll Surg 2014;218:246−52.

[14] Basora Macaya M. Treatment of anemia in patients undergoing bariatric surgery. Rev Esp Anestesiol Reanim 2015;62(Suppl. 1):76−9.

[15] Amaya García MJ, Vilchez López FJ, Campos Martín C. Sánchez VeraP, Pereira cunill JL. Micronutrients in bariatric surgery. Nutr Hosp 2012;27(2):349−61.

[16] Enani G, Bilgic E, Lebedeva E, Delisle M, Vergis A, Hardy K. The incidence of iron deficiency anemia post-Roux-en-Y gastric bypass and sleeve gastrectomy: a systematic review. Surg Endosc 2020;34(7):3002−10.

[17] Parrott J, Frank L, Rabena R, Craggs-Dino L, Isom KA, Greiman L. American Society for Metabolic and Bariatric Surgery integrated health nutritional guidelines for the surgical weight loss patient 2016 update: micronutrients. Surg Obes Relat Dis 2017;13(5): 727−41.

[18] Toh SY, Zarshenas N, Jorgensen J. Prevalence of nutrient deficiencies in bariatric patients. Nutrition 2009;25(11):1150−6. Kehagias I, Karamanakos SN, Argentou M, Kalfarentzos F (2011) Randomized clinical trial of laparoscopic Roux-en-Y gastric bypass versus laparoscopic sleeve gastrectomy for the management of patients with BMI < 50 kg/m^2. Obes Surg 21(11):1650−1656.

[19] Moizé V, Andreu A, Flores L, Torres F, Ibarzabal A, Delgado S, Lacy A, Rodriguez L, Vidal J. Long-term dietary intake and nutritional deficiencies following sleeve gastrectomy or Roux-En-Y gastric bypass in a Mediterranean population. J Acad Nutr Diet 2013;113(3):400−10.

[20] Jericó C, et al. Déficit de hierro y cirugía bariátrica. Endocrinol Nutr 2016;63(1):32−42.

[21] Ten Broeke R, Bravenboer B, Smulders FJ. Iron deficiency before and after bariatric surgery: the need for iron supplementation. Neth J Med 2013;71:412−7.

References   255

[22] Weng TC, Chang CH, Dong YH, Chang YC, Chuang LM. Anaemia and related nutrient deficiencies after Roux-en-Y gastric bypass surgery: a systematic review and meta-analysis. BMJ Open 2015;5(7):e006964.

[23] Soenen S, et al. Normal protein intake is required for body weight loss and weight maintenance, and elevated protein intake for additional preservation of resting energy expenditure and fat free mass. J Nutr 2013;143(5):591−6.

[24] ASMBS. Allied health nutritional guidelines for the surgical weight loss patient. Surg Obes Relat Dis 2008;4(5 Suppl. l):S73−108.

[25] Abellán Galiana P, Antonia Pérez-Lázaro M, Cámara Gómez R, Francisco Merino-Torres J, Ponce Marco JL, Piñón Selles F. Severe protein-calorie malnutrition after gastric bypass. Endocrinol Nutr 2008;55(5):223−5.

[26] Kuin C, den Ouden F, Brandts H, Deden L, Hazebroek E, van Borren M, et al. Treatment of severe protein malnutrition after bariatric surgery. Obes Surg 2019;29(10):3095−102.

[27] Faria SL, Faria OP, Buffington C, Cardeal MA, Ito MK. Dietary protein intake and bariatric surgery patients: a review. Obes Surg 2011;21:1798−805.

[28] Ma P, Ghiassi S, Lloyd A, Haddad A, Boone K, DeMaria E, et al. Reversal of Roux en Y gastric bypass: largest single institution experience. Surg Obes Relat Dis 2019;15(8):1311−6.

[29] Goodman JC. Neurological complications of bariatric surgery. Curr Neurol Neurosci Rep 2015;15(12):79.

[30] Kumar N. Neurologic complications of bariatric surgery. Continuum Life Long Neurol 2014;20(3):580−97.

[31] Koffman BM, Greenfield LJ, Ali II, Pirzada NA. Neurologic complications after surgery for obesity. Muscle Nerve 2006;33(2):166−76.

[32] Juhasz-Pocsine K, Rudnicki SA, Archer RL, Harik SI. Neurologic complications of gastric bypass surgery for morbid obesity. Neurology 2007;68(21):1843−50.

[33] Kazemi A, Frazier T, Cave M. Micronutrient- related neurologic complications following bariatric surgery. Curr Gastroenterol Rep 2010;12(4):288−95.

[34] Ba F, Siddiqi ZA. Neurologic complications of bariatric surgery. Rev Neurol Dis 2010;7(4):119−24.

[35] Thaisetthawatkul P, Collazo-Clavell ML, Sarr MG, et al. A controlled study of peripheral neuropathy after bariatric surgery. Neurology 2004;63(8):1462−70.

[36] Aasheim ET. Wernicke encephalopathy after bariatric surgery: a systematic review. Ann Surg 2008;248(5):714−20.

[37] Elias WJ, Pouratian N, Oskouian RJ, et al. Peroneal neuropathy following successful bariatric surgery. Case report and review of the literature. J Neurosurg 2006;105(4):631−5.

[38] Sechi G, Serra A. Wernicke's encephalopathy: new clinical settings and recent advances in diagnosis and management. Lancet Neurol 2007;6(5):442−55.

[39] Singh S, Kumar A. Wernicke encephalopathy after obesity surgery. Neurology 2007;68(11):807−11.

[40] Thomson AD, Marshall EJ. The natural history and pathophysiology of Wernicke's Encephalopathy and Korsakoff's Psychosis. Alcohol Alcohol 2006;41(2):151−8.

[41] Kumar N. Neurologic presentations of nutritional deficiencies. Neurol Clin 2010;28(1):107−70.

[42] Kumar N. Acute and subacute encephalopathies: deficiency states (nutritional). Semin Neurol 2011;31(2):169−83.

[43] Koike H, Ito S, Morozumi S, et al. Rapidly developing weakness mimicking Guillain-Barre syndrome in beriberi neuropathy: two case reports. Nutrition 2008;24(7−8): 776−80.
[44] Homewood J, Bond NW. Thiamin deficiency and Korsakoff's syndrome: failure to find memory impairments following nonalcoholic Wernicke's encephalopathy. Alcohol 1999;19(1):75−84.
[45] Zuccoli G, Motti L. Atypical Wernicke's encephalopathy showing lesions in the cranial nerve nuclei and cerebellum. J Neuroimaging 2008;18(2):194−7.
[46] Thomson AD, Marshall EJ. The treatment of patients at risk of developing Wernicke's encephalopathy in the community. Alcohol Alcohol 2006;41(2):159−67.
[47] Sechi G. Prognosis and therapy of Wernicke's encephalopathy after obesity surgery. Am J Gastroenterol 2008;103(12):3219.
[48] Carmel R. Current concepts in cobalamin deficiency. Annu Rev Med 2000;51:357−75.
[49] Carmel R, Green R, Rosenblatt DS, Watkins D. Update on cobalamin, folate, and homocysteine. Hematology Am Soc Hematol Educ Program 2003:62−81.
[50] Stabler SP. Vitamin B12 deficiency. N Engl J Med 2013;368(21):2041−2.
[51] Kumar N, Ahlskog JE, Gross Jr JB. Acquired hypocupremia after gastric surgery. Clin Gastroenterol Hepatol 2004;2(12):1074−9.
[52] Kumar N, Gross Jr JB, Ahlskog JE. Copper deficiency myelopathy produces a clinical picture like subacute combined degeneration. Neurology 2004;63(1):33−9.
[53] Jaiser SR, Winston GP. Copper deficiency myelopathy. J Neurol 2010;257(6):869−81.
[54] Kumar N. Copper deficiency myelopathy (human swayback). Mayo Clin Proc 2006; 81(10):1371−84.
[55] Prodan CI, Bottomley SS, Holland NR, Lind SE. Relapsing hypocupraemic myelopathy requiring high-dose oral copper replacement. J Neurol Neurosurg Psychiatry 2006; 77(9):1092−3.
[56] Spinazzi M, De Lazzari F, Tavolato B, et al. Myelo-optico-neuropathy in copper deficiency occurring after partial gastrectomy. Do small bowel bacterial overgrowth syndrome and occult zinc ingestion tip the balance? J Neurol 2007;254(8):1012−7.
[57] Kumar N, Elliott MA, Hoyer JD, et al. "Myelodysplasia," myeloneuropathy, and copper deficiency. Mayo Clin Proc 2005;80(7):943−6.
[58] Kumar N, Ahlskog JE, Klein CJ, Port JD. Imaging features of copper deficiency myelopathy: a study of 25 cases. Neuroradiology 2006;48(2):78−83.
[59] Mallory GN, Macgregor AM. Folate status following gastric bypass surgery (the Great Folate Mystery). Obes Surg 1991;1(1):69−72.
[60] Vargas-Ruiz AG, Hernandez-Rivera G, Herrera MF. Prevalence of iron, folate, and vitamin B12 deficiency anemia after laparoscopic Roux-en-Y gastric bypass. Obes Surg 2008;18(3):288−93.
[61] de Luis DA, Pacheco D, Izaola O, et al. Clinical results and nutritional consequences of biliopancreatic diversion: three years of follow-up. Ann Nutr Metab 2008;53(3−4): 234−9.

Further reading

[1] Green R, Kinsella LJ. Current concepts in the diagnosis of cobalamin deficiency. Neurology 1995;45(8):1435−40.

CHAPTER 19

The importance of a cookbook for patients who have bariatric surgery

Silvia Leite Faria[1], Mary O'Kane[2]

[1]*Gastrocirurgia de Brasilia/University of Brasilia, Brasilia, Federal District, Brazil;* [2]*Leeds Teaching Hospitals NHS Trust, Department of Nutrition and Dietetics, Leeds, United Kingdom*

Chapter outline

Introduction	258
Practical challenges	258
Phased introduction of fluids and textures	259
Introduction of fluids	259
Blended/pureed phase	259
Soft phase	259
Normal food textures	260
Portion sizes and regular meals	260
Eating habits after bariatric surgery	260
Ongoing postoperative care	261
The importance of protein and other food groups	262
Protein intake	262
Other nutrients	265
Calcium	266
Iron	266
Vitamin and mineral supplements	266
Vegetarian/vegan diet	266
Whole food plant-based diet	267
Side effect	268
Dumping syndrome and hypoglycemia	268
Therapeutic approaches to hypoglycemia including diet and medication	268
IFSO cookbook	269
The contents of a bariatric cookbook	269
Cultural differences	269
Menu planning	270
How to select a recipe for a patient after bariatric surgery?	270

Conclusion	270
Best recipes for normal phase by Sílvia Leite Faria	271
References	279
Resources	282

Introduction

Bariatric surgery is the most effective tool for treating severe and complex obesity. Nowadays, more than 47,000 surgeries are performed annually [1]. The most frequently performed surgeries are Roux-en-Y gastric bypass (RYGB) and sleeve gastrectomy (SG). Both surgeries lead to long-term weight loss and weight maintenance [1—3]. These bariatric procedures also present metabolic effects, such as increased hormones that lead to glucose profile improvement, increased satiety, and microbiota changes, all of which have a relation to weight loss [3]. The new rearrangement of the gastrointestinal tract (GIT), called the incretin effect, favors these effects [4].

With such gastrointestinal changes, nutritional support is crucial. Three points merit attention:

(1) Diet progression: As bariatric surgery has effects in the GIT, there will be, as mentioned above, the need to manage the progression of food texture and fluids;

(2) Nutritional deficiencies: Patients referred for bariatric surgery present with a high prevalence of nutritional deficiencies even before the preoperative stage. In the postoperative period, facing decreased caloric intake, lower absorption of nutrients, and less contact of the food consumed with digestive enzymes, patients are at a higher risk of presenting nutritional deficiencies.

(3) Weight loss and weight maintenance: Certain factors are fundamental for weight loss and weight maintenance among patients who have bariatric surgery. A healthy diet, with increased protein intake, and physical activity are some of the most important points.

Practical challenges

Food plays such an important part of our lives, not just to meet our nutritional requirements but also our social needs. Both of these elements remain very important to patients after bariatric surgery. As part of the preparation for surgery, dietitians will work with patients to discuss the impact of surgery both on meeting their nutritional needs and on their usual food intake [5]. It is important that people, who are considering bariatric surgery, have access to information and the opportunity to discuss this. Many people value being able to speak to others who have had bariatric surgery so they can share their different experiences.

Most bariatric surgical procedures will require the patient to use a staged approach to the reintroduction of fluids and different textures of food [6]. Eating slowly and chewing one's food well are key components of food reintroduction. Patients should also avoid drinking before a meal, with a meal, or too soon after a meal.

Phased introduction of fluids and textures
Introduction of fluids
Often patients will start on fluids on the first day or two after their operation. As these form the main source of nutrition, care must be taken to ensure that most of the fluids are nourishing and contain protein, vitamins, and minerals [6]. Generally, many will be milk-based. This will be an issue for those with milk or lactose intolerance or who are vegan. Beans, legumes, and pulses and plant-based protein powders can be used to make alternative drinks. Patients are advised to aim to drink at least 2 L of fluid over the day, sipping slowly and steadily throughout the day. Water, tea, coffee, and sugar-free drinks are also permitted in addition to the nourishing fluids. The number of days to remain on fluids varies according to the surgical procedure they underwent, and the advice received from their bariatric surgery center. The team should help patients find recipes for nourishing drinks, as many patients often report that they become bored drinking the same fluids. In addition, propriety products with high protein content are helpful for this stage.

Blended/pureed phase
When patients start to eat solids, this food needs to be eaten slowly and chewed well; otherwise, there is a risk of this food getting "stuck" or lodged in the gastric pouch. This leads to discomfort and may result in self-induced vomiting to remove it [7]. Consequently, many dietitians will advise starting with food that has been blended or pureed. This helps with the anxiety of food reintroduction, avoids foods becoming lodged, and helps the patient to build self-confidence.

The blended/pureed phase often requires food to be cooked in a different way, for instance, ensuring that meat and poultry are slow-cooked and tender before being blended. Other sources of protein, at this stage, include fish (often in sauce), reduced fat soft cheese, beans, pulses and legumes, soya, and Quorn. Vegetable purees, tuber/root purees (potatoes, cassava, yams), and pureed/stewed fruit can be included. As the meal may look less appetizing, advice about which recipes to include at this stage and how to arrange the presentation of the meal is very helpful.

As portions are small, nourishing fluids continue to be recommended for in-between meals [5,6].

Soft phase
Once patients are comfortable and have managed the blended/pureed phase well, the dietitian will encourage them to move on to the soft phase [5,6]. Although meals may no longer need to be blended, meat and poultry dishes should be soft and

easy to chew. Fish may need to be flaked or with sauce. Other soft textures of protein include cheese, eggs, pulses, and legumes (beans, chickpeas, kidney beans, peas, black-eyed peas, soya beans). Pasta, rice, and bread may not be tolerated at this stage so patients may need help and advice with suitable, alternative meals. Nourishing fluids will continue to be a key part of their diet [5,6].

In this stage, the maximum volume in each meal is 60—70 g (the equivalent of approximately three tablespoons). Consequently, in the first few weeks, the energy and protein intake from meals is low and may only be between 400 and 800 kcal/day. This reinforces the need for supplementation of vitamins, minerals, and protein [5,6,8,9].

Normal food textures
Gradually over the next few weeks, patients will learn which food textures they can tolerate and which ones they should continue to avoid and reintroduce at a later time. There may be some foods, for instance, tough meats that they are unable to tolerate, however, there will be alternatives. A bariatric cookbook should contain tips and ideas for food reintroduction at this stage.

This stage includes the introduction of foods in solid consistency according to tolerance, such as cooked vegetables, well-cooked legumes, fish, and tender cuts of meat and poultry. A protein supplement should be maintained while protein portions at the main meals are small. The volume of each meal is about 120 mL/g or 4—6 tablespoons (main meals). Hydration should be maintained with milk, protein supplement drinks, or water and calorie-free liquids [5,6,9,10].

Gradually the diet should evolve with the introduction of whole grains, fibers, salads, and/or unpeeled fruits. At this stage, the energy value must be adapted to the weight, sex, BMI, and age of the patient. Studies correlate good weight loss results with diets of higher protein content and reduced fats and carbohydrates [8—10].

Portion sizes and regular meals
Research suggests that certain behaviors have been shown to help people with weight maintenance after bariatric surgery [11,12]. These include eating regular meals, not eating when feeling full, and not eating continuously through the day. Initially, when introducing meals, portions are extremely small. However, after a few months, portions will gradually increase. Guidance from the dietitian and bariatric cookbooks will consider the portions for each stage. As meals increase in size, enabling patients to meet their protein requirements from their meals, there may be less dependence on protein drinks and protein snacks in-between meals. Some surgical procedures, however, result in less dietary protein being absorbed [13,14]. Therefore, it is important that patients discuss their specific nutritional needs with their dietitian [5].

Eating habits after bariatric surgery
Recent studies offer some considerations about the eating habits of patients after bariatric surgery [9,10]

- Use mindful eating techniques, that is, avoid activities that can distract attention during the meal (computers, cell phones, and TV). Take more than 20 min for each meal.
- Chew food carefully. Eating large amounts at a time can cause discomfort due to the small size of the stomach.
- Avoid carbonated drinks. The carbon dioxide present in these drinks increases intraabdominal pressure and causes discomfort.
- Avoid sugary drinks and juices. These high-calorie drinks are related to lower weight loss. In addition, they can lead to the occurrence of dumping syndrome.
- Reduce fatty, high-fat foods (high-fat meats, fried foods, butter, processed foods). These foods are related to higher caloric intake and lower weight loss
- Avoid drinking with meals. Calorie-free liquids can be consumed 30 min before or from 30 to 60 min after each meal.

These behaviors should be reinforced in a bariatric cookbook.

Ongoing postoperative care

As their diet progresses, patients will be instructed to adapt to a normal diet containing all food groups. It is important that they know the main dietary sources of protein so that they can give preference to protein foods, as high sugar and high fat foods, for example, biscuits, cookies, cakes, and crisps are more easily ingested and available [15–17].

The pyramid below (Fig. 19.1) shows that, in the diet of a patient who has had bariatric surgery, proteins must make up 50% of the volume of each meal and that patients can vary the food groups, always seeking to include carbohydrates that have a low glycemic index. Nutritional supplements are part of this routine.

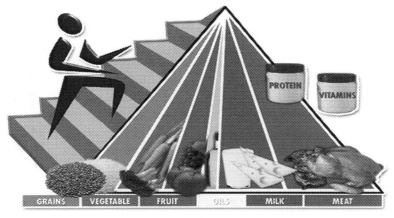

FIGURE 19.1

Pyramid and food groups.

The importance of protein and other food groups

Patients, after bariatric surgery, should, with time, progress to a normal diet. This means that they should include food from all food groups, consuming an adequate amount and distribution of macronutrients, protein, carbohydrates, and fat. The macronutrients are mainly three: proteins, carbohydrates, and fats. Fiber is important for the digestive tract, to regulate intestine rhythm and promote good bowel habits to protect our body from possible toxins that can come with the food and also to improve our gut microbiota.

To receive all macronutrients (and also micronutrients, such as vitamins and minerals), patients should eat foods from all food groups and with a variety of colors (five colors a day is a healthy reference).

Food groups, that are essential for our health, are illustrated in Fig. 19.1 and Table 19.1. Each group has a specific role in our body.

Furthermore, patients should include an adequate amount of water (35 mL per kg of body weight fractionally) and vitamin and mineral supplements [18].

Eating habits of patients form another key point for the success of the surgery. To have a snacking or grazing habit does not lead to a healthy weight. Cookies, nuts, candies, and other energy-dense foods can be consumed without affecting satiety [15,19,20].

Liquids, rich in calories, such as juices, vitamin drinks, smoothies, and especially alcohol, should also be avoided because they do not improve satiety. Alcoholic drinks are high in calories and can cause patients to have nutritional deficiencies, leading to B-complex vitamin deficiencies. Furthermore, alcohol is absorbed quickly after RYGB and SG procedures, leading to higher levels of alcohol in the blood and thus harming the liver [21,22].

Protein intake

This nutrient plays an important role in providing our body with all the essential amino acids for its normal and adequate functioning. Proteins are needed daily, as

Table 19.1 Pyramid and food groups.

Food group	Importance	Examples
Protein	Source of essential amino acids, composition of tissues, nerves, skin, and muscles	Meat, chicken, eggs, milk, cheese, beans, peas, whey or plant protein supplements
Fruits and vegetables	Source of fibers, vitamins, and minerals	Banana, watermelon, pineapple, orange, apple, tomato, lettuce, broccolis, carrots, onions
Carbohydrates	Main source of energy for the body	Bread, rice, potatoes, pasta, couscous, bulgar wheat,
Fats	Regulate hormones and are a source of liposoluble vitamins (A, D, E, and K)	Olive oil, avocado, butter, soya oil, rapeseed oil

every day our cells replicate and we produce hormones, blood cells, immunological cells, and others. So, when we do not achieve an adequate amount of protein, our body starts to take protein from our muscles and begins to decrease the production of important visceral proteins. This situation is called protein malnutrition. Initial signs of protein deficiencies may appear as general weakness, loss of muscle, hair loss, and brittle nails [23−25].

Besides these features, a loss of muscle mass can lead to decreased resting metabolic rate (RMR). Muscles burn a higher quantity of calories than fat mass. Decreased RMR can lead to weight regain. Thus, adequate protein intake is recognized as one of the pillars of bariatric surgery success [24,26].

Our concern is that patients are not able to achieve their minimum daily requirement of protein after bariatric surgery. The recommendation is a minimum intake of 60 g protein per day (during the first 6 months). The optimum daily intake is 1.1−1.5grams per kg of ideal body weight. This means that women will need to consume near 80 g per day and men near 100 g per day [27,28].

Table 19.2 shows important sources of protein and the portion size required to give at least 15 g protein per serving. Table 19.3 shows vegetable sources of protein giving 10−15 g protein per serving.

Table 19.2 Serving portions of meat, poultry, fish, and dairy products to achieve 15 g protein.

Protein Table (each portion has 15g of protein)	
FOOD source	**Quantity**
Meat	
Beef/lamb meatballs with tomato sauce	3 meatballs (not fried)
Grilled beef steak	½ a steak
Beef rolls	1 small roll
Roast beef/cooked pork/lamb	1 small slice
Roasted beef ribs	1 serving spoon
Beef stew	1 serving spoon
Grilled beef (knuckle)	½ a slice
Ground beef	1 serving spoon
Roast mince (with flour and mint)	4 small pieces
Jerked beef	2 small pieces
Stewed beef tongue	1½ medium-sized slices
Pork (sliced thin)	2 tablespoons
Pork ribs	1 medium-sized piece
Hamburger (just the meat)	1 hamburger

Continued

Table 19.2 Serving portions of meat, poultry, fish, and dairy products to achieve 15 g protein.—cont'd

Protein Table (each portion has 15g of protein)	
FOOD source	**Quantity**
Poultry	
Roast Turkey	1 medium-sized slice
Roast chicken (wings)	2 wings
Roast chicken (skinned drumstick)	1 large drumstick
Cooked chicken (skinned drumstick)	1 medium-sized drumstick
Cooked chicken (skinned thigh)	1 small piece
Chicken breast (shredded or with sauce)	¼ of a medium-sized breast
Turkey hamburger	1 hamburger
Offal	
Chicken gizzards	3 medium-sized pieces
Cooked chicken liver	2 medium-sized livers
A slice of beef liver	1 spoon-size potion
Beef liver steak	1 steak
Beef liver (sliced thin)	1 serving spoon
Cooked chicken hearts	1 serving spoon
Fish and seafood	
Roasted/cooked salmon	1 fillet
Canned sardines	1 can
Canned tuna fish	½ a can
Cooked codfish	1 spoon-size portion
Fish fillet (with sauce or grilled)	1 small fillet
Cooked fish steak	½ a steak
Braised octopus	6 tablespoons
Lobster	2 pieces
Crab (siri type)	3 small crabs
Steamed shrimp (unshelled)	3 tablespoons
Crabs	3 tablespoons
Eggs, milk and dairy products	
Natural yogurt or curds	1 pot of 200 g
Skimmed cow milk	1 glass (250 mL)
Pasteurized cow milk	1 glass (250 mL)
Powdered cow milk	2 heaping tablespoons
Omelette (with 2 eggs)	1 omelette
Omelette with cheese	1 small omelette
Boiled chicken egg	2 boiled eggs
Scrambled chicken egg	5 tablespoons

Table 19.2 Serving portions of meat, poultry, fish, and dairy products to achieve 15 g protein.—cont'd

Protein Table (each portion has 15g of protein)	
FOOD source	Quantity
Egg whites	3 egg whites
Cheese curds	1 skewer
Cottage cheese	2 tablespoons
Provolone, mozzarella or minas frescal cheese	2 medium-sized slices
Parmesan cheese	2 tablespoons
Ricotta cheese	3 tablespoons

Table 19.3 Vegetable servings providing 10–15 g of protein per serving.

Vegetable Proteins (About 10–15 g of protein per serving.)	
Food source	Quantity
Cooked peas	6 tablespoons
Pinto beans	2 ladles
Black beans	2 ladles
Chickpeas	5 tablespoons
Lentils	6 tablespoons
Textured soy protein (braised)	1 serving spoon
Tofu	4 slices

So, when evaluating a menu or selecting a recipe, these important points should be remembered:

(1) Protein content: at least 10 g (more than 20 g is better for main meals)
(2) Sugar content: avoid all sugar or at least limit it to less than 4 g per meal
(3) Fiber: rich fiber meals increase satiety so try to include whole grains, oats, bran cereal, beans or legumes, fruits, and whole-grain bread
(4) Fats: no more than 3 g for each 100 kcal of food consumed
(5) Carbohydrates: avoid an excess of sugary carbohydrates;
(6) Avoid high-caloric meals because they hinder weight loss goals

Other nutrients

A bariatric cookbook should include recipe suggestions that help to promote a good oral intake of calcium and iron.

Calcium

Calcium is an essential mineral that helps to form and maintain healthy teeth and bones. A proper level of calcium in the body over a lifetime can help prevent osteoporosis. After bariatric surgery, due to decreased food ingestions and lower acid production, patients present a higher risk of calcium deficiency. Vitamin D levels should also be checked, because of its important role in calcium regulation. Dairy foods, such as milk, yogurt, and cheese, are good sources of calcium, as are sardines and green colored vegetables.

Besides these sources, additional supplements of calcium and vitamin D are recommended after bariatric surgery [5,29]. Doses are adjusted in accordance with food consumption and lab exams.

Iron

Iron is an essential mineral. Its absorption is adversely affected after bariatric surgery. The reduced level of acid production and lower food ingestion can lead to iron deficiencies and iron deficiency can lead to anemia. Signs and symptoms of iron deficiency include hair loss, pallor, tiredness, and fatigue [23,30]. Fertile and pregnant women, adolescents, and athletes are at higher risk of presenting iron deficiency because of increased requirements.

Main food sources of iron include meat, chicken, fish, gizzards, liver, eggs, beans, pistachio, raisins, sunflower seeds, and pumpkin seeds. Most patients will need iron supplementation, following bariatric surgery, depending on the signs and symptoms they present and their laboratory exams [5,29].

Vitamin and mineral supplements

Healthcare professionals, working in bariatric surgery, are aware of the need for life long vitamin and mineral supplements [5,29]. Healthcare professionals, working outside of this area, may wrongly assume that once the person is eating a wide range of foods, that vitamin and mineral supplements are no longer needed. Patients may also think this too and may need reminding that vitamin and mineral supplements should be continued lifelong [5,6,13].

Vegetarian/vegan diet

Recent studies show more than 500% rise in the number of people seeking vegetarian diets in the United States [31,32]. To follow this diet, it is necessary to exclude all types of meat from one's menu, whether foods derived from animals, such as eggs and milk, are included or not. A vegetarian diet can be followed for ethical reasons, or out of compassion for animals, or concern for the environment, or due to a food allergy, or one's religion, or for health reasons. Regardless of the reason, it is important to follow a healthy and adequate diet, trying new flavors, and varying the foods consumed as much as possible.

The vegan diet does not include any animal products at all, so eggs, diary, and honey are also avoided. The main concern about a vegan diet is related to possible nutritional deficiencies. Plant-based sources of protein (such as soy, tofu, quinoa, beans, cereals, etc.) do not contain all the amino acids needed by the human body. Moreover, this type of diet may not provide adequate amounts of iron, vitamin B12, other B vitamins, and zinc. In addition, plant-based sources of protein are also rich in fiber, which hinders the absorption of vitamins and minerals [31].

For these reasons, a patient following a vegan diet will need nutritional supervision to prevent greater risks of nutritional deficiencies. It is very probable, patients, on a vegan diet, will need higher doses of supplements, including vegan protein supplements.

Whole food plant-based diet

There is no definite consensus about what a whole-food plant-based (WFPB) diet consists of. It is not, strictly speaking, a rigid diet—it is more a lifestyle. This is because plant-based diets can differ considerably according to whether or not a person includes animal products in their diet. There are, however, basic principles of a whole food, plant-based diet, namely [32].

An emphasis on whole, minimally processed foods. A limitation or elimination of animal products.

A focus on plants, including vegetables, fruits, whole grains, legumes, seeds, and nuts that serve as the basis of the diet. An exclusion of refined foods, like white flour, added sugars, and processed oils.

Special attention is given to food quality and the promotion, by many of this diet's followers, of locally sourced, organic food whenever possible.

Consequently, this diet is frequently confused with vegetarian or vegan diets. Although they appear to be somewhat similar, they are not the same.

Those who follow vegan diets abstain from eating any and all animal products, including dairy products, meat, poultry, seafood, eggs, and honey. Generally, vegetarians eliminate all meat and poultry from their diets; however, some of them eat eggs, seafood, or dairy products.

In contrast, the WFPB diet exhibits more flexibility. Followers eat mostly plants, but animal products are not totally excluded. They may consume small amounts of eggs, poultry, seafood, meat, or dairy products.

Decreasing the consumption of processed foods is an advantage and reveals a healthy attitude that can improve microbiota and help maintainenance of a stable weight after losing excess weight. The disadvantages include an increase in costs and the possible appearance of nutritional deficiencies among patients who do not use higher doses of vitamins and minerals. Sarcopenia (lower muscle mass) can occur even among those who follow a WFPB diet or a vegan diet. Nutritionists should closely observe these patients, evaluating their needs and preferences and prescribing supplements accordingly.

Side effect
Dumping syndrome and hypoglycemia

Dumping Syndrome (DS) may be experienced by some people following bariatric surgery. DS is classified as either early or late. Early DS occurs from 30 to 60 min after eating and includes symptoms of bloating, diarrhea, nausea, and lightheadedness. It occurs due to undigested calorie-dense liquids or solids that provoke hyperosmolarity of the intestinal content causing fluid to be drawn into the intestinal lumen leading to intestinal distention, fluid sequestration, decreased intravascular volume, and hypotension. Patients should be instructed to recognize the signs and symptoms and avoid high-calorie liquids and solids. Early DS is more frequent among patients who have a RYGB [33]. In general, 70% of RYGB patients experience DS [34–36].

Postprandial DS, called hyperinsulinemic hypoglycemia, is a complication related to nonbanding procedures. Symptoms can occur from 1 to 3 h after meals, particularly meals rich in high glycemic carbohydrates. It can happen due to the role of the incretin hormone glucagon-like peptide-1 (GLP-1) as a critical contributor to the inappropriate insulin secretion. Hypoglycemic symptoms can be broadly classified as autonomic (e.g., palpitations, lightheadedness, sweating) or neuroglycopenic (e.g., confusion, decreased attentiveness, seizure, loss of consciousness). More severe hypoglycemia associated with neuroglycopenia is rare but can occur from 1 to 3 years post-RYGB [37,38].

Therapeutic approaches to hypoglycemia including diet and medication

Dietary changes are the first-line treatment for DS. Patients should be advised to eat smaller and more frequent meals (about five–six per day) Patients should save fluids for after meals, separating their intake of "dry" from "wet" nutrients by more than 1 h (because liquids accelerate gastric transit), lying down after meals, decreasing their carbohydrate intake, and preferentially eating complex carbohydrates rather than simple ones [34].

Alcohol, coffee, and beverages with caffeine should be avoided. Patients may feel worse with milk and dairy products, so eliminating them has been helpful for many patients. Meals should be composed of carbohydrates (with a low glycemic index), lipids, protein, and fiber (mixed meals). Adding soluble fiber before or during the meals can help to slow the pace of the food through the gastrointestinal tract. Avoidance of sweets and simple carbohydrates is an essential element of the bariatric diet used to sidestep DS symptoms. To include fiber supplementation with meals to diminish the pace of food in the gastrointestinal tract is a good strategy (guar gum, glucommanan, and pectin). If the dietetic intervention fails to cure these events, medications should be used for improvement. As a parallel treatment, physicians can use acarbose, octreotide, and diazoxide [3,39].

IFSO cookbook

For the International Congress IFSO 2019, the challenge was issued of developing an international cookbook for patients after bariatric surgery. A competition, open to IFSO members, was launched. Members were invited to send in their recipes, detailing the ingredients, cooking instructions, and nutritional composition and supply a photograph. A considerably large number of entries were received.

There were entries from all five IFSO chapters. The criteria used to judge the entries included nutritional composition, originality, the degree of difficulty in following the recipe, and its quality and presentation. Selecting the best recipes was a challenge as some of the ingredients were not known by all judges as they reflected local foods not available in other countries. This added to the judges' interest and all learned more about the cuisines of different countries. In assessing the nutritional composition, efforts were made to ensure that the calculations were accurate. For instance, in some recipes, the protein content was too high as the cooked weight of an ingredient, rather than the raw weight, had been used for the recipe analysis. A small number of recipes had high sugar or fat content and were seen as inappropriate to be included. All recipes were evaluated and the best were chosen to be included in the cookbook. The IFSO cookbook, launched at IFSO 2019, is available for purchase from IFSO.

The contents of a bariatric cookbook

There are many bariatric cookbooks on sale. These have a mixture of authors ranging from registered dietitians to people who have had bariatric surgery. It is not possible to review all of these books or make specific recommendations. However, the healthcare professionals in bariatric surgery centers will be able to recommend appropriate cookbooks to their patients. In addition, some centers offer bariatric cooking classes.

People who have had bariatric surgery have specific needs and, therefore, emphasis is given to some factors that influence people's diets and food intakes after bariatric surgery.

Cultural differences

Cookbooks give a fantastic opportunity to sample different cuisines. It is worth noting, however, that it may not be easy to follow the recipes that have been written for the audience of a different country. Different weights and measures may be used.

For instance, what is a cup of flour in imperial or metric weights? Is crushed red pepper the same as crushed chili flakes? What can be used in the place of Freekah if it is not available in my country? Will Cilbir taste nice, once cooked? To those of us, not used to Turkish cuisine, Cilbir sounded unusual as it was poached eggs with yogurt, crushed red pepper, thyme, and mint topping. It tasted delicious and was cooked by the winner in the IFSO 2019 competition.

Before purchasing a cookbook, it may be helpful for people to look at a sample of the book, read reviews, and speak to other people, including their healthcare professionals to determine whether the cookbook meets their needs. Often people will have already purchased other cookbooks before surgery to help with their weight loss journey. It is worth reminding people that once they have expanded the range of textures they have managed, they can start to use these books again and include other healthy recipes.

Menu planning

Research shows planning ahead and having a routine is helpful for weight management. Planning ahead helps us to save time and also decrease food wastage. Cookbooks, with their range of meals, can aid menu planning and the elaboration of a shopping list. Many include suggestions for batch cooking and freezing meals and contain a list of commonly used store cupboard items.

How to select a recipe for a patient after bariatric surgery?

When you want to evaluate a menu or select a recipe, you should remember these important points:

(1) Respect the phase the patient is going through—liquid, puree, or normal diet.
(2) Do not emphasize just calories: pay attention to macronutrients, the glycemic index, and the fiber content.
(3) Protein content is a key point. A recipe should include at least 10 g (more than 20 g is better for main meals).
(4) Sugar content: avoid all sugar or at least limit it to less than 4 g per meal.
(5) Fiber: fiber-rich meals increase satiety, so whole grains, oats, bran cereal, beans or legumes, fruits, and whole-grain bread should be included.
(6) Fats: no more than 3 g for each 100 kcal of food consumed.
(7) Carbohydrates: avoid any excess of refined carbohydrates;
(8) Avoid high-caloric meals because they can hinder your goal to lose weight

Conclusion

The success of bariatric surgery depends on healthy eating habits and behaviors. The selection of good, high protein recipes can help patients to select good options and may help patients to adhere to healthy eating habits and lifestyles. Patients may need support and guidance from dietitians in this area.

Best recipes for normal phase by Sílvia Leite Faria

(1) Meatballs with tomato sauce (Fig. 19.2)

Preparation time: 50 min | Yield: eight portions—approx. 250 g each.
Nutritional information per serving: Caloric value: 240 kcal | Protein: 25 g | Fats: 12 g | Carbohydrates: 10 g | Fibers: 1.5 g.

Ingredients
- 650 g of ground rump steak or lean minced steak
- 3 slices of crumbled bread without crusts
- 1/2 cup of skim milk
- 1 slightly beaten egg yolk
- 1 tablespoon of olive oil
- 2 crushed garlic cloves
- 1 cup of tomato sauce
- 1/2 cup of water

Preparation
1. In a large bowl, mix the meat, bread, milk, and egg yolk, with pepper and salt to taste, until forming a very homogeneous mixture. Form meatballs the size of ping-pong balls and flatten them a little. Sprinkle with flour.
2. Heat the oil in a large skillet over moderate heat. Sauté the garlic and fry the meatballs for 10 min, until golden brown. Cook over low heat for 12 min, turning the meatballs from time to time.
3. Add the sauce and water and leave for another 5 min. Serve immediately.

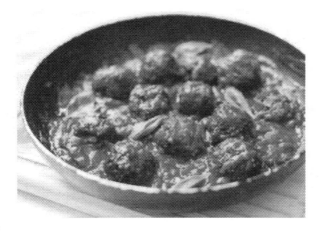

FIGURE 19.2

Meatballs with tomato sauce.

CHAPTER 19 Cookbook for patients who have bariatric surgery

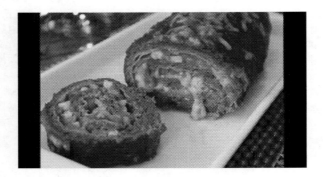

FIGURE 19.3

Ground beef roulade.

(2) Ground beef roulade

Preparation (Fig. 19.3) time: 60 min | Yield: six portions—approx. 180 g each. Nutritional information per serving: Caloric value: 127 kcal | Protein: 22 g | Fats: 3 g | Carbohydrates: 3 g | Fibers: 1.5 g.

Ingredients.

Meat
- 500 g of minced meat
- 1 teaspoon of chia seeds
- 1 onion, chopped into small cubes
- 1 crushed garlic clove
- 1 grated carrot
- Oregano to taste
- Salt and black pepper to taste

Filling
- 1 zucchini cut into thin strips
- 4 slices of turkey breast
- Pieces of white cheese
- Cherry tomato to taste

Preparation
1. Put the minced meat, the chopped onion, the garlic, the carrot, and the spices in a bowl and mix everything very well with your hands until the mixture is homogeneous.
2. Open a piece of plastic wrap and on top of it spread out this meat mixture as if you were covering the wrapping paper, forming a rectangular shape. To help spread the mixture and to form the rectangular shape, knead it with your fingertips, being careful not to get spread it too thin. The ideal height is about the thickness of a finger.
3. Put a layer of zucchini, a layer of turkey breast, a layer of white cheese, and a layer of tomatoes over the meat.

4. Now with the help of the plastic film, roll the whole rectangle of meat, forming a cylinder. Squeeze this a little to avoid the filling falling out and bake it in a preheated oven at 200°C.
5. The time of baking will depend on your oven. In mine, it took 30 min until it was ready, when the upper crust was golden.

(3) Whey pancakes (Fig. 19.4)

Preparation time: _10 min | Yield: four pancakes—approx. 50 g each

Nutritional information per serving: Caloric value: 110 kcal | Protein: 18 g | Fats: 1 g | Carbohydrates: 7.5 g.

Ingredients:
- 1 cup of fine oat flakes
- 2 scoops of vanilla or chocolate whey (a scoop has 20 g of protein, 2 g of carbs, and 1 g of fat)
- 6 tablespoons of milk
- 1/2 teaspoon of vanilla extract
- 4 egg whites

Preparation:

To make these whey pancakes, start by beating all the ingredients in a blender or processor until you get a homogeneous dough.

Grease a frying pan with margarine, put it on medium-low heat, and pour in a ladle of dough. Cook the dough on both sides **until the pancake is golden brown** and move it to a plate. Repeat the procedure until you have used all the dough.

When you serve these whey pancakes, made with oat flakes, you can sweeten them with honey and add a side dish of fruit, the most popular being banana. Try it and tell us what you think.

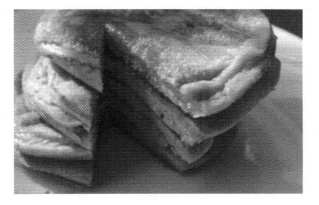

FIGURE 19.4

Whey pancakes.

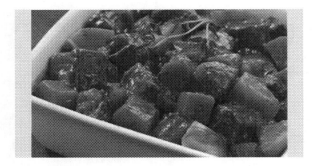

FIGURE 19.5

Meat with carrots.

(4) Meat with carrots
Preparation (Fig. 19.5) time: 120 min | Yield: six portions—approx. 280 g each.
Nutritional information per serving: Caloric value: 290 kcal | Protein: 35 g | Fats: 10 g | Carbohydrates: 10 g | Fibers: 3 g.
Ingredients
- 1 kg of chuck steak cleaned and cut into cubes
- 3 cloves of crushed garlic
- 1/2 tablespoon of oil
- Salt to taste
- 400 g of sliced carrot
- 2 diced onions
- Green seasonings (parsley, chive, scallion, etc.) to taste

Preparation
1. Season the meat with garlic and salt. Pour the oil into a pan and sauté the meat until it browns well.
2. Mix in the carrots (add a little more water). After the mixture is cooked, stir in the onions and green seasonings, mix well, and turn off the heat.

(5) Chicken chilli
Preparation (Fig. 19.6) time: 40 min | Yield: six portions—approx. 230 g each.

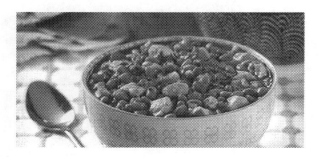

FIGURE 19.6

Chicken chilli.

Nutritional information per serving: Caloric value: 180 kcal | Protein: 15 g | Fats: 8 g | Carbohydrates: 7 g | Fibers: 2 g.

Ingredients
- 1 teaspoon of olive oil
- 400 g of turkey mince chicken breast (can be the prepackaged type)
- 1 medium onion, chopped
- 1/2 cup of chopped celery
- 1 large chopped carrot
- 380 g of cooked beans
- 2 cans of peeled tomatoes
- 1/2 can of water
- 1 teaspoon of chilli powder
- 1 teaspoon of salt
- 1/2 teaspoon of garlic powder
- 1 teaspoon of cumin powder
- 1/4 teaspoon of ground black pepper
- 1 teaspoon of sugar (if necessary)

Preparation
1. Pour the olive oil into a large saucepan and fry the onion and the shredded chicken breast.
2. Add all the other ingredients (except sugar) and leave the mixture on low heat for approximately 20–30 min, stirring occasionally.
3. Taste and adjust the salt. If you prefer more pepper, add a little more chilli powder. Add sugar if the chilli is acidic.
4. Serve in a soup plate and add some cheese or cilantro (or other preferences).

(6) Shepherd's (Fig. 19.7) pie with sweet potatoes

Preparation time: 60 min | Yield: four portions—approx. 110 g each.
Nutritional information per serving: Caloric value: 180 kcal | Protein: 20 g | Fats: 10 g | Carbohydrate s: 8g | Fibers: 1 g.

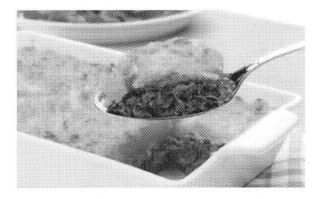

FIGURE 19.7

Shepherd's pie with sweet potato.

Ingredients
- 1 cup of lean beef cut into cubes (can be rump, tenderloin, knuckle, topside or bottom round)
- 1 cooked sweet potato (you do not need to remove the peel)
- 3 onion rings
- 2 slices of tomato
- 1 egg white
- Grated cheese to taste
- Olive oil

Preparation
1. In a frying pan, sauté the onion and tomato with a drizzle of olive oil.
2. Add the meat and let it cook for a while.
3. Put the mixture aside.
4. Mix the potato with the egg white and, with the help of a fork, crush it to the texture of a puree.
5. Place a layer of potato on a tray, pour the cooked meat over it and cover the meat with more puree.
6. Add some grated cheese and bake in the oven until it browns.
To make the dish even healthier, serve it with a salad of dark green leafy vegetables (arugula, watercress, chard, etc.), along with carrots, beets, and cucumbers.

(7) Oat- (Fig. 19.8) crusted chicken fillets

Preparation time: 40 min | Yield: four portions—approx. 80 g each.
Nutritional information per serving: Caloric value: 170 kcal | Protein: 18 g | Fats: 7 g | Carbohydrates: 8 g | Fibers: 1 g.

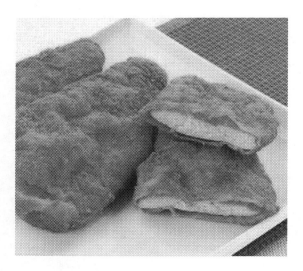

FIGURE 19.8

Oat-crusted chicken fillets.

Ingredients
- 4 chicken fillets (300 g)
- 1 cup of oat flour or thin oat flakes
- 2 egg whites
- 1 teaspoon of salt
- 2 garlic cloves
- the juice of 1 lemon
- 1 tablespoon of mustard
- 1 tablespoon of oil

Preparation
1. Season the fillets with salt, lemon, oil, and mustard. Let these seasonings settle in for at least 30 min.
2. Dip the fillets in the egg white and then in the oat flour or oat flakes.
3. Line a baking sheet with baking paper and spread out the fillets.
4. Bake in the oven at medium heat for 40 min.

(8) Pasta (Fig. 19.9) with chicken
Preparation time: 50 min | Yield: three servings—approx. 170 g each.
Nutritional information per serving: Caloric value: 350 kcal | Protein: 35 g | Fats: 20 g | Carbohydrates: 5 g | Fibers: 0.5 g.

Ingredients
- 4 tablespoons of oil
- 1 chopped onion
- 2 chopped garlic cloves
- 4 tablespoons of tomato paste
- 300 g shredded chicken breast, cooked with seasonings
- Salt, pepper and chopped parsley to taste
- 1/2 cup of grated Parmesan cheese

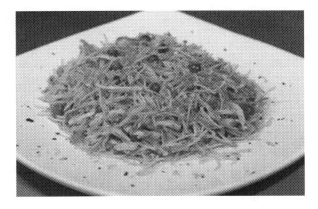

FIGURE 19.9

Pasta with chicken.

Preparation
1. Heat the oil in a saucepan and brown the onion and garlic.
2. Add the tomato paste and chicken, cooking for 5 minutes, then season the mixture with salt and pepper, adding the parsley.
3. Place the rice noodles of your choice in a serving dish and cover them with the sauce.
4. Sprinkle with grated cheese and serve.

(9) Chicken (Fig. 19.10) breast with cheese spread
Preparation time: 40 min | Yield: eight portions—approx. 90 g each.
Nutritional information per serving: Caloric value: 150 kcal | Protein: 15 g | Fats: 9 g | Carbohydrates: 3 g | Fibers: 0.5 g.
Ingredients
- 2 chicken breasts
- 1 chopped garlic clove
- 1 chopped onion
- green seasonings (to taste)
- potato sticks
- 1 glass of cheese spread

Preparation
1. Cook the chicken breasts in salted water
2. Shred them into small pieces
3. Sauté the chicken, seasoned with garlic, onion, and the green seasonings
4. Pour into a pyrex dish.

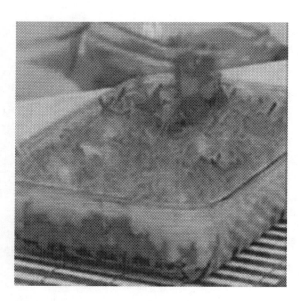

FIGURE 19.10

Chicken breast with cheese spread.

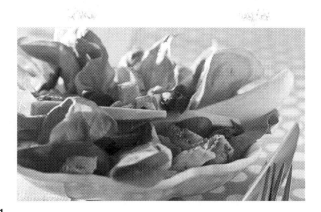

FIGURE 19.11

Green salad with tuna.

      5. Pour the cheese spread on top. Heat in the oven or microwave until the cheese melts.

      6. Serve with rice and potato sticks.

(10) Green (Fig. 19.11) salad with tuna

Preparation time: 20 min | Yield: three portions—approx. 170 g each.

Nutritional information per serving: Caloric value: 160 kcal | Protein: 20 g | Fats: 9 g | Carbohydrates: 2.5 g | Fibers: 2 g.

Ingredients

- 1/2 bunch of arugula (rocket leaves)
- 1/2 a head of smooth lettuce
- 1/2 a head of purple curly lettuce
- 1 can of drained canned tuna
- 1 cup of sliced palm hearts
- 1 cup of boiled quail eggs cut in half

Preparation.

Wash the leaves and place them on the edges of a salad bowl. In the center, place the tuna, palm hearts, and quail eggs. Serve when ready.

References

[1] Angrisani L, Santonicola A, Iovino P, et al. IFSO worldwide survey 2016: primary, endoluminal, and revisional procedures. Obes Surg 2018;28(12):3783−94. https://doi.org/10.1007/s11695-018-3450-2.

[2] Gagner M. Obesity and weight management editorial. The Future of Sleeve Gastrectomy. European Endocrinology 2016;12(1):37−8. https://doi.org/10.17925/EE.2016.12.01.37.

[3] Mingrone G, Bornstein S, Le Roux CW. Optimisation of follow-up after metabolic surgery. Lancet Diabetes Endocrinol 2018;6(6):487−99. https://doi.org/10.1016/S2213-8587(17)30434-5.

[4] Wabitsch M. Gastrointestinal endocrinology in bariatric surgery. In: Endocrine development, vol. 32. S. Karger AG; 2017. p. 124–38. https://doi.org/10.1159/000475735.
[5] Parrott JM, Craggs-Dino L, Faria SL, O'Kane M. The optimal nutritional programme for bariatric and metabolic surgery. Curr Obes Rep 2020. https://doi.org/10.1007/s13679-020-00384-z. Accessed ahead of print 26 May 2020.
[6] Aills L, Blankenship J, Buffington C, Furtado M, Parrott J. ASMBS allied health nutritional guidelines for the surgical weight loss patient. Surg Obes Relat Dis 2008;4: S73–108. https://doi.org/10.1016/j.soard.2008.03.002.
[7] Sarwer DB, Dilks RJ, West-Smith L. Dietary intake and eating behavior after bariatric surgery: threats to weight loss maintenance and strategies for success. Surg Obes Relat Dis 2011;7(5):644–51. https://doi.org/10.1016/j.soard.2011.06.016.
[8] Jastrzebska-Mierzyńska M, Ostrowska L, Razak Hady H, Dadan J, Konarzewska-Duchnowska E. The impact of bariatric surgery on nutritional status of patients. Videosurg Other Miniinvasive Tech 2015;1:115–24. https://doi.org/10.5114/wiitm.2014.47764.
[9] Leahy CR, Luning A. Review of nutritional guidelines for patients undergoing bariatric surgery. AORN J 2015;102(2):153–60. https://doi.org/10.1016/j.aorn.2015.05.017.
[10] Dagan SS, Goldenshluger A, Globus I, Schweiger C, Kessler Y. Nutritional recommendations for adult bariatric: clinical practise. Adv Nutr 2017;8(12):382–94. https://doi.org/10.3945/an.116.014258.382.
[11] Sanborn VE, Spitznagel M-B, Crosby R, Steffen K, Mitchell J, Gunstad J. Cognitive function and quality of life in bariatric surgery candidates. Surg Obes Relat Dis 2018;14:1396–401. https://doi.org/10.1016/j.soard.2018.06.010.
[12] Mitchell JE, Christian NJ, Flum DR, et al. Behavioral variables and weight change 3 years after bariatric surgery. JAMA Surg. 2016;8:752–7. https://doi.org/10.1001/jamasurg.2016.0395.
[13] O'Kane M, Parretti HM, Hughes CA, et al. Guidelines for the follow-up of patients undergoing bariatric surgery. Clin Obes 2016;6(3):210–24. https://doi.org/10.1111/cob.12145.
[14] Shoar S, Poliakin L, Rubenstein R, Saber AA. Single anastomosis duodeno-ileal switch (SADIS): a systematic review of efficacy and safety. Obes Surg 2018;28(1):104–13. https://doi.org/10.1007/s11695-017-2838-8.
[15] Faria SL, Kelly EDO, Faria OP, Ito MK. Snack-eating patients experience lesser weight loss after roux-en-Y gastric bypass surgery. Obes Surg 2009:1293–6. https://doi.org/10.1007/s11695-008-9704-7.
[16] Faria SL, Faria OP, Lopes TC, Galvão MV, De Oliveira Kelly E, Ito MK. Relation between carbohydrate intake and weight loss after bariatric surgery. Obes Surg 2009; 19(6):708–16. https://doi.org/10.1007/s11695-008-9583-y.
[17] Goodpaster KPS, Marek RJ, Lavery ME, Ashton K, Merrell Rish J, Heinberg LJ. Graze eating among bariatric surgery candidates: prevalence and psychosocial correlates. Surg Obes Relat Dis 2016;12(5):1091–7. https://doi.org/10.1016/j.soard.2016.01.006.
[18] Armstrong LE, Johnson EC. Water intake, water balance, and the elusive daily water requirement. Nutrients 2018;10(12):1–25. https://doi.org/10.3390/nu10121928.
[19] Pizato N, Botelho PB, Gonçalves VSS, Dutra ES, de Carvalho KMB. Effect of grazing behavior on weight regain post-bariatric surgery: a systematic review. Nutrients 2017; 9(12):1–12. https://doi.org/10.3390/nu9121322.

References

[20] Ruffault A, Vaugeois F, Barsamian C, et al. Associations of lifetime traumatic experience with dysfunctional eating patterns and postsurgery weight loss in adults with obesity: a retrospective study. Stress Health 2018;34(3):446−56. https://doi.org/10.1002/smi.2807.

[21] Bishop FM. Self-guided Change: the most common form of long-term, maintained health behavior change. Health Psychology Open 2018:1−14. https://doi.org/10.1177/2055102917751576.

[22] Iossa A, Ciccioriccio MC, Zerbinati C, Guida A, Di Giacomo L, Silecchia G. Alcohol ingestion symptoms after sleeve gastrectomy: intoxication or drunkenness? A prospective study from a Bariatric Centre of Excellence. Eat Weight Disord 2019. https://doi.org/10.1007/s40519-019-00813-6 (0123456789).

[23] Levinson R, Silverman JB, Catella JG, Rybak I, Jolin H, Isom K. Pharmacotherapy prevention and management of nutritional deficiencies post Roux-en-Y gastric bypass. Obes Surg 2013;23(7):992−1000. https://doi.org/10.1007/s11695-013-0922-2.

[24] Ito MK, Siqueira V, Gonçalves S, et al. Effect of protein intake on the protein status and lean mass of post-bariatric surgery patients: a systematic review. Obes Surg 2016. https://doi.org/10.1007/s11695-016-2453-0.

[25] Kassir R, Debs T, Blanc P, et al. Complications of bariatric surgery: presentation and emergency management. Int J Surg 2016;27:77−81. https://doi.org/10.1016/j.ijsu.2016.01.067.

[26] Faria SL, Kelly E, Faria OP. Energy expenditure and weight regain in patients submitted to roux-en-Y gastric bypass. Obes Surg 2009;19(7):856−9. https://doi.org/10.1007/s11695-009-9842-6.

[27] Via MA, Mechanick JI. Nutritional and micronutrient care of bariatric surgery Patients : current evidence update. Curr Obes Rep 2017:286−96. https://doi.org/10.1007/s13679-017-0271-x.

[28] Mechanick JI, Apovian C, Brethauer S, et al. Clinical practice guidelines for the perioperative nutrition, metabolic, and nonsurgical support of patients undergoing bariatric procedures − 2019 update: cosponsored by American Association of Clinical Endocrinologists/American College of Endocrinology. Surg Obes Relat Dis 2020;16(2):175−247. https://doi.org/10.1016/j.soard.2019.10.025.

[29] Parrott J, Frank L, Rabena R, Craggs-Dino L, Isom KA, Greiman L. American society for metabolic and bariatric surgery integrated health nutritional guidelines for the surgical weight loss patient 2016 update: micronutrients. Surg Obes Relat Dis 2017;13(5):727−41. https://doi.org/10.1016/j.soard.2016.12.018.

[30] Via MA, Mechanick JI. Nutritional and micronutrient care of bariatric surgery patients: current evidence update. Curr Obes Rep 2017;6(3):286−96. https://doi.org/10.1007/s13679-017-0271-x.

[31] Sherf-Dagan S, Hod K, Buch A, et al. Health and nutritional status of vegetarian candidates for bariatric surgery and practical recommendations. Obes Surg 2018;28(1):152−60. https://doi.org/10.1007/s11695-017-2810-7.

[32] Lynch H, Johnston C, Wharton C. Plant-based diets: considerations for environmental impact, protein quality, and exercise performance. Nutrients 2018;10(12):1841. https://doi.org/10.3390/nu10121841.

[33] Scarpellini E, Arts J, Karamanolis G, Laurenius A, Siquini W, Suzuki H, et al. International consensus on the diagnosis and management of dumping syndrome. Nature Reviews 2020;16:448−66. https://doi.org/10.1038/s41574-020-0357-5.

[34] Ritz P, Vaurs C, Barigou M, Hanaire H. Hypoglycaemia after gastric bypass: mechanisms and treatment. Diabetes Obes Metabol 2016;18(3):217−23. https://doi.org/10.1111/dom.12592.
[35] Elrazek AEMAA, Elbanna AEM, Bilasy SE. Medical management of patients after bariatric surgery: principles and guidelines. World J Gastrointest Surg 2017. https://doi.org/10.4240/wjgs.v6.i11.220.
[36] Ramadan M, Loureiro M, Laughlan K, Caiazzo R, Iannelli A, Brunaud L, Czernichow S, Nedelcu M, Nocca D. Risk of dumping syndrome after sleeve gastrectomy and roux-en-Y gastric bypass: early results of a multicentre prospective study. Gastroenterol Res Pract 2016;2016:2−7. https://doi.org/10.1155/2016/2570237.
[37] Berg P, McCallum R. Dumping syndrome: a review of the current concepts of pathophysiology, diagnosis, and treatment. Dig Dis Sci 2016;61(1):11−8. https://doi.org/10.1007/s10620-015-3839-x.
[38] Tack J, Deloose E. Complications of bariatric surgery: dumping syndrome, reflux and vitamin deficiencies. Best Pract Res Clin Gastroenterol 2014. https://doi.org/10.1016/j.bpg.2014.07.010.
[39] Craig CM, Liu LF, Deacon CF, Holst JJ, McLaughlin TL. Critical role for GLP-1 in symptomatic post-bariatric hypoglycaemia. Diabetologia 2017;60(3):531−40. https://doi.org/10.1007/s00125-016-4179-x.

Resources

[1] IFSO. Cook Book. Available from: https://www.ifso.com/cook-book/.

Index

'*Note*: Page numbers followed by "f" and "t" indicate figures and tables respectively.'

A

Abdominal sepsis, 88
Accelerometers, 31
Acute kidney injury (AKI), 108
Adiposity-based chronic disease, 87
Adjustable gastric banding (AGB)
    benefits, 76
    complications, 76−77
    silicone band, 76
Adolescent obesity
    dietary tips, 191t
    multidisciplinary team (MDT) approach, 188
    nutritional assessment
        family and home environment, 189
        nutritional deficiencies, 188
        parenting style, 189
        preoperative multivitamin regimen, 188−189
        recommended laboratory parameters, 188
    nutritional monitoring
        academic environment, 194−196
        age-appropriate laboratory parameters, 194, 195t
        hunger assessment, 194
        hypothalamic obesity (HyOb), 196
        Prader−Willi Syndrome (PWS), 196
        reproductive health, 196
    nutritional needs
        copper, 193
        daily recommended intake, 191t
        iron, 193
        omega-3 fatty acids, 193
        protein, 192
        vitamin A, 193
        vitamin B1, 192
        vitamin B6, 192
        vitamin B9, 192
        vitamin B12, 192
        vitamin D/calcium, 193
        zinc and magnesium, 193
    nutrition education, 189−190
    postoperative diet food, 190t
    prevalence, 187
Adult distress respiratory syndrome (ADRS), 107
American Society for Metabolic and Bariatric Surgery (ASMBS), 187
American Society for Parenteral and Enteral Nutrition (ASPEN), 88, 101

Anemia, 5
    folic acid deficiency, 243
    inaccurate diagnosis, 241
    iron deficiency
        blood loss, 241
        hemoglobin level, 241
        intolerance/ineffectiveness, 242
        iron absorption, 240−241
        malabsorptive technique, 240−241
        prevalence, 240−241
    pregnancy, 214
    vitamin B12 deficiency, 242−243
Anthropometric assessment
    body fat percentage, 19−20
    body mass index (BMI), 19, 20t
    midarm muscle area (MAMA), 21
    midarm muscle circumference (MAMC), 20−21
    midupper arm circumference (MUAC), 20
    skinfold anthropometry, 21
    waist circumference (WC), 20
Arterial waveform analysis-based techniques, 69
Atherogenic dyslipidemia, 52
Atrial fibrillation, 107−108
Authoritarian parenting style, 189

B

Bariatric smoothies, 159
Bariatric surgery
    biliopancreatic diversion (BPD)/duodenal switch (DS)
        excess weight loss (EWL), 82
        gastric resection, 81
        ileo-ileostomy, 80f−81f
        one-anastomosis gastric bypass (OAGB), 82
        single-anastomosis duodeno-ileal switch (SADI-S), 83
        subtotal gastrectomy, 80
        total bowel length, 81
    calcium supplements, 266
    cultural differences, 269−270
    diet progression, 258
    dumping syndrome (DS), 268
    eating habits, 260−261
    fluids and textures
        blended/pureed phase, 259
        fluids introduction, 259
        normal food textures, 260

Index

Bariatric surgery (*Continued*)
　nutritional deficiencies, 258
　soft phase, 259—260
　IFSO cookbook, 269
　iron supplements, 266
　menu planning, 270
　monitoring recommendations, 71—72, 72f
　mortality, 88
　patient evaluation, 6—8, 7t
　patient preparation, 9—12
　posthypoglycemia, 268—269
　postoperative care
　　protein, 262
　　protein intake, 262—265, 265t
　　pyramid and food groups, 261f, 262t
　　vegetable servings, 265t
　postoperative complications. *See* Postoperative complications
　practical challenges, 258—261
　restrictive procedures, 75
　　adjustable gastric banding (AGB), 76, 77f
　　sleeve gastrectomy (SG), 77
　Roux-en-Y gastric bypass (RYGB), 78
　vegetarian/vegan diet, 266—267
　very low-calorie diet (VLCD), 40—43
　vitamin and mineral supplements, 266
　weight loss and maintenance, 258
　whole-food plant-based (WFPB) diet, 267—268
Basal metabolic rate (BMR), 24
Biliopancreatic diversion (BPD)/duodenal switch (DS)
　excess weight loss (EWL), 82
　gastric resection, 81
　ileo-ileostomy, 80f—81f
　nutritional recommendations. *See* Hypoabsorptive procedures (HAP)
　one-anastomosis gastric bypass (OAGB), 82
　postoperative nutritional deficiencies, 226
　single-anastomosis duodeno-ileal switch (SADI-S), 83
　subtotal gastrectomy, 80
　total bowel length, 81
Binge-eating disorder, 96
Bioimpedance, 100
　analysis, 30
　technologies, 70—71

C

Calcium. *See also* Vitamin D
　adolescent obesity, 193
　deficiency, 10
　malabsorption, mixed procedures, 175—176
　obese elderly patients, 202
　postoperative, 228—229, 229b
　recommended dietary allowance (RDA), 181
Carbajo's technique, 83. *See also* One-anastomosis gastric bypass (OAGB)
Carbohydrate
　laparoscopic adjustable gastric band (LAGB), 122
　metabolism, 38
　Roux-n-Y gastric bypass, 147
Carbonated liquids, 159
Central venous catheters (CVCs), 91—92
Childhood obesity
　multidisciplinary team (MDT) approach, 188
　nutritional deficiencies, 188—189
　Prader—Willi Syndrome (PWS), 196
　protein, 192
　vitamin D/calcium, 193
Cholecalciferol, 165
Cholelithiasis, 39
Clear liquid diets, 159
Cobalamin
　adolescent obesity, 192
　deficiency
　　anemia, 242—243
　　hypoabsorptive procedures (HAP), 163
Constipation, pregnancy, 213
Contraception, 212
Copper
　adolescent obesity, 193
　deficiency
　　hypoabsorptive procedures (HAP), 166
　　laparoscopic adjustable gastric band (LAGB), 126—127
　neurological complications, 249—250
　postoperative, 233—234, 233b—234b
Craniopharyngioma (CP), 196
Critical ill obese patients
　artificial feeding
　　hyperglycemia, 104—105
　　hyperlipidemia, 106
　body weight, 101
　cardiovascular system, 107—108, 109t
　kidney injury, 108
　low-calorie high-protein diets
　　age, 103
　　energy intake, 103
　　hypocaloric parenteral nutrition, 103
　　indirect calorimetry, 102
　micronutrient supplementation, 104
　nutritional requirements, 100—102
　nutritional screening test, 100

nutritional support, 105f
pharmacotherapy, 109–110
protein needs, 102
respiratory complications
  adult distress respiratory syndrome (ADRS), 107
  intubation risk, 106
  mechanical ventilation standards, 107
  obstructive apnea and hypoventilation-obesity syndromes, 106
  prone decubitus, 107

D

Diarrhea
  hypoabsorptive procedures (HAP), 168
  pregnancy, 213
Dietary interventions
  diet classifications, 47–48, 48t
  dyslipidemia, 52
  hypertension, 51–52
  low-calorie diets (LCD), 49
  low carbohydrate ketogenic diet (LCKD), 49–50
  metabolic and bariatric surgery guidelines, 54–58
  nonalcoholic fatty liver disease (NAFLD), 52–53
  type 2 diabetes, 50–51
  very low calories diet (VLCD), 49
Dietary iron, 5
Dietary reference intakes (IDR), 9t
Disengaged parents, 189
Doubly labeled water (DLW) technique, 31
Dual-energy x-ray absorptiometry (DXA), 22–23
Dumping syndrome (DS), 151, 168, 268
Durnin–Womersley equation, 21
Dyslipidemia (DLP)
  dietary interventions, 52, 53t
  metabolic and bariatric surgery guidelines
    American societies, 55
    European societies, 57–58
  very low calories diet (VLCD), 52

E

Eating behavior, hypoabsorptive procedures (HAP), 158–159
Eating disorders, 96
Elderly patient. *See* Obese elderly patients
Electric bioreactance (EB) analysis, 70–71
Encephalopathy, 246
Endoscopic techniques, 46–47
Energy malnutrition, Roux-n-Y gastric bypass, 152–153

Enhanced recovery after bariatric surgery (ERABS) clinical pathways, 116
European Association for the Study of Obesity (EASO), 181
European Society of parenteral and enteral nutrition (ESPEN) guidelines, 90
Excess weight loss (EWL)
  adjustable gastric banding (AGB), 76
  biliopancreatic diversion (BPD)/duodenal switch (DS), 82
  Roux-en-Y gastric bypass (RYGB), 80
  single-anastomosis duodeno-ileal switch (SADI-S), 83
  sleeve gastrectomy (SG), 77–78

F

Fats
  laparoscopic adjustable gastric band (LAGB), 122
  Roux-n-Y gastric bypass, 147
Ferritin, 241
Ferropenia, 180
Fiber, Roux-n-Y gastric bypass, 147
FloTrac/Vigileosystem, 69–70
Fluid overload, 63
Fluid responsiveness, 66, 71
Fluid therapy
  fluid overload, 63
  goal-directed fluid therapy (GDFT), 66–67
  hypovolemia, 63
  intraoperative period, 64–65
  intravascular volume estimation, 63
  intravascular volume status monitoring, 67
  laparoscopy, 65
  monitoring recommendations, 71–72
  physiological changes, 65, 66f
  preoperative factors, 64
  surgical factors, 65–66
Folic acid
  adolescent obesity, 192
  deficiency, 4–5
    anemia, 240
    hypoabsorptive procedures (HAP), 165
    laparoscopic adjustable gastric band (LAGB), 124
    neurological complications, 251
    postoperative, 230–231, 232b
    pregnancy and bariatric surgery, 214
    treatment, 11
  pregnancy and bariatric surgery, 214
  recommended dietary allowance (RDA), 178
Food frequency questionnaires, 26

Food intolerance, 149
Food records, 25
Food substitutes, 41t

G

Gastroesophageal reflux disease (GERD), 137—138
Gastrointestinal symptoms, hypoabsorptive procedures (HAP), 167—168
Gestational diabetes, 215—216
Ghrelin, sleeve gastrectomy (SG), 77—78
Global Leadership Initiative on Malnutrition diagnostic criteria, 18—19, 100
Goal-directed fluid therapy (GDFT)
    arterial waveform analysis-based techniques, 69
    benefits, 67
    bioimpedance-based technologies, 70—71
    dynamic volume response parameters, 67
    Esophageal Doppler devices, 70
    fluid responsiveness, 66
    functional hemodynamic variables, 71
    hemodynamic parameters, 67
    intravascular volume status monitoring, 67
    pulmonary artery catheterization (PAC), 68
    static parameters, 66
    theory, 66
    tissue perfusion optimization, 66
    transesophageal echocardiography (TEE), 68

H

Hepatomegaly, 46—47
High Mallampati score, 106
Hunger assessment, 194
Hydrophilic drugs, 109
Hyperglycemia
    artificial nutrition, 104—105
    critical ill obese patients, 104—105
Hyperinsulinemic hypoglycemia, 168, 268
Hyperlipidemia, critical ill obese patients, 106
Hypertension (HTN)
    dietary interventions, 51—52
    metabolic and bariatric surgery guidelines
        American societies, 55
        European societies, 57
Hyperuricemia, 39
Hypoabsorptive procedures (HAP), 156t
    gastrointestinal symptoms, 167—168
    intestinal segments length, 156—157
    long-term follow up, 168—169, 168t—169t
    postoperative diet and supplementation
        bariatric smoothies, 159
        clear liquid diets, 159
        diet progression, 161t
        mashed/puréed diet, 159
        protein intake, 160
        protein shakes, 159
    preoperative nutritional evaluation, 157
        bone health, 157—158
        eating behavior screening and weight loss, 158—159
        liver function, 158
        micro/macronutrients, 157
        total bowel length (TBL), 156—157
Hypoalbuminemia, 109—110, 245
Hypocaloric diets, 35
Hypoglycemia, 39, 152
Hypothalamic obesity (HyOb), 196
Hypoventilation-obesity syndromes, 106
Hypovitaminosis D, 4, 201—202

I

Incretin effect, 258
Indirect calorimetry, 28, 100—101
Internal hernia, 96
International Federation for Surgery of Obesity (IFSO), 83
Iron
    adolescent obesity, 193
    deficiency, 5
        blood loss, 241
        gastric bypass, 176
        hemoglobin level, 241
        hypoabsorptive procedures (HAP), 165
        intolerance/ineffectiveness, 242
        iron absorption, 240—241
        laparoscopic adjustable gastric band (LAGB), 124
        malabsorptive technique, 240—241
        postoperative, 227—228, 228b
        pregnancy and bariatric surgery, 214
        prevalence, 240—241
        treatment, 11
    obese elderly patients, 202
    supplementation
        pregnancy and bariatric surgery, 214
        recommended dietary allowance (RDA), 180
Isocaloric diets, 35

J

Jejunostomies, 94

K

Korsakoff syndrome, 247—248

L

Laparoscopic adjustable gastric band (LAGB), 46–47
  advantages, 116
  calorie goals, 121
  complications, 116
  dietary recommendations, 118t–119t
  macronutrients
    carbohydrates, 122
    fat, 122
    protein, 121
  micronutrients assessments and recommendations
    copper, 126–127
    folate, 124
    iron, 124
    vitamin B1, 123
    vitamin B12, 123–124
    vitamin D and calcium, 124–125
    vitamins A, E, and K, 125–126
    zinc, 126
  multistage nutritional progressive program, 117
  postoperative nutritional stages, 117–120
    stage 1, 117
    stage 2, 117
    stage 3, 117–120
    stage 4, 120
  and pregnancy, 127
  total body weight loss (TBWL), 116
Laparoscopic sleeve gastrectomy (LSG), 46–47
  body mass index (BMI), 129
  complications and nutritional issues, 135–138
  immediate postoperative period, 130
  indications, 129–130
  narrow tubular stomach, 130
  nutritional recommendations
    balanced bariatric dish portions, 133f
    at discharge, 131, 131t
    enhanced recovery after surgery (ERAS) programs, 130–131
    follow-up, 131–135, 132t
    food introduction guide, 134t
    fresh vegetables and fruits, 133
    immediate postoperative period, 130–131
    protein, 132
  obese elderly patients, 203
  staple line leakage, 137
  symptomatic stenosis, 136
  technical issues, 130
  technique and patient selection, 129–130
  ulcers and upper gastrointestinal hemorrhage, 137–138

Laparoscopy, fluid therapy, 65
LiDCO algorithm, 69
Lipophilic drugs, 109
Low-calorie diet (LCD). *See also* Very low-calorie diet (VLCD)
  bariatric surgery, 40–43
  definition, 35
  indications, 36, 49
Low-calorie high-protein diets
  age, 103
  energy intake, 103
  hypocaloric parenteral nutrition, 103
  indirect calorimetry, 102
Low-calorie special medical purpose foods, 41t
Low carbohydrate diets, 49–50
Low carbohydrate ketogenic diet (LCKD), 49–50

M

Macrocytic (megaloblastic) anemia, 3–4
Macronutrient deficiency, 6
Malabsorption, vitamin B12 deficiency, 4
Malnutrition, 96, 152–153
Marginal ulcer, 95–96
Megaloblastic anemia, 231
Menopause, 217–218
Metabolic acidosis, 108
Metabolic and bariatric surgery guidelines
  American societies
    dyslipidemia (DLP), 55
    general conditions, 54–55
    hypertension (HTN), 55
    nonalcoholic fatty liver disease (NAFLD), 55–56
    type 2 diabetes, 55
  European societies
    dyslipidemia (DLP), 57–58
    general conditions, 56–57
    hypertension (HTN), 57
    nonalcoholic fatty liver disease (NAFLD), 58
    type 2 diabetes, 57
Metabolic cart, 29
Metabolic equivalents (MET), 31
Metabolic surgery, 46–47
Midarm muscle area (MAMA), 21
Midarm muscle circumference (MAMC), 20–21
Midupper arm circumference (MUAC), 20
Mini-gastric bypass (MGB), 83
Myelopathy, 246
Myocardiopathy, 107–108

N

Narrow tubular stomach, 130
Naso-jejunal tubes, 94
Neurological complications
   bariatric surgery, 246
   copper deficiency, 249–250
   folate deficiency, 251
   immediate perioperative period, 246
   mechanisms, 246
   vitamin B6 deficiency, 250–251
   vitamin B12 deficiency, 248–249
   vitamin B1/thiamine deficiency, 247–248
   vitamin D deficiency, 252
   vitamin E deficiency, 251–252
Neuropathy, 246
NICE-Sugar Trial, 104–105
Night-eating disorder, 96
Nonalcoholic fatty liver disease (NAFLD), 40–42, 158
   dietary interventions, 52–53
   low carbohydrate ketogenic diet (LCKD), 53
   metabolic and bariatric surgery guidelines
      American societies, 55–56
      European societies, 58
   very low calories diet (VLCD), 52
Nutritional assessment
   anthropometric assessment. *See* Anthropometric assessment
   body composition analysis
      bioimpedance (BIA), 21–22, 21t
      computed tomography (CT), 22
      dual-energy x-ray absorptiometry (DXA), 22–23
      ultrasound (US), 23
   malnutrition, 18
   risk screening tools, 18–19
   visceral adipose tissue, 19
Nutritional deficiencies
   malabsorptive techniques, 175
   mixed procedures, 175–177
   postoperative vitamin and mineral supplementation
      calcium, 181
      continuous nutritional evaluation, 177
      folate acid, 178
      implications and decision makin, 181–183
      iron, 180
      recommendations, 177
      thiamine, 178
      vitamin A, 179
      vitamin B12, 178–179
      vitamin D, 179
      vitamin E, 180
      vitamin K, 179–180
      zinc, 181
   restrictive procedures, 175
Nutritional education, 174
Nutritional recommendations
   hypoabsorptive procedures (HAP). *See* Hypoabsorptive procedures (HAP)
   laparoscopic adjustable gastric band (LAGB)
      macronutrients, 121–122
      micronutrients, 122–127
      pregnancy, 127
   laparoscopic sleeve gastrectomy (LSG)
      balanced bariatric dish portions, 133f
      at discharge, 131, 131t
      enhanced recovery after surgery (ERAS) programs, 130–131
      follow-up, 131–135, 132t
      food introduction guide, 134t
      fresh vegetables and fruits, 133
      immediate postoperative period, 130–131
      protein, 132
   Roux-en-Y gastric bypass (RYGB)
      alcohol, 147
      balance diet, 145–146, 146f, 146t
      carbohydrates, 147
      clear liquid diet/tolerance phase, 143
      complete liquid diet, 143–144, 144t
      crushed diet, 144, 145t
      dietitian-nutritionist process, 148–149
      fats, 147
      fiber, 147
      immediate postoperative period, 143–146
      long-term recommendations, 146–148
      proteins, 147
      soft diet, 144–145, 145t
Nutritional requirements
   elderly patient. *See* Obese elderly patients
   energy intake (EI), 25–26, 27t
   protein requirements, 32
   total energy expenditure (TEE)
      additional energy costs, 30
      lower physical activity, 30
      physical activity energy expenditure (PAEE), 31
      resting metabolic rate (RMR), 28–30
      thermic effect of food (TFF), 31–32
   women
      maternal overweight and excess weight gain, 211t
      menopause, 217–218
      polycystic ovary syndrome (PCOS), 210
      pregnancy. *See* Pregnancy

Index   289

O

Obese elderly patients
  aging-related changes
    gastric function, 201
    small intestinal function, 201
  calcium, 202
  follow-up and supplementation, 204
  iron, 202
  laparoscopic sleeve gastrectomy (LSG), 203
  nutritional profile, 200−201
  one-anastomosis gastric bypass (OAGB-MGB), 204
  preoperative clinical evaluation, 200
  prevalence, 199
  protein, 202−203
  Roux-en-Y gastric bypass (RYGB), 203
  vitamin B12, 202
  vitamin D, 201−202
Obesity
  definition, 19
  incidence, 99−100
  prevalence, 2
  protein deficiency, 6
Obesity paradox, 100
Obstructive apnea, 106
Omega-3 fatty acids, adolescent obesity, 193
One-anastomosis gastric bypass (OAGB), 82, 82f
  nutritional recommendations. *See* Hypoabsorptive procedures (HAP)
  obese elderly patients, 204
Optic neuropathy, 246
Orthostatic hypotension, 39

P

Pancreatic enzymes replacement therapy, diarrhea, 168
Parenting models, 189
Pedometers, 31
Percentage body fat (PBF), 19
Perioperative complications, 46−47
Peripherally inserted central catheters (PICCs), 92
Permissive parenting style, 189
Phase angle, 22
Physical activity energy expenditure (PAEE), 31
PiCCO algorithm, 69
Picking and nibbling disorder, 96
Plethysmographic waveform variation (PWV), 71
Pneumoperitoneum, 130
Polycystic ovary syndrome (PCOS), 210
Polyradiculopathy, 246
Posthypoglycemia, 268−269
Postoperative complications

eating disorders, 96
enteral nutrition routes
  jejunostomies, 94
  leaks/fistula, 92−93, 93f−94f
  naso-jejunal tubes, 94
  remnant gastrostomy, 93
indications and access routes
  overfeeding and harmful effects, 89
  parenteral nutrition (PN), 90
internal hernia, 96
malnutrition, 96
marginal ulcer, 95−96
nutritional needs, 91
parenteral access route
  central venous catheters (CVCs), 91−92
  peripherally inserted central catheters (PICCs), 92
stenosis, 95
surgical complications, 89
Postoperative nutritional deficiencies
  biliopancreatic diversion with duodenal switch, 226
  copper deficiency, 233−234, 233b−234b
  early detection, 224
  follow-up, 224, 235t
  gastric bypass, 225
  micronutrient deficiencies
    folate deficiency, 230−231, 232b
    iron deficiency, 227−228, 228b
    recommendation grade, 227, 227t
    vitamin B1 deficiency, 231−232, 232b
    vitamin B12 deficiency, 230, 230b
    vitamin D and calcium, 228−229, 229b
    vitamins A, E, K deficiency, 232−233, 233b
  pathophysiology
    nutrient absorption, 225f
    patient factors, 224−225
  prevalence, 226, 226t
  prevention, 223−224
  restrictive techniques, 225
  selenium deficiency, 236
  single anastomosis duodeno-ileal with sleeve gastrectomy (SADI-S), 226
  treatment, 224
  zinc deficiency, 234, 234b
Postprandial hypoglycemia (PPH), 168
Prader−Willi Syndrome (PWS), 196
Prebariatric surgery
  nutritional assessment. *See* Nutritional assessment
  nutritional requirements. *See* Nutritional requirements

Pregnancy
    bariatric surgery
        childbearing age, 212
        contraception, 212
        dietary recommendations, 213
        follow-up, 212
        gestational diabetes, 215–216
        maternal nutritional factors, 213
        micronutrient deficiency, 214t
        nutritional supplements, 213–215
        obesity-related complications, 211, 211t
        sleeve gastrectomy, 212
        surgical complications, 212
    lactation, 209–210, 217
    laparoscopic adjustable gastric band (LAGB), 127
    maternal overweight and excess weight gain, 211t
    neonatal care, 216–217
    weight gain recommendation, 210
Preoperative diets
    low-calorie diet (LCD)
        bariatric surgery, 40–43
        definition, 35
        indications, 36
    very low-calorie diet (VLCD). *See* Very low-calorie diet (VLCD)
Preoperative nutritional deficiencies
    minerals
        iron deficiency, 5
        selenium deficiency, 5–6
        zinc deficiency, 6
    vitamins
        vitamin A deficiency, 5
        vitamin B1 deficiency, 3
        vitamin B9 deficiency, 4–5
        vitamin B12 deficiency, 3–4
        vitamin D deficiency, 4
Prone decubitus, 107
Protein
    adolescent obesity, 192
    deficiency
        hypoabsorptive procedures (HAP), 160
        treatment, 10
    hypoabsorptive procedures (HAP), 160
    laparoscopic adjustable gastric band (LAGB), 121
    malnutrition
        intestinal malabsorption, 244
        prevalence, 244
        prevention, 244–245
        Roux-n-Y gastric bypass, 152
        surgical factors, 244
    treatment, 245
    obese elderly patients, 202–203
    requirements, 32
    Roux-n-Y gastric bypass, 147
Protein shakes, 159
Psychosocial assessment, 18
Pulmonary artery catheterization (PAC), 67–68
Pulse-contour analysis-based techniques, 72
Pulse pressure algorithm (PulseCO), 69
Pylorus sparing technique gastrectomy, 83

R

Rebound phenomenon, 53–54
Recommended dietary allowance (RDA), 182t
    calcium, 181
    folate acid supplementation, 178
    iron deficiency, 176
    iron supplementation, 180
    thiamine supplementation, 178
    vitamin A, 179
    vitamin B12, 178
    vitamin D, 179
    vitamin E, 180
    vitamin K, 179–180
    zinc supplementation, 181
Remnant gastrostomy, 93
Reproductive health, adolescent obesity, 196
Respiratory quotient (RQ), 28
Resting energy expenditure (REE), 24
Resting metabolic rate (RMR), 24
    bioimpedance analysis, 30
    indirect calorimetry, 28
    predictive equations, 29t
Restrictive techniques
    nutritional deficiencies, 175
    postoperative nutritional deficiencies, 225
Rhabdomyolysis (RML), 65–66
Roux-en-Y gastric bypass (RYGB)
    bowel derivation, 142
    internal hernia, 96
    long-term results, 78–79
    nutritional care, 143
    nutritional complications
        dumping syndrome, 151
        food intolerance, 149
        hypoglycemias, 152
        malnutrition, 152–153
        micronutrient deficiencies, 150–151
    nutritional recommendations
        alcohol, 147
        balance diet, 145–146, 146f, 146t
        carbohydrates, 147

clear liquid diet/tolerance phase, 143
complete liquid diet, 143–144, 144t
crushed diet, 144, 145t
dietitian-nutritionist process, 148–149
fats, 147
fiber, 147
immediate postoperative period, 143–146
long-term recommendations, 146–148
proteins, 147
soft diet, 144–145, 145t
obese elderly patients, 200, 203
Roux limb, 142
small pouch, 142
stenosis, 95
supplementation, 153
technique, 79
variations, 141

S

Sarcopenia, 6, 100
Sarcopenic obesity
adverse outcomes, 23
definition, 23
diagnosis, 24
diagnosis criteria, 23t
epidemiologic studies, 24
pathophysiological pathways, 23–24
Selenium deficiency, 5–6, 11, 236
Sepsis, 108
Silicone band, 76
Single anastomosis duodenoileal bypass with sleeve gastrectomy (SADI/S)
nutritional recommendations. *See* Hypoabsorptive procedures (HAP)
postoperative nutritional deficiencies, 226
Single-anastomosis duodeno-ileal switch (SADI-S), 83
Skinfold anthropometry, 21
Sleep apnea hypopnea syndrome (SAHS), 38
Sleeve gastrectomy (SG)
complications, 95f
duodenal switch, 77
hormonal effect, 77–78
laparoscopic sleeve gastrectomy (LSG). *See* Laparoscopic sleeve gastrectomy (LSG)
metabolic effect, 77–78
resection, 77
stenosis, 95
Stenosis, 95, 136
Surviving sepsis campaign, 108
Systemic inflammatory response syndrome, 17–18

T

Thermic effect of food (TFF), 31–32
Thiamine, 178. *See also* Vitamin B1
Thoracic Electrical Bioimpedance (TEB), 70
Total body weight loss (TBWL), 116
Total energy expenditure (TEE)
additional energy costs, 30
lower physical activity, 30
physical activity energy expenditure (PAEE), 31
resting metabolic rate (RMR), 28–30
thermic effect of food (TFF), 31–32
Transesophageal echocardiography (TEE), 68
Transferrin, 5
Type 2 diabetes
dietary interventions, 50–51
metabolic and bariatric surgery guidelines
American societies, 55
European societies, 57

U

Ulcer, 137–138
Ultrasound (US), 23

V

Vasopressin, 64
Vegetarian/vegan diet, 266–267
Very low-calorie diet (VLCD), 49
bariatric surgery, 40–43
body composition changes, 38
carbohydrate metabolism, 38
commercial products, 39–40
contraindications, 36
definition, 35–36
enteral nutrition formulas, 41t
food substitutes, 41t
hypertensive patients, 38
indications, 36
lipid profile, 38
macronutrients, 39t
meal replacement, 37
postsurgical healing process, 42
recommended composition, 39t
regulations, 37
side effects, 38–39
vitamins and minerals, 41t
weight loss, 37
Visceral adipose tissue, 19
VISEP Trial, 104–105
Vitamin A, 179

Vitamin A (*Continued*)
  adolescent obesity, 193
  deficiency, 5
    hypoabsorptive procedures (HAP), 165
    laparoscopic adjustable gastric band (LAGB), 125–126
    recommended dietary allowance (RDA), 179
Vitamin B1
  adolescent obesity, 192
  deficiency
    incidence, 3
    laparoscopic adjustable gastric band (LAGB), 123
    metabolic derangements, 3
    neurological complications, 247–248
    postoperative, 231–232, 232b
    treatment, 10
    Wernicke encephalopathy (WE), 3
Vitamin B12
  adolescent obesity, 192
  deficiency, 3–4
    anemia, 242–243
    gastric bypass, 176
    laparoscopic adjustable gastric band (LAGB), 123–124
    neurological complications, 248–249
    obese elderly patients, 202
    postoperative, 230, 230b
    pregnancy and bariatric surgery, 214
    treatment, 10
  recommended dietary allowance (RDA), 178
Vitamin B6 deficiency, 250–251
Vitamin B9 deficiency, 4–5
Vitamin C deficiency, 5
Vitamin D
  adolescent obesity, 193
  deficiency
    hypoabsorptive procedures (HAP), 165
    hypovitaminosis D, 4
    laparoscopic adjustable gastric band (LAGB), 124–125
    neurological complications, 252
    pregnancy and bariatric surgery, 214–215
    treatment, 10
  obese elderly patients, 201–202
  postoperative, 228–229, 229b
  recommended dietary allowance (RDA), 179
  supplementation

  pregnancy and bariatric surgery, 214–215
  recommended dietary allowance (RDA), 179
VitaminD3, 125
Vitamin E
  deficiency, 5
    hypoabsorptive procedures (HAP), 165–166
    laparoscopic adjustable gastric band (LAGB), 125–126
    neurological complications, 251–252
  recommended dietary allowance (RDA), 180
Vitamin K
  deficiency
    hypoabsorptive procedures (HAP), 166
    laparoscopic adjustable gastric band (LAGB), 125–126
    postoperative, 232–233, 233b
  recommended dietary allowance (RDA), 179–180

W

Waist circumference (WC), 20
Waist height ratio (WHtR), 20
Waist hip ratio (WHR), 20
Weight loss, hypoabsorptive procedures (HAP), 158–159
Wernicke encephalopathy (WE), 3, 247–248
Whole-food plant-based (WFPB) diet, 267–268
Women
  bariatric surgery
    menopause, 217–218
    pregnancy. *See* Pregnancy
  reproductive function
    maternal overweight and excess weight gain, 211t
    polycystic ovary syndrome (PCOS), 210
    pregnancy, weight gain recommendation, 210, 210t

Z

Zinc
  adolescent obesity, 193
  deficiency, 6
    hypoabsorptive procedures (HAP), 166
    laparoscopic adjustable gastric band (LAGB), 126
    postoperative, 234, 234b
    treatment, 11–12
  recommended dietary allowance (RDA), 181

Printed in the United States
By Bookmasters